A GUIDE TO ACHIEVING MEANINGFUL USE

Leverage Your EHR to Redesign Workflows and Improve Outcomes

Helga Rippen, MD, PhD, MPH, FACPM
Denise M. Scott, MM, RN-BC
Carolyn P. Hartley, MLA

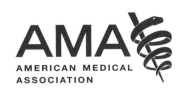

AMA
AMERICAN MEDICAL
ASSOCIATION

Copyright 2013 by the American Medical Association. All rights reserved.

Printed in the United States of America

No part of this publication may be reproduced, stored in a retrieval system, or transmitted, in any form or by any means electronic, mechanical, photocopying, recording, or otherwise, without the prior written permission of the publisher.

US public laws and federal rules and regulations included in this publication are in the public domain. However, the arrangement, compilation, organization, and history of, and references to, such laws and regulations, along with all CPT data and other materials are subject to the above copyright notice.

Internet address: www.ama-assn.org

The American Medical Association (AMA) has consulted sources believed to be knowledgeable in their fields. However, the AMA does not warrant that the information is in every respect accurate and/or complete. The AMA assumes no responsibility for the use of the information contained in this publication. The AMA shall not be responsible for, and expressly disclaims liability for, damages of any kind arising out of the use of, reference to, or reliance on, the content of this publication. This publication is for informational purposes only. The AMA does not provide medical, legal, financial, or other professional advice, and readers are encouraged to consult a professional advisor for such advice.

The Center for Medicare & Medicaid Services is responsible for the Medicare content contained in this publication and no endorsement by the AMA is intended or should be implied. Readers are encouraged to refer to the current official Medicare program provisions contained in relevant laws, regulations, and rulings.

Additional copies of this book may be ordered by calling 800 621-8335 or from the secure AMA Web site at www.amastore.com. Refer to product number OP178913. Ancillary materials are available for download at ama-assn.org/go/OP178913aaa.

AMA publication and product updates, errata and addendum can be found at ama-assn.org/go/ProductUpdates.

Library of Congress Cataloging-in-Publication Data
Rippen, Helga, author.
  A guide to achieving meaningful use: leverage your EHR to redesign workflows and improve outcomes / by Helga Rippen, Denise M. Scott, Carolyn P. Hartley.
    p. ; cm.
  Includes bibliographical references and index.
  Summary: "A Guide to Achieving Meaningful Use demonstrates how physicians can leverage meaningful use to strengthen their practice, not just meet the Meaningful Use Criteria. This book operationalizes Stage 1 and 2 Meaningful Use requirements with early guidance on Stage 3"—Provided by publisher.
  ISBN 978-1-60359-833-0
  I. Scott, Denise M., author. II. Hartley, Carolyn P., author. III. American Medical Association, issuing body. IV. Title.
  [DNLM: 1. Electronic Health Records—organization & administration. 2. Efficiency, Organizational. 3. Quality Assurance, Health Care. WX 175]
  R864
  610.285—dc23
                                                                                          2013006504

ISBN 978-1-60359-833-0
BQ20:13-P-000:05/29

To Kristen and Laurie, my meaningful daughters and powerful advocates of patient-physician communication and care plans and to their children.—CPH

To the hundreds of small, independent primary-care doctors I have worked with who have so bravely embarked on their electronic health record journey. I have seen the struggle you faced through less-than-ideal training and implementation support, the humbling learning curve to introduce technology into your long-standing patient relationships, and your willingness to do it all for the hopeful benefit of your patients. The information shared with you in this book was realized by working with those who took this journey before you. May this guide steer you through the unknowns of the Meaningful Use process and lead you expeditiously to the incentive payment you so deserve.—DMS

To physicians and their staff who are committed to delivering excellent care to their patients in an environment of increasing regulations and reporting requirements while working with EHR systems that are not yet able to meet their needs.—HER

A Guide to Achieving Meaningful Use: Leverage Your EHR to Redesign Workflows and Improve Outcomes — Ancillary Content

As an added bonus, purchasers of this book may download free ancillary content referred to throughout this book. Go to **ama-assn.org/go/OP178913aaa** to download the documents.

Content includes:

- Daily Resources for Meaningful Use Project Managers
- Stage 2 EP Spec Sheets
- CMS CQMs for 2014 CMS EHR Incentive Programs for EPs
- CMS Attestation User Guide for EPs
- CMS EP Attestation Worksheet
- CMS Payment Adjustments & Hardship Exceptions Tipsheet for EPs
- CMS Stage 1 vs Stage 2 Comparison Table for EPs
- CMS Stage 2 Overview Tipsheet
- CMS Stage 1 Changes Tipsheet
- The Medicare and Medicaid EHR Incentive Programs: Stage 2 Toolkit

CONTENTS

v

ACKNOWLEDGMENTS

Families come first for all of us, and so we want to acknowledge them above all others for fixing their own meals, listening to late-night keyboard chatter, and allowing us to slip away into hiding, sometimes into the early hours, to complete this book for you. Remarkably, all three of us remained married, even though all of us have pushed deadlines many times.

We also want to thank our employers, who saw the opportunity for us to make a difference in health care by pulling together an enormously comprehensive Meaningful Use guide.

Thanks also to the Physicians EHR team for late-night readings, editorial suggestions, graphic support, and picking up the slack, especially during the final editing weeks. In particular, thank you to Rahul Patel, Laurie O'Brien, and Marguerite Stout. To Marcus Sharpe, thank you for the clinical and technical support you provided.

We would like to thank Liza Assatourians, Ana English, and Carol Scheele who have graciously and thoughtfully assisted with the peer review. Their significant and valued insights and contribution have made this a better book.

To our AMA acquisitions editor, Elise, you could not be a more encouraging force and are a rare friend indeed. A rich thank you to Lisa Chin-Johnson for paying attention to more details than we ever wanted to acknowledge; and warmest hugs to the marketing team, including our friend Carol Brockman, who finds the most creative ways to place this book into your hands.

Finally, we acknowledge the practices that trusted us to get them through attestation, Stage 1, and had the boldness to ask us to be with you through Stages 2 and 3. We love you back! You taught us more about perseverance, consistency, data management, and velvet-hammer negotiation than you will ever know. Tough love forever!

Helga Rippen, MD, PhD, MPH, FACPM

Helga Rippen has been a leader in bridging technology and health care to maximize value to the patient, clinician, and health care sector for more than 20 years. She has worked with diverse groups such as physicians and consumers on a variety of topics, including electronic health record (EHR) roadmap development and adoption across physician offices, hospitals, and other health care entities. Rippen has worked on health care quality and reporting, disease management, ethics, a national health information infrastructure, usability, privacy, and consumer control. She led the conceptualization, prototype development, and implementation of many consumer tools. Rippen has presented to numerous wide-ranging audiences and has published in many trade and peer-reviewed journals.

Rippen has experience in roles that span all aspects of technology and health care, including treating patients, basic research, product development, implementation, clinical outcomes, and national policy development. She has been able to leverage her expertise, roles, and understanding as an effective change agent, strategist, visionary leader, problem solver, communicator, and implementer. Rippen is the Chief Health Information Officer and Vice President of Westat's INSIGHT, Center for Health Information Technology, providing consulting services to government and private-sector clients. She was the Chief Health Information Officer and Vice President of Health Information Technology (Health IT) for HCA where she led the development of the clinical EHR Program. Rippen served as Senior Advisor for Health IT for the Secretary's office at the US Department of Health and Human Services where she was involved with the creation of the Office of the National Coordinator for Health IT (ONC). Previously, she was Director of the Science and Technology Policy Institute for RAND, supporting the White House Office of Science and Technology Policy, Director of Health IT for Pfizer Health Solutions, and Founder of the Health IT Institute for Mitretek Systems (now Noblis).

Rippen received her medical degree, with honors, from the University of Florida and completed her medical residency training in General Preventive Medicine at Johns Hopkins University, where she also received her Masters in Public Health with a focus on health policy and management. Rippen obtained her PhD in biomedical engineering from Duke University. She is a Fellow of the American College of Preventive Medicine and Board Certified in Public Health and General Preventive Medicine with active medical licenses in Maryland and Virginia. She can be reached at HelgaRippen@westat.com.

Denise M. Scott, MM, RN-BC

Denise Scott brings her nursing perspective from 28 years of acute and ambulatory patient care, more than 10 years of varied experiences in advancing the use of health information technology, and her current work with physicians to use their EHR data to improve the quality of care and transform their practices while cashing their checks for meeting Meaningful Use in the EHR Incentive Program. She is currently the Director of Quality & Informatics at Cooley-Dickinson Practice Associates (CDPA), a multispecialty independent-practice association in western Massachusetts whose community physicians have adopted one common EHR, successfully attested, and are on the transformative road to becoming medical homes. Before joining CDPA, Scott was the Director of Clinical Integration & Quality at a 160+ IPA in central Massachusetts, leading their EHR adoption, quality, and Meaningful Use efforts. To facilitate the IPA physicians' achievement of Meaningful Use, Scott created a ten-webinar series on operationalizing MU measures in a sustainable manner for small practices.

Scott was the Manager, Health Information Technology Services at Masspro and had the great fortune of working on a variety of contracts, including an ONC/CMS secure-messaging project, a New York PCMH transformation and recognition project of more than 200 physicians, and the CMS DOQ-IT project, all precursors to the EHR Incentive Program. Through her work in the use of HIT in physician practices, she has collaborated with physician groups who are some of the nation's early adopters and current leaders in innovative, transformative use of HIT.

During her many years in health care, Scott has significant experience in adopting and leveraging technology in physician offices, workflow analysis and redesign, process improvement, EHR optimization, and pay-for-performance systems and strategies. She continues to guide physician practices through the NCQA PCMH application process to Level 3 recognition.

Since 2010, Scott has been a subcontractor to Booz Allen Hamilton, providing subject-matter expertise on EHR implementation and workflow redesign education. She is one of four lead content designers for ONC's EHR Implementation Boot Camp and cocreator of a virtual class on workflow redesign, educating Regional Extension Center staff across the United States. She is a skilled communicator and motivator with recognized success in leading and facilitating clients to successful outcomes. She has spoken nationally on EHR implementation, workflow redesign, and secure messaging. Her audiences appreciate her ability to interpret the language of policy, explain the objectives and intent of programs to a better level of understanding, and share the reality of everyday challenges and successes in working with physician practices adopting HIT while providing actionable, practical approaches and tools to use in their own efforts.

Scott earned a Masters in Management with a health care–management concentration at Cambridge College, a Bachelor of Arts at Framingham State University, and a nursing diploma from Framingham Union Hospital School of Nursing. She holds a certificate in Health Care Informatics and is ANCC board-certified in Nursing Informatics. Scott is a registered nurse in the Commonwealth of Massachusetts. She can be reached at dmscott44@tds.net.

Carolyn P. Hartley, MLA

Carolyn Hartley, coauthor and the author team's project manager, brings deep knowledge of EHR systems and their implementation and reporting processes to this book on Meaningful Use. She is President, CEO of Physicians EHR, Inc, a Cary, NC–based company that educates and serves as selection, implementation, workflow evaluation, and process redesign project manager, overseeing the front- to back-office operations and all clinical aspects of the data migration in 23 states. She and her health IT team also serve as contracted EHR technical facilitators to national and state medical societies, including the American Society of Clinical Oncology, American College of Cardiology, American Medical Association, American Dental Association, and Texas Association of Community Health Centers (TACHC).

Since 2010, Hartley has been a subcontractor to Westat to coach and provide subject matter expertise to ONC's Vendor Selection and Management Communities of Practice (CoP) and is one of four lead content designers for ONC's EHR Implementation Boot Camp. She is lead or coauthor of 17 textbooks on health information, privacy and security risk management, and health information exchange that have been published by the American Medical Association, American Society of Clinical Oncology, American Dental Association, and American Gastroenterological Association. She is a nationally recognized keynote and breakout-session speaker addressing privacy, security, EHR implementation project management, and workflow analysis and redesign.

Hartley holds a Master of Liberal Arts degree from Baker University with an emphasis in philosophy and medical anthropology and can be reached at Carolyn@physiciansehr.com.

INTRODUCTION

In their article for the *New England Journal of Medicine*, David Blumenthal, MD, MPP, and Marilyn Tavenner, RN, MHA, provided a perspective about the Meaningful Use rule that is cited frequently because of the clarity behind the rule's incentive and purpose.

> The widespread use of electronic health records (EHRs) in the United States is inevitable. EHRs will improve caregivers' decisions and patients' outcomes. Once patients experience the benefits of this technology, they will demand nothing less from their providers. Hundreds of thousands of physicians have already seen these benefits in their clinical practice.
>
> But, inevitability does not mean easy transition. We have years of professional agreement and bipartisan consensus regarding the potential value of EHRs. Yet, we have not moved significantly to extend the availability of EHRs from a few large institutions to the smaller clinics and practices where most Americans receive their health care.
>
> The Meaningful Use rule is part of a coordinated set of regulations to help create a private and secure 21st-century electronic health information system. On June 18, 2010, the Department of Health and Human Services (DHHS) issued a rule that laid out a process for the certification of EHRs so providers can be assured their EHR systems are capable of helping them achieve Meaningful Use. The department has also issued another regulation, which lays out the standards and certification criteria that EHRs must meet in order to be certified. Finally, realizing that the privacy and security of EHRs are vital, the DHHS has been working hard to safeguard privacy and security by implementing new protections contained in the HITECH legislation.
>
> The Meaningful Use rule strikes a balance between acknowledging the urgency of adopting EHRs to improve our health care system and recognizing the challenges that adoption will pose to health care providers. The regulation must be both ambitious and achievable. Like an escalator, HITECH attempts to move the health system upward toward improved quality and effectiveness in health care. But the speed of ascent must be calibrated to reflect both the capacities of providers who face a multitude of real-world challenges and the maturity of the technology itself.[1]

In creating this book, the authors leveraged lessons learned from years of implementation project management, consensus building, data-build and management, policy making, and weekend calls from physicians trying to make sense of their newly installed EHR. We learned not only from the EHR vendors, rule makers, and incentive payers, but also from you, our physician clients, readers who are also our best resources.

The most important lesson you have taught us is one we are proud to pass along to others: Meaningful Use is a process to achieve incentive funds, but it is not the end goal. Rather, the goal of Meaningful Use is to incentivize physicians and health care professionals nationwide to use their EHR and to ensure that EHR vendors provide functionality so that the EHR becomes a tool rather than an obstacle.

This book is not necessarily a book to be read from cover to cover but rather in segments, with sections you can pull out and use with your clinical and administrative teams. We leaned far out on a ledge not only to recap what you could have found if you explored the Centers for Medicare & Medicaid Services EHR Incentive Program pages, but also to provide practical field guidance that you won't find searching the Internet.

A Guide to Achieving Meaningful Use is divided into three parts. Part I focuses on the nuts and bolts of achieving Meaningful Use (Chapter 1) and the value of data (Chapter 2). If you are new to the Meaningful Use process, these chapters will get you well on your way with an abundance of Web site links should you need a deep dive into unique situations. Part II is intended for Meaningful Use project managers who also seek to improve workflow processes and begin using data for business and clinical-reporting purposes. Readers who faced data-collection challenges in Stage 1 reporting will immediately connect with the process redesign chapter. Also included in Part II is a chapter on standards now and those to come, including strategies to secure the infrastructure. Part III is a physician's clinical guide to Meaningful Use written by a physician. Whereas Parts I and II address how to operationalize Meaningful Use, Part III addresses Meaningful Use from a physician's view. What follows is a brief overview of each part.

PART I: NUTS AND BOLTS

In Chapter 1 you will find the nuts and bolts of Meaningful Use. If you are a first-timer, this is a "what to do and how to do it" instruction guide. Included in this chapter is a Meaningful Use gap analysis developed for physician practices, a tool you can use to avoid roadblocks in the middle of attestation. Chapter 1 provides guidance for specialty and multispecialty practices selecting clinical quality measures for reporting purposes.

In Chapter 2 we look at the value that EHRs are bringing to health care and the challenges of adoption. We also challenge you to find innovative ways to use the data you are building in your system. Accurate and dependable clinical data are a necessity for a physician. This chapter also provides guidance on what to expect from your EHR and from the EHR vendor and how to anticipate and plan how your EHR will be used in the future.

PART II: OPERATIONALIZE MEANINGFUL USE

In Chapter 3 you will learn how to build a Meaningful Use infrastructure that supports a secure environment for networking, data capture and management, and patient-portal decisions. There is also a small section on standards that you should know about. This chapter also guides you through the discussions you should have with your EHR vendor. No one wants to learn about "known issues" after diving deeply into the first reporting period.

Chapter 4 focuses on how to redesign your workflows not just for Meaningful Use, but also to ensure that you are capturing critical data that will help in decision making. This chapter compares Meaningful Use workflows by measure and by role and incorporates the process into a patient visit. These workflows are an incredibly difficult process to capture on your own and represent hundreds of hours of trial and error, studies, and successful attestations.

Chapter 5 is your survival chapter and provides strategies for surviving attestation. This includes knowing how to come up with the numbers and documenting the decisions you made along the way so that, in the event of an audit, you can explain how you came up with the numbers that you did. In this chapter, we also provide guidance on how to minimize surprises and how to track when you will receive your incentive funds.

PART III: CLINICAL ASPECTS OF MEANINGFUL USE

Chapter 6 provides advice on a doctor-to-doctor level on building a meaningful patient relationship. Physicians nearly always pride themselves on the relationships they have with their patients and may feel threatened by the initial imposition that a computer brings into the relationship. This chapter provides guidance on how patient portals and clinical summaries help to empower patients.

Chapter 7 presents recommendations on how to improve patient outcomes, from the patient to population levels that best align with the physician practice. As the health care community transitions its perspective to a population view, this chapter makes the case for Meaningful Use measures in public health and disease surveillance and how EHRs can help improve quality of care.

We thought about you as we researched, collected data, and pulled together lessons learned so that this would be the most useful Meaningful Use book in your library.

We hope you'll let us know how you are doing.

REFERENCE

1. Blumenthal D, Travenner M. The Meaningful Use regulation for electronic health records, *N Engl J Med*. 2010;363:501–504. www.nejm.org/doi/full/10.1056/nejmp1006114. Accessed January 30, 2013.

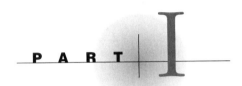

PART I

Nuts and Bolts

Chapters 1 and 2 in Part I of *A Guide to Achieving Meaningful Use* are written for the physician practice that has yet to achieve Meaningful Use (MU) Stage 1 or completed MU attestation, but new workforce members have come on board and need to know more about how the practice reached the numbers it did.

Chapter 1 provides the nuts and bolts of MU, gap analysis tools, and guidance for selecting clinical quality measures for reporting purposes.

Chapter 2 focuses on the value of data in managing a practice, patient health information and demographics, as well as addresses how best to take advantage of data that are stored inside the electronic health record (EHR) software. Practical advice is available as well, if you are contemplating switching to another EHR.

Nuts and Bolts of Meaningful Use Stages 1 and 2

WHAT YOU WILL LEARN IN THIS CHAPTER:

- What the electronic health record incentive program (Meaningful Use) entails
- Step-by-step instructions for meeting Meaningful Use (MU) Stages 1 and 2
- Who is eligible for MU incentives, and what Centers for Meidcare & Medicaid Services (CMS) program is right for you
- Nuts and bolts of MU core measures, menu set measures, and clinical quality measures for Stages 1 and 2
- What you should document for MU attestation
- How to file for MU
- What payment adjustments are and to whom they apply
- What's in store for Stage 3
- What MU means for
  - Physicians
  - Staff
  - Patients
  - Stakeholders
- Steps to take

Key Terms Introduced in This Chapter

Attest
Certified Electronic Health Record Technology
Clinical Quality Measures
Core Measures
Covered Entity
Eligible Professional
Eligible Hospital
Meaningful Use
Meaningful User
Meaningful Use Objective
Measure
Menu Set Measures

The Medicare and Medicaid EHR Incentive Programs provide a financial incentive to eligible professionals (EPs), eligible hospitals (EHs), and critical access hospitals (CAHs) when they achieve "Meaningful Use." EPs can receive up to $44,000 through the Medicare program and up to $63,750 through the Medicaid EHR Incentive Program.

In this chapter, we define *Meaningful Use* (MU) and what it means to be a "meaningful user." We also will describe the value of using certified electronic health record (EHR) technology (CEHRT) to achieve health and efficiency goals. The EHR Incentive Program is not a reimbursement program for purchasing or replacing an EHR, as the recipients of MU funds must demonstrate they can extract specific details from the EHR.[1]

As our primary reference to this and all subsequent chapters, we continually reference three Web sites with continuously updated guidance:

1. www.CMS.gov/EHRIncentivePrograms
    a. This is Centers for Medicare & Medicaid Services' (CMS') official Web site for Meaningful Use.
    b. The MU incentive program is a combination of several pieces of legislation, all of which can be accessed at the Health and Human Services (HHS) health IT portal, www.healthit.gov. Throughout the book, we will reference how they govern the MU incentive program. Rules include:
        Standards and Certification Criteria, Stage 1, and another rule for Stage 2
        Temporary Certification Program (TCP)
        Permanent Certification
        Meaningful Use of Electronic Health Records
        CLIA [Clinical Laboratory Improvement Amendments] Program and Health Insurance Portability and Accountability Act (HIPAA) Privacy Rule: Patients' Access to Test Reports. Stage 2 leverages HIPAA Security Rule and holds EHR vendors accountable for embedding HIPAA technical safeguards in their systems.
    Note the Web sites posted to help keep you current. Throughout this book you will find links to various pages of this Web site.
2. www.HealthIT.gov
    a. This Web site, maintained by the HHS, provides guidance to patients and consumers, health care professionals, and policymakers and researchers.
    b. Use this Web site to find detailed guidance on MU core and menu set measures.
3. www.Healthit.gov/policy-researchers-implementers
    a. This is a portal providing legislative links to regulations and guidance, Office of the National Coordinator for Health Information Technology (ONC) initiatives, news, events and resources, and Health Information Technology for Economic and Clinical Health Act (HITECH Act) program initiatives.
    b. Use this Web site to learn more about policymaking, funding announcements, and links to legislation.

The purposes of this chapter are to both pull together the nuts and bolts from these Web sites and many other credible sources and present leading practices that we have learned from supporting hundreds of physicians through MU attestation. To achieve attestation, you must make a claim or series of claims that, by using your system and information in your medical charts, you were able to meet the requirements in each measure.

To begin, let's take a look at how we got to MU.

A NATION'S BRIEF PATH TO MEANINGFUL USE

On April 27, 2004, President George W. Bush called for the widespread use of EHRs by creating executive order 13335, an initiative to make EHRs available to most Americans within 10 years. That was the start of a series of government initiatives known as the De-cade of Health Information Technology: Delivering Consumer-centric and Information-rich Health Care.[2]

The Secretarial Summit on Health Information Technology launching the National Health Information Infrastructure 2004: Cornerstones for Electronic Healthcare was well attended by over 1,500 people representing the private and public healthcare industry. In challenging both sectors of the healthcare industry, Secretary Tommy G. Thompson stated, "Health information technology can improve quality of care and reduce medical errors, even as it lowers administrative costs. It has the potential to produce savings of 10 percent of our total annual spending on health care, even as it improves care for patients and provides new support for health care professionals." A report, titled The Decade of Health Information Technology: Delivering Consumer-Centric and Information-Rich Health Care, ordered by President George W. Bush in April, was presented on July 21, 2004, by David Brailer, the National Coordinator for Health Information Technology, whom the president appointed to the new position in May. For more information about health IT policy and research, Strategic Action can be accessed at www.healthit.gov/policy-researchers-implementers.[3]

The impetus for this transition to EHRs was largely based on rising health care costs and the need for both clinical and outcomes data to help improve the quality of care.

- Baby boomers are becoming eligible for Medicare at the rate of 10,000 per day, driving up entitlement benefits.[4]
- People are living longer. Medicare outlays have grown twice as fast as the economy for the last 5 years.[4]
- Healthcare premiums have risen 9% for families per year when inflation was running at 2%.[5]
- New procedures improve the quality of care but also increase costs to consumers.
- Unlike the communications, banking, manufacturing, and transportation industries, the health care industry is just starting to agree on standards that facilitate exchange of information.

Between 2004 and 2008, policy advisors and collaborators, medical organizations, privacy and security collaboratives, standards-setting organizations, patient-advocacy groups, and other health care stakeholders set out to study the pros and cons of how the nation could consolidate hundreds of different sets of standards into a narrow few so that physicians could electronically access a current longitudinal patient record and securely exchange health information with other health care providers and their patients. Federally and pri-vately funded programs sponsored prototypes, and the Certification Commission for Health Information Technology (CCHIT) developed the first EHR certification program, providing physicians with some guidance on what EHR system to purchase. Even so, adoption was slow going. By the time EHRs were getting more user-friendly, the nation's economy had begun to collapse, causing more financial strain on physicians and their practices.

Financial barriers created the most significant hurdle because the physician investment would likely yield monetary benefits to other entities, such as third-party payers. Additional barriers included disruption to the office workflow, lack of training and knowledge, some discomfort with the use of computers, and a perceived shift in the doctor-patient relation-ship. Evidence also suggested that, at the time, a large number of EHR products were too costly for small physician practices, some products were not yet ready for the market, and the amount of technical support needed for ongoing business needs would further burden the practice.[6]

To respond to these barriers, health information technology (health IT or HIT) initiatives were expanded when President Obama and the 111th Congress passed the American Recovery and Reinvestment Act (ARRA) of 2009. Embedded in ARRA was the HITECH Act, authorizing more than $20 billion to roll out an HIT adoption plan that incentivized EPs and EHs if they could demonstrate that they are meaningful users of HIT.

The intent of the HITECH Act was to lay the groundwork for: (1) improved health care quality, safety, and efficiency through the use of HIT, including EHRs; (2) the infrastructure to support the adoption of EHRs; and (3) private and secure electronic health information exchange (HIE).

Figure 1-1 provides an overview of the health information adoption timeline.

FIGURE 1-1

Health Information Technology Adoption Timeline

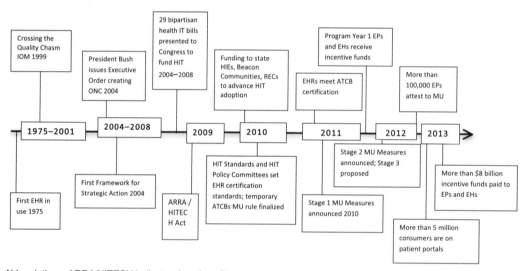

Abbreviations: ARRA/HITECH indicates American Recovery and Reinvestment Act/ Health Information Technology for Economic and Clinical Health Act; ATCB, Accredited Testing and Certification Body; EHR, electronic health record; EP, eligible professional; HIE, health information exchanges; HIT, health information technology; IOM, Institute of Medicine; MU, Meaningful Use; ONC, Office of the National Coordinator for Health Information Technology; and RECs, regional extension centers.

Physicians typically find they must manage a number of challenges when adopting EHRs in their practices.

■ Power outages caused by natural or unnatural events are a given. In anticipation of such events, the practice must determine how it will capture information when electronic access is unavailable.

■ As physicians experience greater mobility using portable tablets and handheld devices, security breaches have skyrocketed. The Ponemon Institute's third annual Benchmark Study on Patient Privacy and Data Security documented that 94% of hospitals reported a breach between 2009 and 2011, with 45% of those hospitals reporting five or more breaches during the two-year period.[7]

■ Process analysis and redesign is a leading practice with hospitals. In the process, hospitals receive a visual map on paper of how workflows are completed so that those workflows can be analyzed for efficiencies and inefficiencies and then be redesigned for the EHR. Without a budget to complete a process analysis, smaller physician practices tend to import paper-based workflows into the EHR and then become frustrated when the EHR does not meet their expectations.

■ HIEs often are initiated by hospitals promising physicians access to the HIE if the physician will upload patient information, but the promise may or may not be accompanied by detailed benefits to the physician.

■ Emerging EHRs designed for specialists may be less expensive or focus on that specialty's needs, but they may not survive entry into the EHR market because of generalist and large EHR companies' domination.

The pathway to an EHR is not easy, nor should any EHR software company tell you a conversion from paper to EHR or from one system to another can be done in a few hours or over a weekend. The reality is that adopting an EHR is a layered, multifaceted task that is best done with help from a peer who has completed the implementation or works with a team who knows EHRs and clinical workflows.

To that end, the MU incentive funds are designed to reward users who have learned to use CEHRT.

GETTING STARTED WITH MEANINGFUL USE

If you haven't purchased an EHR system yet, consider reading the American Medical Association's (AMA) *EHR Implementation: A Step by Step Guide for the Medical Practice*, 2nd edition, by Carolyn P. Hartley and Edward D. Jones. If you haven't yet entered the MU program, this chapter will get you well on your way to understanding what to do and how to do it. But, if you have already registered and attested for MU funds and received first- or second-year funds, this chapter will provide you with the nuts and bolts of Stage 2 and initial direction for Stage 3.

This chapter is for those who:

■ Are just getting started with the Medicare or Medicaid MU incentive programs.

■ Are looking to adopt an EHR and want to know if their vendor will support them on the road to MU.

■ Are in need of a refresher course on the MU process.

■ Want to understand the basics of Stage 2 MU requirements.

Overview of Meaningful Use

As briefly discussed earlier, the HITECH Act embedded in the ARRA of 2009 escalated the adoption of EHRs and ensured that patients and their healthcare professionals could communicate securely in an electronic environment.

The HITECH Act included a number of requirements, including financial incentives under Medicare and Medicaid to hospitals and EPs who demonstrate they are *meaningful users* of CEHRT. A meaningful user must capture health information in a standardized format using a certified EHR and use that information to track key clinical conditions. Stage 1 MU measures focus on five core objectives:

■ Improve quality, safety, and efficiency and reduce health disparities

■ Engage patients and families in their health care

■ Improve care coordination

■ Improve population and public health

■ Ensure adequate privacy and security protections for personal health information

---

Critical Point

Objective is another word for "what to do." For example, core objective #1 [of the EP MU Core Measures (measure 1 of 15) before 2013] has to do with using computerized provider order entry (CPOE) for medication orders.

M*easure* refers to the information (data) you must capture to meet the objective. For core objective #1, the measure is to report that at least 30% of unique patients with at least one medication have had at least one order entered using CPOE.

As required by the HITECH Act, four subsequent regulations have been released that define MU. Table 1-1 provides an overview of each of those four rules and what agency regulates them. In subsequent chapters we will present details about when the rules were developed and what agency regulates the adoption of each rule.

TABLE 1-1

Meaningful Use Regulations and What Each Means

Regulation	What It Does	Who Regulates It?
Incentive Program for Electronic Health Records	Defines the incentive payments allowed to eligible hospitals and EPs under the Medicare and Medicaid Incentive Programs and the minimum eligibility requirements providers must meet to qualify for payments in Stages 1 and 2.	Centers for Medicare & Medicaid Services (CMS)
Standards and Certification Criteria for Electronic Health Records	Rules that identify the standards and certification criteria for certified EHR. This regulation also defines the temporary and permanent certification bodies that can certify that an EHR will meet the core and menu set objectives as well as clinical quality measures.	Office of the National Coordinator for Health Information Technology
Meaningful Use of Electronic Health Records	Provides definition of *meaningful user* in guidelines to health professionals and hospitals on how to adopt and use EHR technology to help improve the quality, safety, and efficiency of patient care.	CMS
Stage 1 and Stage 2 MU Requirements	These are two pieces of legislation, both submitted with a comment period and now posted as final in the Federal Register. 42 CFR Parts 412, 413, 422, et al.	CMS

For more information on regulations and guidance documents, consult the Web site http://healthit.hhs.gov.

Meaningful Use Stages 1, 2, and 3 are designed to incrementally increase the use of EHRs, and explained in the next section.

Overview of the Three Stages for Meaningful Use Participation

There are currently three stages for MU participation, though it is possible that more stages will be added after 2016. In order to successfully attest to MU, you will be required to pull data from your certified EHR (and possibly also from paper charts if they still exist) that demonstrate the ratio of the number of patients in the certified EHR and the number of patients for whom you have entered and used data about that patient encounter.

You may adopt an EHR and be prepared to pull data from your EHR system much faster than HHS's progressive calendar, but the stages nonetheless define the necessary criteria.

- Stage 1 criteria focus on the basic functionalities of an EHR system. A meaningful user must capture health information in a standardized format and use that information to track key clinical conditions. A meaningful user must initiate the reporting of clinical quality measures (CQMs) and public health information and also provide a clinical summary of the encounter to the patient.

- Stage 2 (which begins in 2014) increases overall thresholds and HIE among providers and promotes patient engagement by giving patients secure online access to their health information. Meaningful users will electronically transmit patient care summaries across multiple settings. You cannot enter Stage 2 without first completing Stage 1.

- Stage 3 criteria, beginning in 2016, focus on improving quality, safety, and efficiency, leading to improved health outcomes, decision support for national high-priority conditions, patient access to self-management tools, and access to comprehensive patient data through patient-centered HIEs. You cannot enter Stage 3 without first completing Stages 1 and 2.

Each stage comes with its own set of core measures (required measures) and menu set measures (also required, but elective measures are provided for selection). You also must select CQMs that are cross-referenced with reporting numbers assigned by the National Quality Forum's (NQF) and the Physician Quality Reporting System's (PQRS) reporting criteria. Core and menu measures for Stages 1 and 2 are available in the ancillary material, but they are also available at www.cms.gov/Regulations-and-Guidance/Legislation/EHR IncentivePrograms/Downloads/Stage1vsStage2CompTablesforEP.pdf. Also available in the ancillary material are Stage 2 CQM specification sheets for EPs. Stage 1 CQMs are discussed in Chapter 2, but to find the 2014 (Stage 2) CQMs, go to www.cms.gov/Regulations-and-Guidance/Legislation/EHRIncentivePrograms/Stage_2.html.

At the CMS' Web site, www.cms.gov/EHRIncentivePrograms, you can learn how the PQRI, NQF, and CMS have cross-referenced quality measures allowing you to report for many initiatives using the same set of numbers.[8] For example, CQM's Alternate Core Measure #2, Preventive Care and Screening: Influenza Immunization for Patients 50 Years Old or Older, is also NQF #0041 and PQRS #110.

How to Get Your Meaningful Use Incentive Funds

CMS incentive funding in 2012 paid out more than $8 billion to hospitals and physicians and, in general, was a measureable driver in the adoption of EHRs. If you are an EP or EH as defined in Task 1 of this chapter (see next page), the CMS is making available incentive payments (which can be used to help defray the cost of software, implementation, and upgrades) if you demonstrate you are a meaningful user. To prove you are a meaningful user to the CMS, Stage 1 requires you to capture information in your EHR as structured or reportable data. *Structured data* means that all persons who have access to the EHR enter health information (data) into the same field using the same terms. For example, a certified EHR will allow you to enter height using feet and inches, inches only, or centimeters. While the EHR designers anticipate you will enter data using general observational findings, what actually happens is that some users enter a five-foot-tall woman as 60 inches tall, 5'0", 5 feet 0 inches, or 152.4 cm. Should you need to identify all women with a body mass index (BMI) of 22% to 35%, the system cannot calculate the data as it will not identify consistent (structured) data. The same data-entry principle applies to patient date of birth, preferred language and race, medications, allergies, and problem list (presenting problems).

Launching into MU without a strategic plan will, for many reasons, likely lead to failure. For example, are data entered consistently so that they can be extracted for decision making? Are some physicians frustrated with templates (forms) and developing their own? Are scanned records consistently called by the same indexing strategy so that physicians can find them in the system? We will discuss more about the value of data in Chapter 2.

The following four questions can be used to outline your participation.

- Are you eligible for MU funds?
- Are you a meaningful user?
- Should you apply under the Medicaid or Medicare Incentive Program?
- Of the 25 core and menu set measures and the 44 CQMs, which ones are required and which ones should you select?

What to Do: Determine Your Meaningful Use Eligibility

Task 1: Evaluate whether you are eligible for MU incentive payments. There are two types of health care providers who are eligible to participate in the Medicare and Medicaid EHR Incentive Programs: EHs and EPs. These categories were established in the HITECH Act and are briefly categorized below. *Note:* The remainder of this chapter is directed at EPs. It is not our intent to provide guidance for EHs even though they are described below. Detailed information on MU measures for hospitals is readily available at www.healthit.gov.

Eligible Hospitals
- Medicare EHs
  - Subsection (d) hospitals in the 50 states or Washington, DC, which are paid under the hospital inpatient prospective payment system. Hospitals in Maryland may also participate per law.
  - Critical Access Hospitals (CAHs)
- Medicaid EHs
  - Acute care hospitals with at least 10% Medicaid patient volume. This may include CAHs and cancer hospitals.
  - Children's hospitals

Critical Point

In Stage 1, EPs who are employees of a health care system but also practice in an ambulatory environment may not be eligible for incentive funds because of their employment status. However, in Stage 2, those EPs may be eligible if:

- They demonstrate that they fund the acquisitions, implementation, and maintenance of CEHRT, including the support of hardware and interfaces needed for Meaningful Use.
- They do not receive reimbursement from an EH or CAH.
- They use their CEHRT at a hospital, in lieu of using the hospital's CEHRT.
- They are not hospital-based.

Determination of eligibility will be made through an application process currently in development.

Eligible Professionals. Incentive payments are calculated on an individual-provider basis, not by practices or medical groups. A provider may designate a practice to receive the funds on his or her behalf, but it is up to the provider to make the decision whether to take the funds directly or pass them along to the practice. The practice cannot independently claim the incentive payment or make the decision for the provider, even if the EHR belongs to the practice.[9] As an EP, you must also complete at least 50% of your patient encounters in a practice or location where you use a certified EHR. Hardship exemptions may apply to you. Two starting places for those exemptions include AMA's Incentive Program Web site[15] and HealthIT.gov, key search "hardship exemptions."[10]

Each EP is only eligible for one incentive payment per calendar year, regardless of how many locations at which the EP provides services. EPs who perform more than 90% of their services in a hospital inpatient or emergency department setting (hospital-based) do not qualify for Medicare or Medicaid incentive payments.

- Medicare EPs
  - Doctors of medicine or osteopathy
  - Doctors of dental surgery or dental medicine
  - Doctors of podiatric medicine
  - Doctors of optometry
  - Doctors of chiropractic medicine
- Medicaid EPs
  - Doctors of medicine or osteopathy
  - Nurse practitioners
  - Certified nurse-midwives
  - Doctors of dental surgery or dental medicine
  - Physician assistants who practice in a federally qualified health center (FQHC) or rural health center (RHC) that is led by a physician assistant
  - Doctors in Medicare Advantage (MA) programs

In addition to providing at least 20 hours per week of patient care services, a Medicare Advantage EP must either be employed by a Medicare Advantage organization that is a licensed HMO or be employed by, a partner of, or contracted by a Medicare Advantage organization in which the EP provides at least 80% of that organization's Medicare patient care services to enrollees of the Medicare Advantage organization. Medicare Advantage–EPs cannot directly receive an incentive payment paid directly to the MA organization.

To participate in the Medicaid Incentive Program an, EPs must:

- Have a minimum of 30% Medicaid patient volume (20% minimum for pediatricians) or practice predominantly in an FQHC or RHC and have at least 30% patient volume of needy individuals. For pediatricians, the requirement is 20% of patient volume or a calculation determined by the individual states.
- Offer Children's Health Insurance Program (CHIP). CHIP patients did not originally count toward the Medicaid patient volume criteria in Stage 1, but a change was issued with the Stage 2 rule. States that have offered CHIP as part of a Medicaid expansion under Title 19 or Title 21 can include those patients in their provider's Medicaid patient volume calculation. In Stage 1, only CHIP programs created under a Medicaid expansion via Title 19 are eligible. This change to the patient volume calculation is applicable to all eligible providers, regardless of the stage of the incentive program they are participating in.[11]

Medicaid EPs can participate in nonconsecutive years for a total of six incentive payment years through the end of the program in 2021, with the last year to begin participation being 2016. To qualify for incentive payments, a Medicaid EP must not be hospital-based and must meet certain Medicaid patient volume criteria as noted above. Providers who file for Medicaid as a secondary payer and meet the 30% threshold using secondary payers as the base may also elect to file as a Medicaid EP.[12]

Task 2: Determine if you are a meaningful user. *Step 1:* Determine if you are eligible. Begin by referencing Task 1 to determine if you fall into the category *EP* or *EH.*

Step 2: Meet the three main functions that the HITECH Act requires of you to be considered a meaningful user.

1. Are you using CEHRT in a meaningful way? For example, are you e-prescribing? (See Step 3 below.)
2. Are you using CEHRT for electronic exchange of health information to improve quality of health care? For example, can you securely share electronic health information with another health care provider who has a different EIN or tax ID? In Stage 2, the other health care provider cannot be using the same software version that you use.
3. Are you using CEHRT to submit CQMs and other such measures selected by the Secretary of HHS? You will learn more about certified EHR technology in Chapter 3.

Step 3: Determine if you are using the EHR in a meaningful way. In order to extract data from a system, data must be searchable. Current technology does not favor extracting information contained in a scanned document and bringing it into a database query.

In plain language, this means that data, such as a patient's demographics, blood pressure, height, weight, active medications, and medication allergies, must be entered into the EHR so that the data are "structured" or "discrete." Structured data are typically entered into the EHR when you type numbers or letters into a field that accepts only numbers, letters, or both or when a choice is selected from a drop-down list or check-off box.

Critical Point

An EHR that cannot capture structured data will not meet certification criteria.

Many physician practices have abandoned EHRs that were essentially an electronic filing system of scanned documents. Scanned documents have a place in every EHR as historical data, but generally they are not searchable.

Step 4: Identify whether your EHR is certified. Nearly all EHR vendors are proud to let you know that their EHR software has been certified by the ONC. The ONC Certification body was formerly named the Accredited Testing and Certification Body (ATCB) under the Temporary Certification Rule. Under the Permanent Certification Rule, now in effect, the new accredited testing and certifying bodies are referred to as ONC Certification bodies.

EHR vendors can achieve EHR certification in two formats: (1) as a complete EHR or (2) as a modular EHR. A complete EHR system is required to prove how it will meet all of the MU core and menu measures, as well as a defined minimum number of CQMs.

Most EPs purchase a complete EHR. However, an EP can cobble together several EHR modules, perhaps at a lower price, to achieve MU Stage 1, but an EP also will need a robust reporting engine that can reach up into each of the modules and extract clinical and demographic information for each of the core, menu, and CQMs. Some EPs chose this route for Stage 1.

Critical Point

In purchasing or transitioning into an EHR, be sure to ask whether the EHR has achieved Complete EHR certification or Modular EHR certification. You will need several certified EHR modules and a good reporting engine to query the multiple systems relevant to health quality to meet MU Stage 1 requirements. EHR modules can be less expensive than a Complete EHR, but cross-reference the core, menu, and quality measures with the bundled modular EHRs you purchase. A certified EHR built from modules is only a certified system for Stage 1 reporting if you elect to use all the modules used to achieve 2011 Edition certification. If you choose to use a different module than one included in your vendor's certification process, the EHR is no longer a certified system for Stage 1. Each of the modules must be certified as a package for you to complete attestation, even if the module you chose to use is included in another vendor's certification but not in your system.

In Stage 1 of the ONC testing, a few EHR vendors seeking certification for a complete EHR actually bundled together their core EHR and a few modules and then certified the entire package as a complete EHR. Unfortunately, they did not also bundle the prices together as a complete EHR, so when practices implemented these bundled complete certified systems, they found that they would also have to purchase all the components in order to be using a certified system or purchase an upgrade that included the additional certified components. ONC now requires the EHR vendor to be transparent about any bundles and disclose its pricing for add-on modules on the Certified Healthcare Product List (CHPL) Web site.

To determine if you are using an ONC-Certified system, complete the following tasks.

1. Go to http://oncchpl.force.com/ehrcert?q=CHPL. Click on either the 2011 or 2014 edition (or both for a comprehensive list that covers both 2011 and 2014). You can find this Web site through other HHS portals, such as www.healthit.gov or http://oncchpl.force .com/ehrcert, or simply use your Internet search engine and use the keywords ONC, CHPL for the certified healthcare product list.

2. Select "Ambulatory Practice Type" or "Inpatient Practice Type" to get started on your search. Then, search for your EHR vendor by vendor name, product name, or CHPL Product Number. Most users search by vendor name or product name. Be sure you double check your current version with the EHR version that is certified. If you claim that you are using a currently certified version when you are actually using an earlier version, you will likely be required to return your incentive funds and begin the MU process again.

3. When your search results appear, you will also be able to see "Additional Software Required" to meet MU. This lets you know how the EHR vendor bundled its software to get certified for MU Stage 1.

4. Click on the vendor name and your version number to see a list of all general criteria, ambulatory criteria, and ambulatory clinical quality measures that the EHR vendor met during certification testing. A checkmark indicates the vendor was certified for this core, menu, or quality measure. When you are selecting CQMs to report on, be sure your EHR vendor has been tested and certified for this measure, or you may have difficulty extracting results for MU reporting.

5. When you select "Add to Cart," you are not purchasing anything; rather you are requesting a CMS Certification ID number that you will need when attesting to MU. You will read more on attestation in Chapters 4 and 5.

6. If you are building your own modular EHR, you must continue to select modular products until you have reached 100% of the certification criteria. A certified complete EHR meets 100% of the criteria.

Task 3: Determine whether you qualify for Medicaid and/or Medicare. A Medicaid EP may also qualify for the Medicare Incentive Program but may only apply to participate in one EHR Incentive Program per year. However, CMS will allow a one-time switch. One reason physicians choose to switch between programs is that fewer reporting criteria are required and more dollars are available in years 1 and 2 under Medicaid. They then switch to the Medicare Incentive Program for years 3, 4, and 5. However, to do this, you must meet the Medicaid patient volume criteria and also apply for incentives under your state's Medicaid program. Comparisons to help you make this decision are in Table 1-2.

To qualify for Medicare, you must treat Medicare patients and bill for Part B services on the Medicare Physician Fee Schedule. The Medicare threshold is $24,000 of allowable charges in a calendar year, and MU payments equal to 75% of the $24,000 threshold ($18,000) will be distributed after the provider meets that threshold. If the provider *does not meet the $24,000* of allowable Medicare charges by December 31, the provider who successfully attests to MU will receive 75% of that year's allowables after the claims are calculated for that year.

The Medicare EHR Incentive Program for EPs started in 2011, and EHR incentive payments under Medicare will continue through 2016. See Table 1-3. Depending on the first year you participate, you can receive incentive funds for up to 5 consecutive years. The last year to begin participation in the Medicare EHR Incentive Program is 2014, if you'd like to receive incentive payments and not be subject to the payment adjustments by CMS and required by Congress.

The Medicaid EHR Incentive Program for EPs also started in 2011, and by 2012 nearly all states had a Medicaid incentive program in place. EHR incentive payments will continue through 2021 with 2016 as the last year to register and receive full benefits. EPs can receive up to $63,750 through the Medicaid EHR Incentive Program. See Table 1-4.

TABLE 1-2

Comparison Between Medicare and Medicaid EHR Incentive Programs

Medicare EHR Incentive Program	Medicaid EHR Incentive Program
Run by Centers for Medicare & Medicaid Services	Run by your state Medicaid agency
Maximum incentive amount is $44,000	Maximum incentive amount is $63,750
Payments over five consecutive years	Payments over six years that do not have to be consecutive
Payment adjustments will begin in 2015 for providers who are eligible but decide not to participate	No Medicaid payment adjustments
Providers must demonstrate Meaningful Use (MU) every year once they enter the program to receive incentive payments.	In the first year, providers can receive an incentive payment for adopting, implementing, or upgrading electronic health record technology. Providers must demonstrate MU in the remaining years to receive incentive payments.

TABLE 1-3

Medicare Incentive Payments

	CY 2011	CY 2012	CY 2013	CY 2014	CY 2015	CY 2016	Maximum Payments
MU Stage Timeline	Stage 1						
				Stage 2			
						Stage 3	
Medicare Incentive Payments	$18,000	$12,000	$8,000	$4,000	$2,000		$44,000
		$18,000	$12,000	$8,000	$4,000	$2,000	$44,000
			$15,000	$12,000	$8,000	$4,000	$39,000
				$12,000	$8,000	$4,000	$24,000

Abbreviations: CY indicates calendar year, and MU, Meaningful Use.

Note the column represented by 2018–2021 (in Table 1-4) represents a continuation of the same pattern of payments. Medicaid incentives are established and managed by each state.

Consider the advantages and disadvantages of selecting Medicaid (see Table 1-4) over Medicare. In nearly all cases, MU incentives payments favor the Medicaid provider.

Critical Point

In a practice in which two or more health care professionals are EPs, one EP may apply for Medicare incentive funds and the other for Medicaid. The variable is dependent on the payer population (Medicare or Medicaid and needy) recorded in the EHR. Eligibility overlaps in most instances, but reporting measures under both incentives may add to the MU project manager's workload, as he or she will need to capture measure data for both federal and state reporting in future years.

As of August 24, 2012, the HHS announced it had paid out MU incentive dollars to more than 120,000 EPs and 3,300 EHs. With that number growing by approximately 10,000 per month in 2012, EPs waiting until 2013 or 2014 to adopt an EHR and complete MU attestation under Medicare will find that time is not in their favor. The incentive program for Medicaid offers a more lenient timeframe.

Table 1-3 shows the payment chart for Medicare Incentive Payments. If you waited until 2013 to enter the MU program, your incentive funds dropped from $44,000 to $38,000 payable over 4 years, instead of the 5 payment years available to earlier participants. But if you wait until 2014 to enter the program, the incentive funds drop to a maximum of $24,000 payable over just 3 years.

Compare Tables 1-3 and 1-4 and notice the benefits of selecting Medicaid as your incentive program of choice. The payments are higher, the restrictions less rigid, and the incentives are spread out over a longer period of time. We will discuss the advantages of one over the other in this section.

TABLE 1-4

Medicaid Incentive Payments

	2011	2012	2013	2014	2015	2016	2017	2018–2021	Total Medicaid Payments
MU Stage Timeline	Stage 1								
				Stage 2					
						Stage 3			$63,750
Medicaid Incentive Payments	$21,250	$8,500	$8,500	$8,500	$8,500				$63,750
		$21,250	$8,500	$8,500	$8,500	$8,500			$63,750
			$21,250	$8,500	$8,500	$8,500	$8,500		$63,750
				$21,250	$8,500	$8,500	$8,500	$8,500	$63,750
					$21,500	$8,500	$8,500	$8,500	$63,750
						$21,250	$8,500	$8,500	$63,750

Abbreviations: MU indicates Meaningful Use.

Advantages of Medicaid Over Medicare Meaningful Use Participation

- Reporting requirements for Medicaid are more favorable for the first year an EP enters the program. In year 1, the EP must attest to adopting, implementing, or upgrading a certified EHR.
  - *Adopted* means having acquired and installed. *Adopt* does not mean that you are undecided as to your choice of systems.
  - *Implemented* means that you have commenced utilization; *implementing* involves staff training, documented efforts to redesign workflows, and that EPs are using the system. You must demonstrate actual implementation prior to the incentive payment.
  - *Upgraded* means you have expanded the available functionality.
- Incentive funds exceed those from Medicare.
- Larger incentive amount in year 1 calculated to be 85% of $25,000 for the first year or $21,250 reimbursement for expenses incurred for adopting, implementing, or upgrading. Subsequent reimbursements are for 85% of $10,000 in years 2 through 6 for a maximum of $8,500.
- EPs can receive up to $63,750 over 6 years compared to $44,000 over 5 years for Medicare. Pediatricians with Medicaid patient volume between 20% and 29% of their total patient volume could receive two-thirds of the maximum payment amount ($42,500).
- All states and territories have implemented a state Medicaid MU program.

Advantages of Medicare Over Medicaid

- Administered nationally through CMS with the ONC to operationalize MU
- Information and guidance are readily available at www.cms.gov.
- Funding to states and territories may be challenged by budgets and statewide legislation.

Note: If you are eligible for both Medicare and Medicaid payments, you may choose not to participate. However, you still would be subject to a Medicare penalty if you are not meeting the MU requirements based on timelines designated in the rule. In general, there is either no penalties, or there are loosely defined penalties under the Medicaid payment program.

Now that you have determined whether you will apply for MU under Medicare or Medicaid, it is now time for you to move on to Task 4 and complete a MU Gap Analysis.

Task 4: Conduct a MU gap analysis. A *gap analysis* is a tool that helps you determine what you have and what you need. The gap analysis provided in Table 1-5 not only provides the questions, but also the chapter within this book to find solutions.

A gap analysis also helps identify where barriers should be addressed to achieve your practice goals. We will get into barriers later in this chapter, but for now, we focus just on questions and answers that help assess potential bottlenecks.

T A B L E 1-5
Meaningful Use Gap Analysis and Solutions Tool

Question	Your Answer	Where to Find the Solution	Our Comments	Your Gaps
What eligible professionals (EPs) can attest to Meaningful Use (MU)? For EPs in a Federally Qualified Health Center (FQHC)	Names of EPs, including MDs, DOs, physician assistants, chiropractors, optometrists, podiatrists, certified nurse-midwives Add: Physician assistants and nurse practitioners (NPs)	Chapter 1 provides definitions and eligibility criteria for EPs.	EPs must meet eligibility criteria.	Check if complete. Make notes on what to do in this column.
Do the EPs meet the eligibility criteria?		Chapter 1 provides guidance on eligibility.	Demographic information in your practice management system can help.	
Will you attest under Medicare or Medicaid or some of each?	Medicare Medicaid	Chapter 1 provides pros and cons of both.	You cannot apply for both, but if some EPs see more Medicaid than Medicare, the EP can apply for Medicaid while others in the practice apply for Medicare.	

(*continued*)

TABLE 1-5 (continued)

Meaningful Use Gap Analysis and Solutions Tool

Question	Your Answer	Where to Find the Solution	Our Comments	Your Gaps
Are you part of a super group or a health system that is overseeing what core, menu, and clinical quality measures you will report on?	Is there a governing body overseeing the MU strategy, or are you on your own?		Your answer is driven by who determines menu and clinical quality measures (CQMs) for attestation.	
Is your practice-management system stable?	Have you been using it long enough to work out the software bugs and workflow? Are the new demographic fields included?	Chapter 1 provides the demographic information you must capture. Chapter 4 provides workflows for capturing demographics.	Have you recently moved data into a new practice management (PM) system, and is it working for you?	
Have you determined where you are in the MU stages?	All EPs enter at Stage 1.	Chapter 1 addresses Stage 1. All chapters address Stage 2.	Attestation in year 1, Stage 1 is 90 continuous days for Medicare. Years 2 to 5 are 365 days.	
Have you registered your EPs?		Chapter 1 provides instructions on how to register and what you will need. Chapter 5 provides guidance on attestation.	You may designate a third party to register for you. All EPs register at Centers for Medicare & Medicaid Services (CMS), but Medicaid EPs also register with the state.	
Have you verified that the electronic health record (EHR) vendor and modules you are using are certified?	Write down the version number and CMS certification number.	Chapter 1 provides answers on how to find the certification number.		
Which approach to using an Office of the National Coordinator for Health Information Technology (ONC) certified EHR vendor did your practice select?	Modular, single-source, best of breed	Chapter 2 provides guidance on: Single source—one EHR vendor Best of breed—your PM system and an EHR from another company.	Modular EHRs may require data gathering from each module. A data-reporting program must be used for best-of-breed systems and some single-source systems.	
Who manages demographic input?		Chapter 2 explains value of data. Chapter 4 provides workflow for gathering data.	Ensure there is a field for all demographics, including preferred language, gender, race, ethnicity, date of birth.	

(continued)

TABLE 1-5 (continued)

Meaningful Use Gap Analysis and Solutions Tool

Question	Your Answer	Where to Find the Solution	Our Comments	Your Gaps
Who does computerized provider order entry (CPOE) in the EHR?		Chapter 1 identifies CPOE eligibility. Chapter 4 identifies workflow.	This may be an MD, DO, NP, or nurse under physician's supervision.	
Have you determined your CQMs?		Chapter 1 provides Stage 1 CQMs, core and alternate core measures.	CQMs are discussed in every chapter of this book.	
Have you determined your menu measures?		See Chapter 1. Menu measures also are in Appendix A.		
Are you exempt from any of the core measures?	Review the Stage 1 Meaningful Use Attestation worksheet in the Appendix.	Chapters 1 and 7 provide guidance.		
Can you submit data to a public registry?		See Chapters 1, 4, and 7.		
How does your EHR provide a clinical summary for the patient?		See Chapter 4.		
Does your EHR vendor have a patient portal?			Portals are not required in Stage 1. Vendor portals work best for primary-care providers and FQHCs. Disease-specific portals often work better for specialty practices.	
Have you mapped International Classification of Disease (ICD) and logical observation identifiers names and codes (LOINC) to Current Procedural Terminology (CPT®) codes?	Make a list of diagnostic, laboratory, and procedure orders with your CPT codes to be sure you are capturing these data.		Some physicians use multiple codes for orders. When building a report, query for all the relevant codes.	
Do you have an imaging department within your practice or clinic?	Relevant in Stage 2, not Stage 1.			

(continued)

TABLE 1-5 (continued)

Meaningful Use Gap Analysis and Solutions Tool

Question	Your Answer	Where to Find the Solution	Our Comments	Your Gaps
Does your practice offer an infusion center?			Bar-code readers to match intravenous prescriptions with the patient are not included in Stage 1 but are included in Stage 2 and most likely Stage 3.	
How do you document who received patient education?			Embed patient education materials, if possible, in the EHR.	
Have you completed an annual Health Insurance Portability and Accountability Act (HIPAA) risk assessment?		Consult risk assessments available online.[13]		
Does the EHR vendor require reporting software for data extraction? Does the vendor automate measure calculation for MU?	Is there back-end software to let you know if you are meeting measures?		The EHR vendor will identify software. You want to know costs of licensing. Are you capturing narcotic prescriptions that cannot be sent electronically?	
Core Measure–Specific Gap Analysis				
1. Who can complete CPOE?	Identify who can complete CPOE. Are they entering orders consistently? Does the physician ever amend an order from another provider?	For alternate CPOE measures, see www.cms.gov/Regulations-and-Guidance/Legislation/EHRIncentivePrograms/Downloads/Stage1ChangesTipsheet.pdf	See CPOE infrastructure, this chapter. Is CPOE included in your clinical standard operating procedures (SOPs)?	
2. How do physicians check drug interactions?	Are you maintaining a current list of medications?		This measure is its own core measure and cannot be used to demonstrate clinical decision support (CDS).	
3. Do you maintain updated problem lists?	Are you using *ICD-9* and/or SNOMED-CT® codes to maintain problem lists?		See section on Health information technology (IT) Standards in this chapter.	

(continued)

TABLE 1-5 (continued)

Meaningful Use Gap Analysis and Solutions Tool

Question	Your Answer	Where to Find the Solution	Our Comments	Your Gaps
4. What is your quality assurance (QA) process for e-prescribing permissible prescriptions?			While not required for MU reporting, one designated person to "push" (ie, electronically fulfill) all e-prescriptions helps standardize the process. E-prescribing requirements for controlled substances are determined by state and federal laws. If the state law allowed it as of January 13, 2010, you may count (as a numerator for e-prescribing) controlled substances.[14]	
5. How do you maintain active medication lists?	Implement a process for a patient to verify active and inactive medications.		Maintain patient confidentiality while reviewing this medication list. Potential privacy issues at the front office if you ask for a current medication list while the patient is in waiting room.	
6. How do you capture medication allergy list?	Implement a process to track medication allergies.		EHR vendors should have a field for "No Medication Allergies." Document patient allergies.	
7. Does the front office accurately record demographics?	Implement processes for consistent gathering of data.		Train front-office staff to ask about and input all fields. A quick reference guide helps with this.	
8. When recording and charting vital signs, can you also create a trend line or growth chart?	Cross-train staff capturing medication list with staff capturing height, weight, blood pressure (BP), and body mass index (BMI)?	Chapter 1 focuses on the value of data.	Vital signs are not consistently captured in specialty practices. Ensure electronic medical devices (BP cuffs or scales) enter data accurately. BP measures for patients with hypertension require two visits. If BMI is out of range, document a follow-up plan.	

(*continued*)

T A B L E 1-5 (continued)

Meaningful Use Gap Analysis and Solutions Tool

Question	Your Answer	Where to Find the Solution	Our Comments	Your Gaps
9. Record smoking status	Ensure this field is a structured data field in the EHR. Also, ensure EHR does not scrub data between visits or the two visits will be difficult to track.		Recording status is a Stage 1 core measure. CQM is to counsel patient on smoking cessation. Smoking cessation counseling, a CQM, requires two visits.	
10. How will you select and report CQMs?	Coordinate measures with your patient population to meet the numbers. Your top 10 visit types are a great resource.	Guidance in Chapters 2 and 3	In practices with three or more EPs, this becomes an easier reporting task if EPs agree on clinical quality measures. Required: three core/alternate core and three additional CQMs. Data must be consistently entered into the system to report a CQM.	
11. Have you selected a CDS rule? Stage 2 requires five CDS interventions related to four or more CQMs.	Involve all members of the practice for this measure. CDS rule may include reminders for all patients needing a mammogram, embedded link to clinical guidelines, condition-specific order sets, documentation templates.		E-prescribing and medication alerts do not count here.	
12. Electronic copy of patient record	Develop a policy for providing patients with an electronic summary, if requested.	See clinical policies and procedures, this chapter.	Patient portals may serve as an efficient and secure process for delivering summaries.	
13. What is your process to provide clinical summaries?	Did you set protocols for what can be extracted from the record into the summary? Engage staff to help meet this requirement.	See Standards and Clinical Policies, this chapter.		

(continued)

T A B L E 1-5 **(continued)**

Meaningful Use Gap Analysis and Solutions Tool

Question	Your Answer	Where to Find the Solution	Our Comments	Your Gaps
14. Have you determined an electronic exchange of clinical information partner?	For Stage 1, start with a small exchange. Ask your vendor to provide guidance on this as they will have interfaces already set up.		Start with a small exchange. Sending an e-mail with a protected document is not an electronic exchange between EHR systems. Must be sent to another legal entity.	
15. How do you protect electronic health information?	Have you conducted an updated HIPAA risk assessment and put measures in place to mitigate risks?		Answering "yes" establishes a date in time that identifies the risks you knew and when you knew them.	

After completing the core measures gap analysis and identifying the gaps, this is a good time to also identify the menu measures so that you can cross-reference and manage potential gaps. A gap indicates a process that may hinder successful attestation. You must select five from this list.

Critical Point

One of the five measures in Stage 1 must be a department of public health (DPH) measure (see numbers 9 and 10). In Stage 2, the transmission to DPH must be successful and ongoing for the entire reporting period.

Just as you reviewed the potential gaps in the core measures, complete the gap analysis in Table 1-6 for menu measures.

T A B L E 1-6

Menu Measures Infrastructure Gap Analysis

Question	Your Answer	Where to Find the Solution	Our Comments	Your Gaps
1. Does your practice management (PM) system or e-prescribing system conduct formulary checks?	While the measure applies only to drug formularies when writing prescriptions, HIPAA 5010 transactions became effective January 1, 2012. The 270 (request)/271 (response) transaction applies to eligibility. Consult AMA's 5010 Toolkit for guidance.[15]	See this chapter, standards section.	Payers prefer if patients are prescribed medications on the payer's formulary and that generics are used when possible.	

(*continued*)

T A B L E 1-6 (continued)

Menu Measures Infrastructure Gap Analysis

Question	Your Answer	Where to Find the Solution	Our Comments	Your Gaps
2. Is the process to enter clinical laboratory test results consistent with anyone accessing your patients' records?	Are results returning to you in positive, negative, or numerical format so they can be entered as structured data? Eligibility checks prior to running a laboratory test can save thousands of dollars.		Laboratory results in structured data can be uploaded into flow sheets, especially beneficial to measure the progression or recession of a disease.	
3. Do you have patient lists by condition?	Can you export a list of patients by specific condition?	See standards, this chapter. This may be done using SNOMED-CT and *ICD-9*.	Terrific preventive medicine tool.	
4. How do you send out patient reminders?	Are you sending patients reminders for preventive or follow-up care?		This measure is focused on patients 65 years old or older or 5 years old or younger. Keeping demographics current plays a significant role in data extraction.	
5. Have you implemented a process for patients to electronically access personal health information?	Can you send laboratory results, problem lists, medication lists, and medication allergies in an electronic format for the patient to securely access?		A patient portal and a personal health record (PHR) are good examples for this measure. If you accept content from a PHR and use it to make clinical decisions, the patient's information becomes part of your legal medical record.	
6. How will you track when you provide patient-specific educational materials?	Can the electronic health record's (EHR's) internal logic provide notice that educational materials would be valuable for a particular patient?		This measure is tied directly to the EHR's ability to accurately read medications and problem lists. Eligible professional (EP) may count telemedicine visits as "seen by the EP." Counting telemedicine visits must be done consistently.[16] The EHR does not have to generate the educational materials, but someone must record that the materials were provided.	

(continued)

TABLE 1-6 (continued)

Menu Measures Infrastructure Gap Analysis

Question	Your Answer	Where to Find the Solution	Our Comments	Your Gaps
7. Do you or does your system reconcile medications with each e-Rx?	Does someone in the practice check to see if the name, dosages, frequency, and route of current medications reported by the patient are accurate?			
8. What do you provide when you are transitioning a patient to another location or provider?	Provide a summary of care for each transition of care or referral.	See standards in Chapter 3.	Electronic transmission of care summary required in Stage 2. In Stage 1, the transition summary can be on paper or sent electronically. Significant concerns exist over e-mail transitions as they do not count as an electronic transmission and may not be secure.	
9. Can you successfully submit immunization data to the immunization information systems (IIS)?	Standards and state requirements can complicate this measure.	See standards in Chapter 3.	In Stage 2, the exception is if the transmission is not allowed or the standards are not compatible between the IIS and the EHR.	
10. Do you track syndromic surveillance data and submission?		See standards in Chapter 3.	Syndromic surveillance data focus on particular health threats or problems as part of a prevention and control program. HIV/AIDS prevention programs are examples.	

Now that you've completed your gap analysis, your next task is to review the core measures and select MU menu measures and CQMs.

Critical Point

While we identify Stage 1 measures by number in Table 1-7, we also provide notes on how this measure will be updated in Stage 2. Measures in Stage 2 may not have the same corresponding numbers as those in Stage 1. If you have not yet completed Stage 1, Table 1-5 will help you complete an MU gap analysis.

Throughout the MU program, you will consistently hear about numerators and denominators. During attestation (described in Chapter 5), you will be asked to query the system for a ratio of the number of patients you have seen during the reporting period (denominator), and the number of patients for whom you provided a service or consultation (numerator).

For example, when attesting to menu measure #6 (See Table 1-9), you are asked to "Use certified EHR technology to identify patient-specific education resources and provide those resources to the patient, if appropriate."

For this core measure, CEHRT should allow you to electronically provide patient-specific education resources based on the patient's problem list, medication list, and laboratory results. Providing a link to an Internet search engine does not meet this measure.

The numerator then, is how many patients you provided educational materials (numerator) out of all the patients you saw during this reporting period (denominator.)

Figure 1-2 provides a diagram of how to view numerators and denominators.

Task 5: Understanding the core measures and choosing your menu set measures.
First, determine how you will query the EHR database to complete the 15 core objectives.

■ Begin with a strategic approach to achieve consistent data entry. Chapter 4 provides detailed workflow guidance on all MU core, menu, and additional measures.

■ Determine if there is an exemption in the core objectives in Table 1-7 and the reporting measures in the column on the right side.

■ For additional guidance on exemptions, refer to the MU Glossary and Requirements Table[17] as a quick reference guide for Stage 1 MU measures and exemptions or to CMS'

FIGURE 1-2

Numerators and Denominators

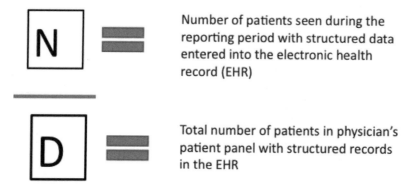

EP Attestation User's Guide online.[18] The Stage 1 Attestation Guide also is available as part of this book's ancillary material. This guide also provides information on Stage 2 objectives and measures.

■ After reviewing all core objectives and corresponding measures in Table 1-7, move to Table 1-8 to select 5 menu set measures that will help you meet Measure #10.

TABLE 1-7

Stage 1 Core Objectives for Eligible Professionals

Stage 1, Section 1: REQUIRED Core Objectives—Must Meet All 15		
#	**Objective or Measure**	**Work Performed by/Notes**
1	Computerized provider order entry (CPOE) for medication orders More than 30% of all unique patients with at least one medication in their medication list seen by the eligible professional (EP) have at least one medication order entered using CPOE. Exclusion: EP who writes fewer than 100 prescriptions during the electronic health record (EHR) reporting period	Attestation: Numerator/Denominator For alternate CPOE measures, see www.cms.gov/Regulations-and-Guidance/Legislation/EHRIncentivePrograms/Downloads/Stage1ChangesTipsheet.pdf.
2	Drug-drug and drug-allergy interaction checks Functionality is enabled for the entire EHR reporting period. Exclusion: None	Attestation: Yes/No (must be "yes")
3	Maintain an up-to-date problem list of current and active diagnoses More than 80% of all unique patients seen by the EP have at least one entry (or an indication that no problems are known for the patient) recorded as structured data (entered into data fields). Exclusion: None	Attestation: Numerator/Denominator
4	E-prescribing (e-Rx) More than 40% of all permissible prescriptions written by the EP are transmitted electronically using certified EHR technology. Exclusion: Any EP who writes fewer than 100 prescriptions during the EHR reporting period	Attestation: Numerator/Denominator
5	Maintain active medication list More than 80% of all unique patients seen by the EP have at least one entry (or an indication that the patient is not currently prescribed any medication) recorded as structured data. Exclusion: None	Attestation: Numerator/denominator

(*continued*)

T A B L E 1-7 (continued)

Stage 1 Core Objectives for Eligible Professionals

Stage 1, Section 1: REQUIRED Core Objectives—Must Meet All 15		
#	**Objective or Measure**	**Work Performed by/Notes**
6	Maintain active medication allergy list More than 80% of all unique patients seen by the EP have at least one entry (or an indication that the patient does not have any medication allergies) recorded as structured data. Exclusion: None	Attestation: Numerator/Denominator
7	Record demographics More than 50% of all unique patients seen by the EP have demographics recorded as structured data (must include preferred language, gender, race, ethnicity, and date of birth (DOB)) Exclusion: None	Attestation: Numerator/Denominator
8	Record and chart changes in vital signs For more than 50% of all unique patients age 2 and over seen by the EP, height, weight, and blood pressure are recorded as structured data (also calculate, plot, and display body mass index (BMI)) Exclusion: Any EP who sees no patients 2 years or older or who believes that all three vital signs of their patients have no relevance to their scope of practice	Attestation: Numerator/Denominator This changes per the Stage 2 rule but can change for Stage 1 reporting before 2014, if desired by EP.
9	Record smoking status for patients 13 years or older More than 50% of all unique patients 13 years old or older seen by the EP have smoking status recorded as structured data. Exclusion: Any EP who sees no patients 13 years or older	Attestation: Numerator/Denominator
10	Report ambulatory clinical quality measures (CQMs) to Centers for Medicare & Medicaid Services (CMS)/states. For Stage 1, submit clinical measures electronically. See Table 1-8. Must fulfill three core set of CQMs and choose another three from a set of 38 Exclusion: None	Your three core measures are drawn first from the required core measures discussed in Table 1-8A. Your certified EHR technology (CEHRT) should be able to calculate these, but they may not apply because of your patient population. In that case, you will continue to select CQMs from the alternate core measure group until you are able to report on a total of three core CQMs. See discussion on core, menu, and CQM measures this chapter. For Stage 2, EPs will **not** be required to report CQMs as part of their Meaningful Use attestation. However, in 2014 and beyond, they will be

(continued)

TABLE 1-7 (continued)

Stage 1 Core Objectives for Eligible Professionals

Stage 1, Section 1: REQUIRED Core Objectives—Must Meet All 15		
#	Objective or Measure	Work Performed by/Notes
10		required to participate in quality reporting programs, such as physician quality reporting system (PQRS), accountable care organizations (ACOs), e-prescribing (eRx), and Childrens Health Insurance Program Reauthorization Act (CHIPRA). See Tables 1-8 and 1-9(A&B).
11	Implement one clinical decision support rule relevant to specialty, along with the ability to track compliance with that rule. You must decide what that rule is and implement it in the system. Rule/alert that is intelligently provided through software at time of care (for example, a patient with a specific prostate-specific antigen (PSA) level should be screened for prostate cancer; a standing order of complete blood count (CBC)) for all patients arriving for chemotherapy. Exclusion: None	EP must determine which rule to use; performed by EHR system Must be in addition to drug-to-drug and drug-to-allergy interaction alerts Attestation: Yes/No
12	Provide patients with an electronic copy of their health information, upon request More than 50% of all patients who request an electronic copy of their health information are provided it within 3 business days. CCD (continuity-of-care document) should include diagnostic test results, problem list, medication list, medication allergies). Electronic copy must be in electronic form (could be patient portal, patient health record (PHR), CD, USB, PDF via e-mail per patient preference, etc). Exclusion: Any EP who has no requests from patients or their agents for an electronic copy of their health information during the reporting period	EHR system enables report of continuity of care record/continuity care document (CCR/CCD) created by information captured by physician (EP) Attestation: Numerator/Denominator Effective 2014 this objective will change to: Provide patients the ability to view online, download, and transmit their health information. The measure is 50% of patients have the ability to view online, download, and transmit their health information.
13	Provide clinical summaries for patients for each office visit Clinical summaries provided to patients for more than 50% of all office visits within 3 business days CCD should include diagnostic test results, problem list, medication list, allergies. Exclusion: Any EP who has no office visits during the EHR reporting period	Physician captures relevant information. Nurse/medical assistant (MA) can pull report. Front- and back-office staff may distribute. Attestation: Numerator/Denominator Clinical summaries transition from 3 business days to 1 business day in Stage 2.

(continued)

T A B L E 1-7 (continued)

Stage 1 Core Objectives for Eligible Professionals

Stage 1, Section 1: REQUIRED Core Objectives—Must Meet All 15		
#	Objective or Measure	Work Performed by/Notes
14	Capability to exchange key clinical information among providers of care and patient-authorized entities electronically Performed at least one test of certified EHR technology's capacity to electronically exchange key clinical information Test must be performed; does not have to be a successful test Exclusion: None	Attestation: Yes/No
15	Protect electronic health information Conduct or review a security risk analysis and implement security updates as necessary and correct identified security deficiencies as part of its risk management process. Exclusions: None	Attestation: Yes/No (must attest "yes" or you will fail attestation; "yes" also means you have completed an annual risk analysis)

Now select five menu measures, including 1 public-health measure. To avoid significant workflow charges, these menu measures should reflect your patient population.

T A B L E 1-8

Stage 1, Meaningful Use Menu Set

Stage 1, Section 2: Meaningful Use Menu Set—Select Five (Must Include One Public-Health Initiative)		
#	Objective	Measure
1	Implement drug-formulary checks	Functionality is enabled for entire reporting period
2	Incorporate clinical laboratory test results as structured data	>40% of all clinical laboratory tests results ordered by the eligible professional (EP) during the electronic health record (EHR) reporting period whose results are either in a positive/negative or numerical format are incorporated in certified EHR technology
3	Generate lists of patients by specific conditions to use for quality improvement, reduction of disparities, research, or outreach	Generate at least one report listing patients with a specific condition
4	Send reminders to patients per patient preference for preventive/follow-up care	>20% of all unique patients ($\geq$ age 65 y or $\leq$ age 5 y) were sent an appropriate reminder during the EHR reporting period
5	Provide patients with timely electronic access to their health information within 3 business days of the information being available to the EP	>10% of all unique patients are provided timely electronic access to their health information, subject to the EP's discretion to withhold certain information

(continued)

#	Objective	Measure
Stage 1, Section 2: Meaningful Use Menu Set—Select Five (Must Include One Public-Health Initiative)		
5	Not another e-copy upon request; patient must be able to access the continually up-dated information any time (patient portal or personal health record (PHR))	
6	Use certified EHR technology to identify pa-tient-specific education resources and provide to patient, if appropriate	>10% of all unique patients are provided pa-tient-specific education resources
7	Medication reconciliation	EP performs medication reconciliation for >50% of transitions of care in which the patient is tran-sitioned into the care of the EP
8	Summary of care record for each transition of care/referrals	Summary of care record provided for >50% of transitions of care and referrals
9	Capability to submit electronic data to immuni-zation registries/systems*	Perform at least one test of certified EHR tech-nology's capacity to submit electronic data to immunization registries, except where prohib-ited, and follow up submission if the test is suc-cessful
10	Capability to provide electronic syndromic surveillance data to public-health agencies*	Perform at least one test of certified EHR tech-nology's capacity to provide electronic syn-dromic surveillance data to public-health agen-cies, except where prohibited, and follow up submission if the test is successful

*At least one public-health objective must be selected.

1. Find five menu measures from Table 1-8 that most closely represent an activity you do in your practice. If you use an EHR that checks formularies when you e-prescribe, this may be one you select. Go through the list to find four more. At least one of the measures must be a public-health measure, such as items 9 and 10 in Table 1-8. Select one of those and include it with the remaining four menu measures.

2. Write down the five menu measures you have selected here:

_____
_____
_____
_____
_____

You've selected five menu measures. Great!

You have completed selecting core and menu measures. Now, let's take a look at select-ing CQMs.

1. Using the checklist here, run a report in your EHR system to determine if any of these CQMs produces a denominator.

T A B L E 1-9A

Required Core CQMs for Core Measure #10

NQF Measure Number and PQRS Implementation Number	CQM Title	Denominator Results
NQF 0013	Hypertension: Blood Pressure Management	
NQF 0028	Preventive Care and Screening Measure Pair: (a) Tobacco Use Assessment, (b) Tobacco Cessation Intervention	
NQF 0421/PQRS 128	Adult Weight Screening and Follow-Up	

Abbreviations: CQM indicates clinical quality measure; NQF, National Quality Forum; and PQRS, Physician Quality Reporting System.

2. Write down the CQMs from Table 1-9A that produced a denominator and numerator. If the denominator produced 0, then move on to the alternate core measures. These are the measures you will use for core measure #10.

_____

_____

_____

Next, if the denominator was zero for any of the core set CQMs above, during attestation, the system will prompt you to select another CQM from the alternate core set CQMs. Before attestation, you should already know whether the EHR system is producing "0" denominators so that you can be prepared to report on the "alternate core measures." **Note:** If you achieved results for the three core set CQMs in Table 1-9A, you do not have to move on to alternate core set CQMs in Table 1-9B. This means you only report a total of six CQMs during attestation. If you were unable to produce a denominator from items in Table 1-9A, then proceed to Table 1-9B until you reach a total of three CQMs for core measure #10. The attestation system will continue to ask for numerators and denominators until you achieve three CQMs for core measure #10.

1. Using the checklist in Table 1-9B, run a report in your EHR system to determine if any of these CQMs also produces a denominator and numerator.

T A B L E 1-9B

Alternate Core Set CQMs

NQF Measure Number and PQRS Implementation Number	CQM Title	Denominator Results
NQF 0024	Weight Assessment and Counseling for Children and Adolescents	
NQF 0038	Childhood Immunization Status	
NQF 0041/PQRS 110	Preventive Care and Screening: Influenza Immunization for Patients 50 Years Old or Older	

Abbreviations: See Table 1-9A.

2. If you needed to select an additional CQM, write down the CQMs from the alternate core CQMs in Table 1-9B that produced a denominator until you are able to achieve at least three core CQMs for core measure #10. Record results for all CQMs you searched until you received three. Be sure to print screenshots for each of the CQMs that produced zero results and keep those screens with your MU documentation.

_____

_____

_____

Figure 1-3 provides an at-a-glance picture of how to select your CQMs for core measure #10.

FIGURE 1-3

Clinical Quality Measures Decision Tree

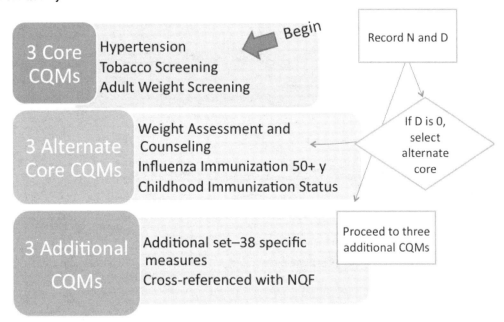

Abbreviations: CQMs indicates clinical quality measures; D, denominator; N, numerator; and NQF, National Quality Forum.

So far, you learned how to determine core and alternate core CQMs. Now, you need to select three additional CQMs from Table 1-10. These are neither core nor menu measures but are additional CQMs for Stage 1 reporting.

1. Review the Stage 1 CQMs in Table 1-10 and select the ones that most closely represent your patient population.
2. Determine if your EHR vendor will support this CQM. Follow this process:
   • Go to http://oncchpl.force.com/ehrcert. Select Ambulatory Practice Type.
   • Move your curser to the Search by Name or CHPL Product Number.
   • Click on the down arrow to Product Name, then enter the product name in the "Search for" field.
   • Click "Search." The Web site will take you to a list of products that matches your search criteria.

- Now, click on the name of the product *and* version number that correspond with the version you are using. **Caution:** The product and version *must* meet the version you are currently using. You will see it highlighted in blue.
- If there is a check mark in front of the criteria, the EHR vendor successfully demonstrated its capability to capture this information. You may use this CQM.
- If there is no checkmark, the EHR vendor either chose not to demonstrate or did not pass testing for these criteria. You also will notice that each of these ambulatory CQMs is from the NQF.

In Stage 2, you will not need to report CQMs as a separate MU measure, but you are required to electronically report NQF measures to CMS. For that reason, MU consultants advise ambulatory practices to carefully consider CQMs so that they can use them again when reporting for future stages.

Specialists undecided about CQMs to select can begin by evaluating the top 10 visit types for their practice and compare them to the CQMs. This comparison represents the highest likelihood that they can capture the measures. Using the top 10 visit types also works well for primary-care physicians who also treat patients with diabetes, hypertension, asthma, and cardiovascular disease.

CMS has issued a Stage 2 Clinical Quality Measures (CQM) Tip Sheet[19] to help prepare for the Stage 2 CQM reporting. In Table 1-10, we provide Stage 1 CQMs to assist with the initial process.

TABLE 1-10

Stage 1 Clinical Quality Measures

Criteria	Functional Requirement That System Must Achieve
National Quality Forum (NQF) 0001 Asthma Assessment	Percentage of patients 5–40 years of age with a diagnosis of asthma and who have been seen for at least two office visits, who were evaluated during at least one office visit within 12 months for the frequency (numeric) of day-time and nocturnal asthma symptoms
NQF 0002 Pharyngitis—Children	**Title:** Appropriate Testing for Children With Pharyngitis. **Description:** Percentage of children 2–18 years of age who were diagnosed with pharyngitis, dispensed an antibiotic and received a group A streptococcus (strep) test for the episode
NQF 0004 Alcohol and Drug Dependence	**Title:** Initiation and Engagement of Alcohol and Other Drug Dependence Treatment: (a) Initiation, (b) Engagement. **Description:** The percentage of adolescent and adult patients with a new episode of alcohol and other drug (AOD) dependence who initiate treatment through an inpatient AOD admission, outpatient visit, intensive outpatient encounter, or partial hospitalization within 14 days of the diagnosis and who initiated treatment and who had two or more additional services with an AOD diagnosis within 30 days of the initiation visit
NQF 0012 Prenatal Care: HIV Screening	**Title:** Prenatal Care: Screening for Human Immunodeficiency Virus (HIV). **Description:** Percentage of patients, regardless of age, who gave birth during a 12-month period who were screened for HIV infection during the first or second prenatal care visit
NQF 0013 Hypertension: Blood Pressure Measurement	**Title:** Hypertension: Blood Pressure Measurement. **Description:** Percentage of patient visits for patients aged 18 years and older with a diagnosis of hypertension who have been seen for at least two office visits, with blood pressure (BP) recorded.

(continued)

T A B L E 1-10 (continued)

Stage 1 Clinical Quality Measures

Criteria	Functional Requirement That System Must Achieve
NQF 0014 Prenatal Care: Anti-D Immune Globulin	**Title:** Prenatal Care: Anti-D Immune Globulin. **Description:** Percentage of D (Rh) negative, "unsensitized" patients, regardless of age, who gave birth during a 12-month period who received anti-D immune globulin at 26–30 weeks' gestation
NQF 0018 Controlling High Blood Pressure	**Title:** Controlling High Blood Pressure. **Description:** The percentage of patients 18–85 years of age who had a diagnosis of hypertension and whose BP was adequately controlled during the measurement year
NQF 0024 Youth Weight Assessment	**Title:** Weight Assessment and Counseling for Children and Adolescents. **Description:** Percentage of patients 2–17 years of age who had an outpatient visit with a primary-care physician (PCP) or an obstetrician-gynecologist (OB/GYN) and who had evidence of body mass index (BMI) percentile documentation, counseling for nutrition, and counseling for physical activity during the measurement year
NQF 0027 Tobacco Use Cessation	**Title:** Smoking and Tobacco Use Cessation, Medical Assistance: a. Advising Smokers and Tobacco Users to Quit; b. Discussing Smoking and Tobacco Use Cessation Medications; c. Discussing Smoking and Tobacco Use Cessation Strategies. **Description:** Percentage of patients 18 years of age and older who were current smokers or tobacco users, who were seen by a practitioner during the measurement year, and who received advice to quit smoking or tobacco use or whose practitioner recommended or discussed smoking or tobacco use cessation medications, methods, or strategies
NQF 0028 Preventive Care: Tobacco Use Assessment and Cessation	**Title:** Preventive Care and Screening Measure Pair: a. Tobacco Use Assessment, b. Tobacco Cessation Intervention. **Description:** Percentage of patients aged 18 years and older who have been seen for at least two office visits who were queried about tobacco use one or more times within 24 months b. Percentage of patients aged 18 years and older identified as tobacco users within the past 24 months and have been seen for at least two office visits, who received cessation intervention
NQF 0031 Breast Cancer Screening	**Title:** Breast Cancer Screening. **Description:** Percentage of women 40–69 years of age who had a mammogram to screen for breast cancer.
NQF 0032 Cervical Cancer Screening	**Title:** Cervical Cancer Screening. **Description:** Percentage of women 21–64 years of age who received one or more Pap tests to screen for cervical cancer
NQF 0033 Chlamydia Screening for Women	**Title:** Chlamydia Screening for Women. **Description:** Percentage of women 15–24 years of age who were identified as sexually active and who had at least one test for chlamydia during the measurement year
NQF 0034 Colorectal Cancer Screening	**Title:** Colorectal Cancer Screening. **Description:** Percentage of adults 50–75 years of age who had appropriate screening for colorectal cancer
NQF 0036 Appropriate Medications for Asthma	**Title:** Use of Appropriate Medications for Asthma. **Description:** Percentage of patients 5–50 years of age who were identified as having persistent asthma and were appropriately prescribed medication during the measurement year. Report three age stratifications (5–11 years, 12–50 years, and total).

(continued)

T A B L E 1-10 (continued)

Stage 1 Clinical Quality Measures

Criteria	Functional Requirement That System Must Achieve
NQF 0038 Childhood Immunization Status	**Title:** Childhood Immunization Status. **Description:** Percentage of children 2 years of age who had four diphtheria, tetanus, and acellular pertussis (DTaP); three polio (inactivated poliovirus [IPV]), one measles, mumps and rubella (MMR); two *Haemophilus influenzae* type B (Hib); three hepatitis B (Hep B); one chicken pox (varicella zoster virus [VZV]); four pneumococcal conjugate (PCV); two hepatitis A (Hep A); two or three rotavirus (RV); and two influenza (flu) vaccines by their second birthday. The measure calculates a rate for each vaccine and nine separate combination rates.
NQF 0041 Influenza Immunization	**Title:** Preventive Care and Screening: Influenza immunization for Patients ≥50 Years Old. **Description:** Percentage of patients aged 50 years and older who received an influenza immunization during the flu season (September through February)
NQF 0043 Pneumonia Vaccination	**Title:** Pneumonia Vaccination Status for Older Adults. **Description:** Percentage of patients 65 years of age and older who have ever received a pneumococcal vaccine
NQF 0047 Asthma Pharmacologic Therapy	**Title:** Asthma Pharmacologic Therapy. **Description:** Percentage of patients 5–40 years of age with a diagnosis of mild, moderate, or severe persistent asthma who were prescribed either the preferred long-term control medication (inhaled corticosteroid) or an acceptable alternative treatment
NQF 0052 Use of Imaging Study: Low Back Pain	**Title:** Low Back Pain: Use of Imaging Studies. **Description:** Percentage of patients with a primary diagnosis of low back pain who did not have an imaging study (plain X ray, magnetic resonance imaging (MRI), computed tomography (CT) scan) within 28 days of diagnosis.
NQF 0055 Diabetes: Eye Exam	**Title:** Diabetes: Eye Exam. **Description:** Percentage of patients 18–75 years of age with diabetes (type 1 or type 2) who had a retinal or dilated eye exam or a negative retinal exam (no evidence of retinopathy) by an eye care professional
NQF 0056 Diabetes: Foot Exam	**Title:** Diabetes: Foot Exam. **Description:** The percentage of patients aged 18–75 years with diabetes (type 1 or type 2) who had a foot exam (visual inspection, sensory exam with monofilament, or pulse exam)
NQF 0059 Diabetes Control: Hemoglobin A_{1c} >9.0%	**Title:** Diabetes: Hemoglobin A_{1c} Poor Control. **Description:** Percentage of patients 18–75 years of age with diabetes (type 1 or type 2) who had hemoglobin $A_{1c} > 9.0\%$.
NQF 0061 Diabetic Patients With Elevated Blood Pressure <140/90 mm Hg	**Title:** Diabetes: Blood Pressure Management. **Description:** Percentage of patients 18–75 years of age with diabetes (type 1 or type 2) who had blood pressure <140/90 mm Hg.
NQF 0062 Nephropathy Screening—Urine	**Title:** Diabetes: Urine Screening. **Description:** Percentage of patients 18–75 years of age with diabetes (type 1 or type 2) who had a nephropathy screening test or evidence of nephropathy.
NQF 0064 Diabetes Control: LDL <100 mg/dL	**Title:** Diabetes: Low Density Lipoprotein (LDL) Management and Control. **Description:** Percentage of patients 18–75 years of age with diabetes (type 1 or type 2) who had LDL-C < 100 mg/dL)

(*continued*)

T A B L E 1-10 (continued)

Stage 1 Clinical Quality Measures

Criteria	Functional Requirement That System Must Achieve
NQF 0067 Antiplatelet Therapy	**Title:** Coronary Artery Disease (CAD): Oral Antiplatelet Therapy Prescribed for Patients with CAD. **Description:** Percentage of patients aged 18 years and older with a diagnosis of CAD who were prescribed oral antiplatelet therapy
NQF 0068 Ischemic Vascular Disease: Asparin or Other Antithrombotic	**Title:** Ischemic Vascular Disease (IVD): Use of Aspirin or Another Antithrombotic. **Description:** Percentage of patients 18 years of age and older who were discharged alive for acute myocardial infarction (AMI), coronary artery bypass graft (CABG), or percutaneous transluminal coronary angioplasty (PTCA) from January 1 to November 1 of the year prior to the measurement year, or who had a diagnosis of ischemic vascular disease (IVD) during the measurement year and the year prior to the measurement year and who had documentation of use of aspirin or another antithrombotic during the measurement year
NQF 0070 Coronary Artery Disease: Beta-Blocker Therapy Post Myocardial Infarction	**Title:** Coronary Artery Disease (CAD): Beta-Blocker Therapy for CAD Patients With Prior Myocardial Infarction (MI). **Description:** Percentage of patients aged 18 years and older with a diagnosis of CAD and prior MI who were prescribed beta-blocker therapy
NQF 0073 Blood Pressure Management: Ischemic Valve Disease	**Title:** Ischemic Vascular Disease (IVD): Blood Pressure Management. **Description:** Percentage of patients 18 years of age and older who were discharged alive for acute myocardial infarction (AMI), coronary artery bypass graft (CABG) or percutaneous trans luminal coronary angioplasty (PTCA) from January 1 to November 1 of the year prior to the measurement year, or who had a diagnosis of ischemic vascular disease (IVD) during the measurement year and the year prior to the measurement year and whose recent blood pressure is in control (<140/90 mm Hg).
NQF 0074 Coronary Artery Disease: Lipid-Lowering Therapy	**Title:** Coronary Artery Disease (CAD): Drug Therapy for Lowering LDL-Cholesterol. **Description:** Percentage of patients aged 18 years and older with a diagnosis of CAD who were prescribed a lipid-lowering therapy (based on current American College of Cardiology/American Heart Association (ACC/AHA) guidelines)
NQF 0075 IVD: Complete Lipid Panel and LDL Control	**Title:** Ischemic Vascular Disease (IVD): Complete Lipid Panel and LDL Control. **Description:** Percentage of patients 18 years of age and older who were discharged alive for acute myocardial infarction (AMI), coronary artery bypass graft (CABG) or percutaneous transluminal angioplasty (PTCA) from January 1 to November1 of the year prior to the measurement year, or who had a diagnosis of ischemic vascular disease (IVD) during the measurement year and the year prior to the measurement year and who had a complete lipid profile performed during the measurement year and whose LDL-C <100 mg/dL
NQF 0081 Heart Failure: ACE/ARB Therapy for LVSD (LVEF <40%)	**Title:** Heart Failure (HF): Angiotensin-Converting Enzyme (ACE) Inhibitor or Angiotensin Receptor Blocker (ARB) Therapy for Left Ventricular Systolic Dysfunction (LVSD) **Description:** Percentage of patients aged 18 years and older with a diagnosis of heart failure and LVSD (LVEF< 40%) who were prescribed ACE inhibitor or ARB therapy

(continued)

TABLE 1-10 (continued)

Stage 1 Clinical Quality Measures

Criteria	Functional Requirement That System Must Achieve
NQF 0083 Heart Failure: Beta Blocker for LVSD	**Title:** Heart Failure (HF): Beta-Blocker Therapy for Left Ventricular Systolic Dysfunction (LVSD). **Description:** Percentage of patients aged 18 years and older with a diagnosis of heart failure who also have LVSD (LVEF <40%) and who were prescribed beta-blocker therapy.
NQF 0084 Heart Failure: Warfarin Therapy	**Title:** Heart Failure (HF): Warfarin Therapy Patients With Atrial Fibrillation. **Description:** Percentage of all patients aged 18 years and older with a diagnosis of heart failure and paroxysmal or chronic atrial fibrillation who were prescribed warfarin therapy
NQF 0086 Primary Open Angle Glaucoma	**Title:** Primary Open Angle Glaucoma (POAG): Optic Nerve Evaluation. **Description:** Percentage of patients aged 18 years and older with a diagnosis of POAG who have been seen for at least two office visits who have an optic nerve head evaluation during one or more office visits within 12 months
NQF 0088 Diabetic Retinopathy: Macular Edema	**Title:** Diabetic Retinopathy: Documentation of Presence or Absence of Macular Edema and Level of Severity of Retinopathy. **Description:** Percentage of patients aged 18 years and older with a diagnosis of diabetic retinopathy who had a dilated macular or fundus exam performed that included documentation of the level of severity of retinopathy and the presence or absence of macular edema during one or more office visits within 12 months
NQF 0089 Diabetes Management: Retinopathy Screening	**Title:** Diabetic Retinopathy: Communication With the Physician Managing Ongoing Diabetes Care. **Description:** Percentage of patients aged 18 years and older with a diagnosis of diabetic retinopathy who had a dilated macular or fundus exam performed with documented communication to the physician who manages the ongoing care of the patient with diabetes mellitus regarding the findings of the macular or fundus exam at least once within 12 months
NQF 0105 Depression Management	**Title:** Antidepressant Medication Management: (a) Effective Acute Phase Treatment, (b) Effective Continuation Phase Treatment. **Description:** The percentage of patients 18 years of age and older who were diagnosed with a new episode of major depression, treated with antidepressant medication, and who remained on an antidepressant medication treatment
NQF 0385 Colon Cancer: Chemotherapy	**Title:** Oncology Colon Cancer: Chemotherapy for Stage III Colon Cancer Patients. **Description:** Percentage of patients aged 18 years and older with Stage IIIA through IIIC colon cancer who are referred for adjuvant chemotherapy, prescribed adjuvant chemotherapy, or have previously received adjuvant chemotherapy within the 12-month reporting period
NQF 0387 Breast Cancer: Hormonal Therapy	**Title:** Oncology Breast Cancer: Hormonal Therapy for Stage IC-IIIC Estrogen Receptor/Progesterone Receptor (ER/PR) Positive Breast Cancer. **Description:** Percentage of female patients aged 18 years and older with Stage IC through IIIC, ER or PR positive breast cancer who were prescribed tamoxifen or aromatase inhibitor (AI) during the 12-month reporting period
NQF 0389 Prostate Cancer: Avoid Overuse of Bone Scan	**Title:** Prostate Cancer: Avoidance of Overuse of Bone Scan for Staging Low Risk Prostate Cancer Patients. **Description:** Percentage of patients, regardless of age, with a diagnosis of prostate cancer at low risk of recurrence receiving interstitial prostate brachytherapy, *or* external beam radiotherapy to the prostate, *or* radical prostatectomy, *or* cryotherapy who did not have a bone scan performed at any time since diagnosis of prostate cancer

(*continued*)

Criteria	Functional Requirement That System Must Achieve
NQF 0421 Adult Weight Screening	**Title:** Adult Weight Screening and Follow-Up. **Description:** Percentage of patients aged 18 years and older with a calculated BMI in the past 6 months or during the current visit documented in the medical record *and* if the most recent BMI is outside parameters, a follow-up plan is documented.
NQF 0575 Diabetes Control: Hemoglobin A_{1c} <8.0%	**Title:** Diabetes: Hemoglobin A_{1c} Control (<8.0%). **Description:** The percentage of patients 18–75 years of age with diabetes (type 1 or type 2) who had hemoglobin A_{1c} <8.0%

3. Cross-reference the list of vendor CQMs with three CQMs of your choosing from the list in Table 1-10.
4. You have successfully selected three additional set CQMs. Write them here.

_____

_____

_____

5. Check your CQM score to be sure you will achieve your minimum (six) or maximum (up to nine). (3 Core + 3 Additional) or (3 Core + up to 3 Alternate Core + 3 Additional)
   • If you successfully selected three CQMs from Table 1-8A without having to go on to Table 1-8B, you will report only six CQMs (three core set CQMs and three additional set CQMs).
   • If the denominator was zero in any of Table 1-8A's CQMs, you must report enough additional measures from Table 1-8B until you reach a total of three core set or alternate core set CQMs.

Task 6: Establish baseline for numerators and denominators. To determine numerators and denominators for each measure, refer to Chapters 4, 5, and 7. Also consult the CMS' MU EP Attestation User Guide (also includes Stage 1 measures), which is available on the ancillary material for this book. Each core and menu measure provides direction on how to calculate the numerator and denominator.

Practice managers and MU consultants continuously reference frequently asked questions posted for each measure at www.healthit.gov.

Task 7: Enroll and register. To enroll in a state's Medicaid program, follow the directions provided by each state's registration process. Go to www.cms.gov/EHRIncentivePrograms and select Medicaid State Information. At the bottom of the page, you will find state Medicaid launch times and related Web sites.

To enroll in the Medicaid incentive program, you will need to access the following documents. In this section, we also provide you with guidance on how to obtain these documents, in the event you don't yet have them.

■ National Provider Identifier (NPI)
■ National Plan and Provider Enumeration System (NPPES) Web user account
■ Provider Enrollment, Chain, and Ownership (PECOS) ID (only if a Medicare professional)
■ EHR Certification Number for Attestation (can bypass for registration)

Some physicians work at more than one location and want to assign benefits to another location. If you are reassigning your benefits, you will need:

■ Payee Tax Identification Number
■ Payee NPI

If you or your practice has retained the services of a third party to register and manage your MU incentive processes, the third party will gather the above information for you. The third party must have an identity and access management system (IAM) Web user account (user ID/password) and be associated to the EP's NPI.

Find Your Enrollment Numbers

How to obtain an NPI/NPPES

1. Apply through a Web-based application process. The Web address to the NPPES is https://nppes.cms.hhs.gov.
2. If requested, give permission to have an Electronic File Interchange Organization (EFIO) submit the application data on behalf of the health care provider.
3. Fill out and mail a paper application form to the NPI Enumerator. This form is now available for download from the CMS Web site (www.cms.gov/cmsforms/downloads/CMS10114.pdf), or by request from the NPI Enumerator.
   Phone: 1-800-465-3203 or TTY 1-800-692-2326
   E-mail: customerservice@npienumerator.com
   Mail: NPI Enumerator, PO Box 6059, Fargo, ND 58108-6059

How to create an NPPES Web user account

1. Successfully obtain an NPI.
2. Register for NPPES at https://nppes.cms.hhs.gov/NPPES/CreateLoginForExistNPIPage.do.
3. Fill in required fields, verify information, and click "Submit."

How to register for PECOS (Medicare professionals only)

1. Checklist of required items for individual practitioners registering on PECOS:
   • An active NPI
   • NPPES user ID and password; Internet-based PECOS can be accessed with the same user ID and password that a physician or nonphysician practitioner uses for NPPES
   • Personal identifying information
     • Legal name on file with the Social Security Administration
     • Date of birth
     • Social Security Number
   • Education information, including:
     • Name of school
     • Graduation year
   • Professional license information, including:
     • Medical license number
     • Original effective date
     • Renewal date
     • State where issued

- Certification information, including:
  - Certification number
  - Original effective date
  - Renewal date
  - State where issued
- Specialty/secondary specialty information
- Drug Enforcement Agency (DEA) number
- If applicable, information regarding any final adverse actions, such as:
  - A Medicare-imposed revocation of any Medicare billing privileges
  - Suspension or revocation of a license to provide health care by any state licensing authority
  - Revocation or suspension by an accreditation organization
  - A conviction of a federal or state felony offense (as defined in 42 CFR 424.535(a)(3)(A)(i)) within the last 10 years preceding enrollment, revalidation, or re-enrollment
  - An exclusion or debarment from participation in a federal or state health care program
- Practice location information, including:
  - Practitioner's medical practice location
  - Special payment information
  - Medical record storage information
  - Billing agency information (if applicable)
  - Any federal, state, and/or local (city/county) professional licenses, certifications, and/or registrations specifically required to operate as a health care physician or nonphysician practitioner
- Electronic Funds Transfer documentation (mechanism by which providers and suppliers receive Medicare Part A and Part B payments directly into a designated bank account)

2. Go to Internet-based PECOS at https://pecos.cms.hhs.gov and complete, review, and submit the electronic enrollment application providing the aforementioned information.
3. Print, sign, and date the two-page Certification Statement and mail the original signed Certification Statement from Internet-based PECOS and supporting documents to the Medicare contractor within 7 days of your electronic submission. **Note:** A Medicare contractor will not process an Internet enrollment application without the signed and dated Certification Statement.

STAGE 2 MEANINGFUL USE MEASURES

The MU Stage 2 rule was released on August 23, 2012, and became effective on October 23, 2012.

Starting in 2014, EPs and EHs who have been participating in the EHR Incentive Program for 2 or more years will be required to meet Stage 2 criteria. Stage 2 includes objectives and measures to improve patient care through better clinical decision support, care coordination, and patient engagement. These measures are discussed in greater detail in Chapters 4 through 7.

Any new EP or EH entering the MU system must begin with Stage 1 before moving on to Stage 2.

DOCUMENTATION IN THE EVENT OF AN AUDIT

At the time of publication, Figliozzi and Company, the CMS-contracted auditor tasked with performing MU audits, had moved from reviewing an analysis of data submitted online during attestation to asking more in-depth questions. These questions are not posted on a Web site but are only made available to individual providers who have called asking for help. The auditing inquiries can be extensive and generally ask for some of the following details and documents.

- Produce a copy of the technology, including version number, of the EHR system and the certification number you obtained from the CHPL Web site. Also produce documentation that indicates your practice purchased the EHR system you are using.
- For measures that required a Yes/No response, provide the following screen shots indicating you have used the system to complete the following:
  - Core #2 Drug Interaction Checks
  - Core #11 Clinical Decision Support Rule
  - Core #14 Electronic Exchange of Clinical Information
  - Core #15 Protect Electronic Health Information
  - Menu Set #1 Drug Formulary Checks
  - Menu Set #3 Patient Lists
  - Menu Set #10 Syndromic Surveillance Data Submission
- Send documentation that indicates you have completed a risk analysis, the date that it was conducted, and your written plans to mitigate the identified risks.
- When comparing the numerators and denominators provided for attestation to the numerators and denominators in supporting documentation, explain the reason for the variance. (The auditors will provide a list of the variances.)

Critical Point

Capture screen shots, especially for MU measures that require a Yes/No response. Write the decisions you made when defining unique patients. Document more than you think you will need, and you will have no reason to fear an audit.

In anticipation of possible audits, keep records, notes, and screen shots. Document everything. If you wonder for any reason whether to document or not, choose to print the screen, keep notes, log everything. In the event of an audit, you will be able to defend the decisions you made, even though the decisions were made years prior. Maintain documentation for 6 years, as required by law.

MEDICARE PAYMENT ADJUSTMENTS

Medicare payment adjustments are required by statute to take effect in 2015 (fiscal year for eligible hospitals/calendar year for EPs) for EPs and eligible hospitals who are not meaningful users.

If you did not meet the criteria to be a meaningful user and cannot participate in the MU incentive reimbursements, then you are **not** subjected to Medicare payment adjustments.

Stage 2 MU rules finalized a process by which payment adjustment can be determined by an EHR reporting period prior to the payment adjustment year 2015. This means that any Medicare EP or EH that successfully registers and attests to MU no later than October

1, 2014, will avoid payment adjustment in 2015. MU attestations to state Medicaid agencies by EPs who are eligible for either Medicare or Medicaid but opted for Medicaid will be accepted to avoid the Medicare penalty. (There is no payment adjustment for Medicaid payments to EPs or hospitals.)[20,21] This means that there are no reimbursement penalties to EPs and EHs if they file under Medicaid.

Consult Appendix B to find a payment adjustments and hardship exemptions tipsheet for EPs.[22]

Critical Point

If you are not eligible for incentive payments, either through Medicare or Medicaid, you will not be affected by payment adjustments in 2015.

Have you gathered information during a payment year? A payment year is the first year of Medicare payment in either a fiscal or calendar year. Hospitals report using a fiscal year (October to September); EPs report using a calendar year. Subsequent years will follow the fiscal or calendar years.

Critical Point

In 2014, the reporting period for all EPs attesting to either Stage 1 for the first time or Stage 2 is 90 days.

In Chapter 2, you will learn why the capture of data is important to you and how data can be used to make clinical and business decisions. With a better understanding of what data can do for you, the outcomes may help you better define your data management strategy.

SUMMARY

What's in It for Physicians?

■ Incentive funds to help pay for the cost of technology, implementation, and upgrades and access to data that help the clinical team makes better quality-of-care decisions

What's in It for Staff?

■ A better EHR system, but initially quite a few headaches until the staff establishes a system for consistently entering data

What's in It for Patients?

■ Patients and payers are the initial winners, but once physicians see the EHR as little more than a tool, the benefits to patients are greater access to the physician, improved loyalty, especially as patients begin to take on more financial responsibility for health care decisions. Patients selecting a physician will be able to conduct Web-based searches that allow them to select physicians with the best outcomes and patient reviews.

ACTION ITEMS

Find your CMS EHR certification number. A certification number is required for each year that you attest to MU, including for Stages 1, 2, and 3.

1. Go to the ONC CHPL Web site: http://onc-chpl.force.com/ehrcert
2. Select practice type (ambulatory or inpatient)

REFERENCES

1. Centers for Medicare & Medicaid Services. EHR incentive Programs. www.cms.gov/Regulations -and-Guidance/Legislation/EHRIncentivePrograms/index.html?redirect=/EHRIncentivePrograms /30_Meaningful_Use.asp. Accessed January 20, 2013.

2. US Department of Health and Human Services. The Decade of Health Information Technology: Delivering Consumer-centric and Information-rich Health Care. July 21, 2004. www.providers edge.com/ehdocs/ehr_articles/the_decade_of_hit-delivering_customer-centric_and_info-rich _hc.pdf. Accessed January 20, 2013.

3. The National Health Information Infrastructure. News. http://aspe.hhs.gov/sp/nhii. Accessed January 20, 2013.

4. American Enterprise Institute. 5 Facts From the 2011 Medicare Trustees Report. www.aei.org /article/health/entitlements/medicare/5-facts-from-last-years-medicare-trustees-report. Accessed January 20, 2013.

5. The Henry J Kaiser Family Foundation. Health Care Costs: A Primer.www.kff.org/insurance/7670 .cfm. Accessed January 20, 2013.

6. Menachermi N. Barriers to Ambulatory EHR: who are "imminent adopters" and how do they differ from other physicians? *Inform Prim Care*. 2006;14(2):101–108.

7. McCann Erin. Health care data breaches on the rise, with potential $7 B price tag. *Healthcare IT News*. December 6, 2012. www.healthcareitnews.com/news/healthcare-data-breaches-trend -upward-come-potential-7b-price-tag. Accessed January 20, 2013.

8. Centers for Medicare & Medicaid Services. Clinical Quality Measures (CQMs). www.cms.gov /EHRIncentivePrograms. Accessed January 20, 2013.

9. Centers for Medicare & Medicaid Services. An Introduction to the Medicare EHR Incentive Program for Eligible Professionals. www.cms.gov/Regulations-and-Guidance/Legislation/EHRIncen tivePrograms/Downloads/Beginners_Guide.pdf. Accessed January 20, 2013.

10. ———. CMS.gov/EHRIncentivePrograms. Accessed January 20, 2013.

11. ———. Frequently Asked Questions (FAQ7537). www.cms.gov. https://questions.cms.gov/faq .php?id=5005&faqId=7537. Accessed January 20, 2013.

12. ———. www.cms.gov/Regulations-and-Guidance/Legislation/EHRIncentivePrograms/downloads /FAQsRemediatedandRevised.pdf. Accessed April 24, 2013.

13. Physician EHR. HIPAA Security Sample Risk Assessments for a Small Physician Practice. www.physiciansehr.com. Also available at www.HealthIT.gov. Accessed January 20, 2013.

14. US Department of Justice. Controlled substances by CSA Schedule. www.deadiversion.usdoj.gov /schedules/orangebook/e_cs_sched.pdf. Accessed January 20, 2013.

15. American Medical Association. 5010 Toolkit: The Physician's Practical Guide to Implementing HIPAA Version 5010. www.ama-assn.org/resources/doc/washington/5010-toolkit.pdf. Accessed January 23, 2013.

16. Centers for Medicare & Medicaid Services. Frequently Asked Questions (10664). www.cms.gov /ehrincentiveprograms. Accessed January 20, 2013.

17. American Medical Association. Meaningful Use Glossary and Requirements Table. www.ama -assn.org/resources/doc/hit/meaningful-use-table.pdf. Accessed January 20, 2013.

18. Centers for Medicare & Medicaid Services. Attestation User Guide For Eligible Professionals. www.cms.gov/Regulations-and-Guidance/Legislation/EHRIncentivePrograms/downloads/EP_Attestation_User_Guide.pdf. Accessed January 20, 2013.

19. ———. 2014 Clinical Quality Measures Tipsheet. Updated August 2012. www.cms.gov/Regulations-and-Guidance/Legislation/EHRIncentivePrograms/Downloads/ClinicalQualityMeasuresTipsheet.pdf. Accessed January 23, 2013.

20. US Department of Health & Human Services. News Release, EHR Stage 2 Final Rule, August 23, 2012. www.hhs.gov/news/press/2012pres/08/20120823b.html. Accessed January 20, 2013.

21. Centers for Medicare & Medicaid Services. Fact Sheets. www.cms.gov/apps/media/fact_sheets.asp. Accessed January 23, 2013.

22. ———. Payment Adjustments and Hardship Exemptions Tipsheet for Eligible Professionals. www.cms.gov/Regulations-and-Guidance/Legislation/EHRIncentivePrograms/Downloads/PaymentAdj_HardshipExcepTipSheetforEP.pdf. Accessed January 20, 2013.

The Need for EHRs and the Value of Data

WHO SHOULD READ THIS CHAPTER?

This chapter is for physicians and office staff acquiring a sense of what data can do for them and why it is important for the future of health care and the practice. It is written for the non-IT personnel, but it can be used as a reference tool for the computer-savvy individual in the practice, who is or might be taking on the new role as the electronic health record and Meaningful Use project manager.

What you will learn in this chapter:

- Benefits of an EHR, not only for applying for Meaningful Use, but also for increased efficiency and improved clinical data
- Managing risks and turning them into benefits
- How to optimize your EHR
- What to expect from your EHR system
- The value of data for physicians and their stakeholders
- Managing the implementation for optimum data management
- What's in it for
  - Physicians
  - Staff
  - Payers
  - Public health
- Exercises and action items

Key Terms Introduced in This Chapter

Data
Electronic Medical Record
Electronic Health Record
Health Information Exchange
Health Information Technology (Health IT)
Meaningful Use
Meaningful User
Standards
Stakeholders
Regulation

OVERVIEW OF DATA'S ROLE IN MEANINGFUL USE

In the months before achieving Meaningful Use (MU), eligible professionals (EPs) often spend a lot of time entering data into the system without knowing what to do with the data entered. Managing data, including how data are entered, used, stored, and accessed, is a lifetime career for some professionals. Most physician practices want to get data into the system as easily and accurately as possible *and* stay in business during the process.

In this chapter, we focus not only on the benefits and challenges of electronic health records (EHRs), but also on the value of data. We will look at several key considerations:

- How EHRs have changed the way physicians access and use data
- Benefits and challenges of an EHR from the patient's and the physician's point of view
- How to decide whether to keep, update, or change your EHR to meet MU measures
- The value of data to physicians
- How to make physicians and practice staff more efficient, thus allowing for more time to focus on patients

EHR software has come a long way since July 2004 when President George W. Bush launched the Decade for Health Information Technology discussed in Chapter 1. Healthcare providers know a lot more about what needs to be in the EHR system today than in 2004, both from using EHRs and from reporting to EHR developers what would make their experiences more meaningful and relevant to the clinical team and to delivery of patient care.

Technology innovation continues to redefine what an EHR can do. As soon as physicians find a stumbling block, a creative inventor begins a search for new technology. New health information technology (HIT) innovations since 2004 have been numerous, creative, and sometimes ahead of their time. For example:

- Increasingly sophisticated voice- and handwriting-recognition applications facilitate data collection.
- Natural language processing (NLP), an emerging technology, will eventually translate dictation into the EHR and allow the data to be searchable.[1]
- Improved technology, such as enhanced virtual private networks and enhanced mobility, allows physicians to access and capture details of clinical notes from any location.
- Secure patient portals allow physicians to upload clinical summaries to patients so that they can better manage their personal health information and communicate using the portal's secure e-mail features.
- Computerized provider order entry (CPOE) has become the physician's medication, procedure orders, and medication-alert system.
- Cloud computing supports the distribution of data between applications, such as EHR modules, for physicians selecting certified EHR modules for MU.
- Physicians are learning how to leverage their EHRs to participate directly in clinical trials.
- New platforms allow a physician to see an image on a handheld device.
- Patients can send a digital photo of a wound or rash to a patient portal and the physician can respond with instructions for recommended treatments.

THE VALUE OF DATA IN EMERGING MARKETS

To most companies, data are gold because they can be aligned with something else, such as a new product launch, to embed data in an application, or to confirm whether physicians are using a product. For example:

- Pharmaceutical companies are increasingly paying for more clinical data as they learn how to effectively mine it for postmarketing surveillance and to provide insights into how well a drug is working.
- Security and transmission of metadata are coming under scrutiny from cyber-security experts, and security regulations are being imposed on healthcare professionals using handheld devices.
- Physicians can collate complex data and use them to demonstrate, for example, successful births in an in vitro fertilization clinic.

When it comes to defining a meaningful user, the possibilities are limited only by creativity and money. Earlier generations in the banking, retail, and transportation industries worked through electronic-exchange solutions so that today a consumer can process a financial transaction from almost anywhere in the world. Now it's healthcare's turn to improve access to data. We begin a discussion on the benefits and challenges of data by providing a case study of how one family depends on data for their son, Robby.

BENEFITS OF AN EHR TO PATIENTS: A CASE STUDY*

Margaret, whose son, Robby, has asthma. She and her family live in a midsize community where residents consult family doctors and a few local specialists rather than drive the 40 miles to where offices of specialists and surgeons are adjacent to a level 1 trauma center. That's where the neonatologists took care of Robby when he was born. It's not that Margaret doesn't need specialists from time to time, but she and her family have chosen a smaller community to raise and care for their children.

Over the years, Robby's asthma has been stabilized with diet and medication. He and his dad warm-up together before Robby's soccer games, expanding his lung capacity so that he can play sports with the other kids.

Several years ago, some of the healthcare providers, led by the community's cardiologist, formed a local health information exchange (HIE). Robby's pediatrician advised Margaret to build a personal health record for all her children and asked her to approve adding Robby's medical chart to her practice's patient portal, which is securely connected to the community hospital. She signed the authorization, and the pediatrician regularly updates the portal with the children's immunizations and visit summaries.

The portal allowed Margaret to log in to the pediatrician's office from work to make appointments. She wouldn't always get her first choice, but at least she wasn't on the phone holding up the scheduler or herself with callbacks. Her family liked knowing the doctor could quickly access Robby's medical chart at night, when he was more likely to have problems.

Toward the end of third grade, Robby had an asthmatic episode when bulldozers began moving dirt for the school's new gymnasium, stirring up a lot of dust on the playground. His teachers had been instructed what to watch for, so when Robby's wheezing got out of control, the school nurse called the paramedics, who then rushed him to the community hospital.

*Note that this case study is based on actual information and events, however, the names and details have been changed to protect the privacy and identity of the family. Nevertheless, the situation described is familiar and common to many families.

Margaret and the school nurse had gone through this drill before, and together they had worked through an emergency plan if something happened while Robby was at school. Because of that plan, the nurse knew the precise next steps. After calling the paramedics, the nurse called Margaret, who immediately left work and headed to the hospital's emergency room (ER).

By the time the paramedics arrived at the hospital, the ER physician had already logged into Robby's chart, provided instructions by the paramedics, accessed his past medical history and current medications, and noted his allergy to penicillin.

This episode would result in an overnight stay to be sure Robby's lungs had stabilized. When he was discharged, the hospital sent a link to the pediatrician so that she would have details of the episode and treatment when Margaret and Robby came in for a follow-up visit.

Because Robby's dad has a flexible spending account (FSA) at work the hospital's insurance claim triggered a transaction that automatically transferred the co-pay from the FSA into the family's checking account. Note that this is how an FSA sponsored by the federal government functions for transactions, which may be different from other FSA programs. For reimbursements not connected to a claim, Robby's family will submit receipts for reimbursement.

Not many communities are synchronized with this level of HIE yet, but separate health-information transactions *are* available today and successfully used by consumers, employers, payers, and healthcare providers.

EHR BENEFITS TO PHYSICIANS

Most health care professionals recognize that an EHR system is designed to mirror a paper chart but to be much more efficient. When housed in an electronic format, a chart doesn't get lost in the facility and isn't left lying around in the office.

With an EHR, physicians can immediately access a patient's current medications, allergies, and adverse reactions to food or drugs; recall the patient's visit and problem lists, and order laboratory tests or procedures directly from the EHR system. If laboratory results do not come back in a timely fashion, the system will send a reminder to the physician. On-call physicians report the convenience of having access to a patient's chart through a secure virtual private network

In the context of the case study, because Robby's physician is using a certified EHR system, the physician and her partners were able to receive incentive funds from the Centers for Medicare & Medicaid Services (CMS) for demonstrating they were meaningful users of certified EHRs. They could use these funds to help offset some of the previous costs invested into updating their EHR system. Discussions of what it means to be a meaningful user and the requirements of a certified EHR are provided in Chapter 1.

Because Robby's electronic medical record (EMR) also contains protected health information (PHI) from multiple sources, including the report from the hospital's neonatologist, his current medical conditions (often called "problem lists" in MU attestation), and a description of the nebulizer used at home or elsewhere and the recommended dose for a child his age and weight, the paramedics and the ER physicians were able to practice accurate medical decision making and provide the appropriate treatment for his asthma attack. Although there are risks to using an EHR, the benefits generally outweigh the risks if the practice takes the time to identify and manage those risks. We will discuss risk management later in this chapter and in Chapter 3.

Besides the benefits to individual physicians and patients, the benefits of EHRs also extend to the greater community of healthcare professionals. Consider a practice that aligns itself with one or more hospitals. The practice benefits from receiving an electronic discharge summary, and the hospital(s) benefits from having access to patient records, as long as both parties achieve a consensus on data that will be exchanged.

When referring a patient to a specialty practice, the practice benefits by receiving electronic consult notes, the patient doesn't have to recount the reason for the visit to a specialist, and the specialist benefits from receiving laboratory results, information about current medications, and other findings relevant to patient care.

CHALLENGES TO EHR ADOPTION

Though the benefits of adopting an EHR are many, there are also many challenges in making the migration. Some are short-lived, while others require long-term management.

EHRs can be quite expensive, and the capital outlay to oversee or manage the implementation process can be as much or more than the actual cost of the software system. The system and its interfaces will need to be maintained and updated, a cost that is often passed along to the physician's practice.

The implementation process will be disruptive to the practice *and* the practice's revenue. A wise practice manager will have set aside a budget for the EHR and for implementation and will also have to manage expectations on how quickly the practice will return to pre-EHR productivity. A return on investment strategy will help the practice measure how long it took to return to productivity and also forecast increased revenues from efficiency.

EHR software is not a perfect science. For example, MU attestations require the system to calculate numerators and denominators, but those calculations may produce results that are obviously faulty. In this case, the EHR's project manager may be able to provide solutions.

An EHR that is right for primary care may not be right for a specialty practice, even though the EHR vendor says it is. Ask to speak to another physician in that same specialty who is using the vendor's product.

Medical necessity for a procedure is likely to be challenged if the physician "clones" or copies progress notes from a previous visit into the current visit without justifying why a procedure or treatment plan is required for the current billing. Until CMS indicated that "cloning" documentation could be a reason for audit, some EHR vendors had touted this as a benefit of EHRs without explaining the outcomes if justification was not also offered.

Some staff members will need to be retooled to perform another task. Computer-savvy medical records clerks may become internal trainers or offer computer support services.

People with extended knowledge of an EHR tend to be sought after for employment by the vendor or another practice or hospital. This may not be a challenge to them but could present a challenge to the practice because of the potential loss of a valued employee.

Privacy and security policies and procedures will need to be updated to accommodate electronic use, disclosure, and storage of PHI.

These challenges, along with others your practice may have identified, indicate the need for a strategic plan and an operational commitment to make the transition run as smoothly as possible. What follows are steps that will help you think through your data management plan.

SELECTING THE RIGHT EHR FOR YOUR NEEDS

To become a meaningful user and make data relevant for quality clinical decisions, the practice will first need to select an EHR that is right for its practice.

What to Do: Determine Whether an EHR System Is Right for Your Practice Environment

Task 1: Determine your needs. Your EHR needs will vary depending on whether your practice is primary care, multispecialty, primary-care with multispecialty, or specialty specific.

If you are a primary-care provider:

- Regional extension centers (RECs) across the country have been tasked to help priority primary-care physicians, critical access hospitals, and federally qualified health centers make EHR selections and to assist with EHR implementation. "A 'primary-care provider' is any doctor of medicine (MD) or osteopathy (DO), any nurse practitioner (NP), any nurse midwife, or any physician assistant with prescriptive privileges in the locality where s/he practices family medicine, internal medicine, pediatric medicine, or obstetrics and gynecology. A priority primary-care physician (PPCP) is a provider who practices in one of the following settings:
  - Individual and small practices of 10 providers or less
  - Community health centers, primary-care clinics, or rural health clinics
  - Public and critical access hospitals
  - Other settings that predominantly serve uninsured, underinsured, and medically underserved populations."[2]
- The list of RECs is updated constantly. By using keyword searches, you can find experienced consultants or go to a trusted source and ask for recommendations.
- Online software-selection companies, such as SoftwareAdvice.com, EMRApproved.com, or EMRConsultant.com, may also provide useful selection guidance.
- Selection advice may be offered for free or at low cost, but generally only after you've narrowed the selection to two EHR vendors.
- Networking capabilities, such as the availability of broadband, will influence your decision.
- To be a meaningful user, you must purchase an EHR that is certified by an Authorized Testing and Certification Body (ATCB).[3]

If you are a specialty or multispecialty practice, your search will be much different:

- Some EHR systems are specifically designed for primary-care providers, but the EHR companies then work with a team of specialists to add modules to support specified specialty needs. This has led to add-on modules for obstetricians, gynecologists, pediatricians, orthopedists, urologists, and cardiologists, as these tend to be partners in a multispecialty practice. One significant benefit to a multiple-specialty EHR is that all clinical users within the practice can access the same patient record without having to build an interface between EHR systems.
- While some EHR companies focus on adding specialty modules to meet market demands, some specialties' modules are sometimes not robust enough for the specialty. Oncology, nephrology, behavioral health, outpatient surgery, ophthalmology, orthopedics, and plastic surgery are specialties that typically require more detailed CPOE and clinical notes, such as:
  - Tumor staging in oncology
  - Interfacing with dialysis centers in nephrology

- Confidentiality, intervention, and privacy in behavioral health
- Managing outpatient surgical procedures
- Managing regimented protocols for orthopedic surgery

Task 2. Determine if a current EHR can fully meet your needs. If you are already using an EHR, you may need to switch to a different system if the legacy EHR has not yet achieved MU certification, and you will be eligible for MU funds.

- Changing EHR systems is, unfortunately, not as simple as exporting data from one file into another. Online discussions and studies by the Medical Group Management Association (MGMA) and the California HealthCare Foundation (CHCF)[4] indicate that the reasons behind nearly 50% of physicians deciding to switch to another EHR are the exact reasons indicated in Task 1.
- You need an EHR system certified by an Office of the National Coordinator for Health Information Technology (ONC)-Authorized Certification Body (ACB) in order to receive MU incentive funds. The ATCB program, as defined by ONC, is a process to ensure that EHR technologies meet adopted standards, certification criteria, and other technical requirements to achieve MU of those records in systems. In the 2012 Report, *On the Road to Meaningful Use of EHRs*, published by the CHCF,[4] 71% of California physicians reported that they have some sort of EHR, but only 30% reported that they have EHRs that can meet all 12 of the MU objectives measured in the study.
- Providers posting online discussions, such as those posted at LinkedIn's EHRIN,[5] discuss the need for clinical protocols defined by their specialty and describe the frustration of having to build those protocols if the EHR vendor doesn't have a history of working with the specialty. To that end, some EHR companies servicing one particular specialty have re-emerged with a clearer focus, not only on the specialty, but also the subspecialties, such as pediatric oncology or interventional nephrology. Specialty-specific systems also have taken note of the ATCB certification process and embedded new fields, such as height, weight, and immunization status, to help their clients meet MU Stage 1 measures.

Task 3. If you are a specialist, evaluate a specialty-specific EHR. An EHR system may be designed specifically for one specialty and its subspecialties because of the complexity of clinical decision making, diagnostics, integrated care management, procedure orders, and workflow processes. Even if you decide not to purchase a specialty-specific system, you will have benefited from learning what other providers want in a system.

By design, specialty-specific EHR software anticipates that the physician will be sending and receiving secure PHI to and from primary-care providers and hospital systems, because this represents the specialty's referral network. The emergence of HIEs, while still a work in progress, has helped define the needs of healthcare professionals in a region.

Critical Point

MU measures may be used as a guideline for purchasing and using an EHR. MU is a system of measurements to help standardize EHR systems and incentivize physicians to become meaningful users of technology. Usability and relevant clinical functionalities should support your EHR decision.

MEASURE THE RISKS AND BENEFITS OF SWITCHING TO A NEW EHR

EHR implementation, whether for a specialty or a primary-care physician, is not an overnight or five-day event, irrespective of some vendor promises. The process will be exhilarating for some and frustrating for others, depending on many variables, such as computer literacy, the depth of content and amount of training, workflow and technological compatibility with practice-management systems, database and template (also called *forms*) customization, and day-to-day use.

But for physicians who have survived and thrived in the transition to an EHR, the benefits are real. Some of those benefits not mentioned earlier in this chapter include:

- An updated professional "image" as being a technology leader
- The minimization of administrative tasks, such as time lost searching for charts or waiting for a fax to be placed into the record
- No handwriting to decipher or misunderstand, particularly in prescription management
- Better communication among caregivers
- Flow sheets, especially in specialty-specific EHRs, can integrate results into a single location, so that the physician can measure improvement or spot a downward trend.
- Increased patient involvement, particularly after the first year of use when the computer often becomes part of the patient-interview process
- Patient reminders to obtain preventive care
- Improved patient safety, as it relates to EHR notification of adverse reactions to medications, food, and allergies. The patient safety challenge here is that a poorly documented encounter contains discoverable data entry. Physicians need to depend on information at the point of care. If the physician data are not entered or are entered inaccurately, the physician begins to mistrust the EHR and must take on the added burden of guessing what could be missing. Nothing drives this point home more clearly than when a physician needs to defend clinical decisions to a patient, a family member, or a jury.

The transition to an EHR can also trigger some vulnerabilities and risks. As you identify them in your practice, manage the risks and turn them into a meaningful experience. Table 2-1 provides an overview of some of those risks, with a high-level strategy to turn the risk into a benefit.

TABLE 2-1

Turn Your EHR Risks Into Benefits

EHR Risks	How to Turn Risks Into Benefits
Physicians dislike typing because it diminishes productivity. Thus, they may return to the paper chart.	Look into using a digital-transcription company that imports the dictated clinical summary, using an HL7 interface, directly into the patient's chart. Health Level 7 or HL7 interface, described in Chapter 3, is the most widely used standard to facilitate communication between two or more clinical applications. Other options include a remote scribe, which follows step-by-step simple-to-complex dictated orders. For example, the physician may dictate, "Insert 155 pounds into the weight field." Voice- or handwriting-recognition software can be very helpful, if the physician invests time to train the application to respond to his or her voice and handwriting pattern.

(*continued*)

T A B L E 2-1 (continued)

Turn Your EHR Risks Into Benefits

EHR Risks	How to Turn Risks Into Benefits
Patient safety may be compromised in a hybrid record. If the practice is part paper and part electronic health record (EHR), the risk is that an important document will be in neither place or just in the EHR when the provider is still using paper record.	Define the designated legal record during the transition. For example, until all departments (front office, back office, clinical) go live, decide that the legal record will be the paper chart. Or, on go-live, all designated paper-record content will be abstracted and entered into the EHR 24 hours before the patient arrives. After three visits, the practice will retire the chart to an offsite storage facility.
Physicians refuse to adopt an EHR. The risks include not only loss of incentive funds and eventual reimbursement penalties, but also a longer time to catch up down the road.	A highly productive physician may need a scribe to assist with the documentation process. Physicians are scientists and respond to data. Ensure that time-savers, such as favorite order sets, are available. Show the reluctant physician results from EHR-adoption studies, such as improved productivity, improved reimbursement, and better documentation.
Physicians attempt to translate paper-based workflows into the EHR. If a physician wishes to import cumbersome paper workflows into the EHR, most EHR systems will allow this, which results in too many clicks or too much movement between screens and reduced productivity. Such inefficiencies will exaggerate personality conflicts and organization disarray.	During training, ask the trainer to instruct super-users on the logic behind data entry and management, but then develop an internal training manual that provides shortcuts for data entry.
Providers do data entry using multiple templates. For example, a dermatologist creating a template may not include height, weight, or blood pressure in a template because that information may not be immediately critical to the office visit or procedures. However, these figures are core Meaningful Use (MU) measures, so the dermatologist would not meet the measure if those figures are not captured. Often, this can result in incomplete reports because the data cannot roll up. This is especially important in measuring clinical quality outcomes.	Appoint a clinical customization team to oversee and direct the development of templates (also called *forms*). The clinical team can then also direct clinical policies and procedures so that data are captured in a standardized manner.
Medical identity theft might increase. "Notably, 30% of physician practices . . . do not use antivirus software, and 34% do not use network firewalls."[6]	Antivirus software is not only good business, but it is also a Health Insurance Portability and Accounting Act (HIPAA) security requirement and is included as part of your HIPAA risk assessment. If you are not using antivirus software and a firewall, you are not mitigating risks and therefore may be subject to penalties under the False Claims Act if you applied for and received incentive funds.
An EHR system is subject to failure.	Make sure to include a disaster recovery plan. This includes system backups available offsite and paper processes during down times.

Implementation of most EHR software takes time before, during, and after the EHR vendor team completes go-live, collects the remainder of the purchase price, and turns the project over to the EHR's maintenance and technical support teams. While most practices look to the practice administrator or practice manager to take the lead as internal project manager, the learning curve can be significant. Practice managers tend to be fairly busy operating the practice and often prioritize activities every day.

The implementation process is best managed and shortened with strategic planning and leadership from healthcare professionals, a skilled project manager, and information technology (IT) support staff. If you are not using an external project manager, the risks in Table 2-1 may serve as an add-on to the strategic plan offered by the EHR vendor.

Resources That Meaningful Use Project Managers Use Every Day

CMS.gov/EHRIncentivePrograms
The process of rule-making is complex, but CMS does a fairly good job of updating this Web site with Q&A, guidance and many links to embedded documents. Because of the volume of information posted, the links may be broken, but CMS actively tries to correct these. We are on this site two to three times a day. Here are some examples of frequently downloaded information:

- Eligible Professional Meaningful Use Table of Contents Core and Menu Set Objectives, available at www.cms.gov/Regulations-and-Guidance/Legislation/EHR IncentivePrograms/downloads/EP-MU-TOC.pdf
- Attestation User Guide—For Eligible Professionals, available at CMS: www.cms.gov /Regulations-and-Guidance/Legislation/EHRIncentivePrograms/downloads/EP _Attestation_User_Guide.pdf

HealthIT.hhs.gov and HealthIT.gov
HealthIT.Hhs.gov is a veritable portal of information that provides guidance on Health Information Technology for Economic and Clinical Health (HITECH) Act funding opportunities, federal advisory committees, regulations and guidance, ONC initiatives, news, and events.

HealthIT.gov is a publicly accessed Web site for patients and families, providers and professionals, and policy researchers and implementers. Content on this Web site has been reviewed by experts in both the private and public sector prior to being posted. The site offers short and quickly understandable content with embedded links, and is a great landing source for MU questions and answers.

AT&T Healthcare Community Online Physician Portal at www.corp.att.com/healthcare/physicianportal/
Another excellent resource for EHR and vendor solutions to achieve Meaningful Use that project managers can refer to is the AT&T Healthcare Community Online Physician Portal (a strategic alliance between the AMA and AT&T). For more information, go to www.corp.att.com/healthcare/physicianportal/.

HITECHAnswers.net
One of the most actively engaging sites in the marketplace, this well-regarded team hosts "MU Live!" Internet radio and vetted products to assist providers to adopt and implement EHRs and meet MU.

ESCALATED TIMELINE

If you adopted an EHR software system prior to February 19, 2009, when the HITECH Act became law, you most likely received more individualized attention and had time to adjust and tweak the system, as well as revise your workflow processes. However, the HITECH Act dramatically spiked the adoption rate of EHRs.

Since that time, EHR vendors, consultants, quality-improvement organizations, and federal agencies have stepped up their activities. They often are also overwhelmed with implementation tasks, meeting certification standards for Stage 2, completing due diligence for *International Classification of Diseases* (*ICD*)-10 transition, and so forth. As a result, many vendors have had to choose between new installations, problem-solving troubled implementations, and moving forward to help healthcare professionals implement and achieve MU. Coupled with a shortage of skilled implementation project managers, many physicians justifiably feel they have been left to problem solve the EHR conundrum on their own.

Even though some providers adopted EHRs as early as 1975,[7] the pace of adoption has really skyrocketed since 2004. Thus, there is a good deal of implementation knowledge out there, and the benefits of learning from other implementations will help manage your risks. Therefore, a strategic plan for how the practice will capture, use, disclose, transmit, and measure data is only as good as the risks it intends to mitigate.

What an EHR Can and Cannot Do for You[8]

EHR software is designed to provide clinicians with clinical information at the click of a mouse or trackpad on a dashboard or drop-down template. As smart technology, EHRs [will] eventually be able to provide the health care professional with longitudinal information about a patient's care, such as what medications the patient received in the emergency room last weekend or what adverse reactions the patient had to a previously prescribed medication.

As smart technology, an EHR can help your practice:

- Reconcile medications the patient is taking prior to prescribing a new drug.
- Select a medication from your favorites list and electronically send it to the patient's pharmacy.
- Provide clinical decision support [by, for example, helping you access a published colleague's treatment protocols]
- Access a published colleague's treatment protocols.
- Store sample letters and correspondence for customization.
- Provide educational material relevant to the patient's disease category or pending lab [*sic*] test.
- Allow more than one clinician to view a record at a time.
- Eliminate redundant operational workflows, such as
  - copying patient-education materials,
  - sending patient reminders, and
  - copying lab [*sic*] results from faxes into flowsheets.
- Readily access a patient chart.
- Provide billing advice, including recommending applicable evaluation and management (E&M) codes[a]
- Send appointment recalls to patients.
- Order a lab [*sic*] test and have the results returned to the nurse or provider queue for review.

However, even the best EHR cannot take the place of the physician and clinical workforce. The EHR cannot provide compassion and care to a patient or family member. It cannot be an active listener. It cannot examine the inside of a child's ear to determine whether the child has an ear infection. Nor can it predict an onset of flu. But it can produce data that can alert a public health agency of emerging issues locally, statewide, and nationwide.

An EHR cannot resolve organizational issues; in fact, it will exacerbate personality conflicts and organizational disarray.

The point is that an EHR is a tool to be used by a skilled physician and clinical workforce that not only know how to enter data, but also can assess and evaluate data to make clinical decisions.

[a]An experienced coder remains one of the best allies to keep on your team.
Reprinted with permission from AMA. Copyright 2011 American Medical Association.

DATA AND THEIR VALUE TO PHYSICIANS AND STAKEHOLDERS

Flesh-and-blood decision making is at the core of a physician's clinical decision making.[1] "We were taught how to organize a patient's history: his chief complaint, associated symptoms, past medical history, relevant social data, past and current therapies," writes Jerome Groopman, MD, in *How Doctors Think.* "Then we were instructed in how to examine people: listening for normal and abnormal heart sounds; palpating the liver and spleen; checking pulses in the neck, arms, and legs; observing the contour of nerve and splay of the vessels in the retina."[1]

When using a paper chart, the physician jots notes onto the patient's chart, makes mental notes throughout the day, and then at the end of the day (sometimes the end of the week) completes dictations and closes out the patient's chart. Considering there may have been 25 to 40 patients each day, recollecting and documenting the visit means sorting through an elaborate web of details stored in the physician's head alongside any personal data the physician also must store, such as birthdays, concerts, or sporting events.

The EHR, when implemented effectively, supports the daily data upload for reimbursement processing and significantly improves the documentation. In the traditional fee-for-service model, this process obtained some financial rewards and perhaps improved outcomes for the patients.

An EHR can take the data to a much deeper level when physicians use the EHR's reporting features to make inquiries into the stored data. For example, a good EHR should be able to query the database and answer the following questions:

- How many female patients between 18 and 60 years have we treated this year for ovarian cysts?
  - Is this an increase over last year?
  - Which treatment worked best: medication or procedures or both?
  - How many of those patients turned out to have ovarian cancer?
- What zip codes do the majority of our patients come from? What do we treat them for? This will help determine if the practice needs to open a satellite practice, open or expand a specialty, or hire a new physician.
- How can we customize our referral and outreach efforts?

From a public-health perspective, EHRs become an invaluable source of data for:

- Detecting adverse drug reactions
- Comparing adverse drug reactions to the patient's underlying conditions[9]
- Monitoring the safety of approved medical products through the Sentinel Initiative, established by the Food and Drug Administration[10]
- Predicting how many falls are likely to occur in a hospital or skilled nursing facility[11]
- Detecting the onset of the flu season
- Identifying the emergence of new diseases or potential acts of bioterrorism
- Improving diabetes management[12]
- Improving asthma care and compliance[13]

Data elements required for an EHR described in Table 2-2 and also in greater detail in Chapter 4 are fairly broad in the Stage 1 EHR Certification Standards, but data generally can be grouped into two main categories: *administrative* and *clinical.* Data in paper documentation are considered to be "document-centric." In a paper chart, the physician flips through documents in the paper chart, hoping to find notes that will assist in patient care. EHRs are data-centric. For years data management associations, such as Health Level 7 (HL7), American Health Information Management Association (AHIMA) and American Society for Testing and Materials (ASTM) International have collaborated to determine data values to be included in the Continuity of Care Document (CCD), a standard that should be used by all EHR vendors in developing EHR software. While data elements for EHR vendor certification are discussed in greater detail in Chapter 3, Table 2.2 provides an overview of the data elements included in the CCD.

The purpose of this table is to demonstrate the commonalities that all EHR vendors share in preparation for HIE, in which confidential health information can be shared between treating physicians.

TABLE 2-2

Data Elements for EHR Documentation

Section	Data Element	What this means to you
Personal Information Module	Timestamp	Shows who had access and what they accessed
Patient Information Event Entry	Person's ID, Address, Phone number, email/URL,	Allows for patient verification
Personal Information	Person's name, gender, DOB, Marital Status, Religious Affiliation, Race, Ethnicity,	Provides information needed for clinical decision making
Language spoken module	Usually a text field, including sign language	Lets the practice know if they will need an interpreter
Support Module	Associated person's name, contact information,	Who is responsible for the patient and what kind of support does the patient have?
Health care Provider Module	Time stamp, type of provider (consulting, primary care, referring provider); provider address and contact information, organization, and ID assigned to the patient.	Provides a tracking mechanism for providers making referrals, waiting for consult notes and provides contact information and ID for those referrals.

(continued)

TABLE   2-2 (continued)

Data Elements for EHR Documentation

Section	Data Element	What this means to you
Insurance Provider Module	Group number, health insurance type	Helps guide the clinical team on orders and treatment that are on the patient's formulary.
Payment Provider Event Entry	Patient's group number and insurance type	Helps determine eligibility and pre-authorizations
Payer	Health Plan insurance information, ID, address, contact info	
Member	Member ID, relationship to subscriber, address, contact information	
Subscriber information	Contact information, ID, DOB	
Allergy/Sensitivity Module	Adverse event, date, type, product, severity,	
Condition Module	Problem entry, type, name	
Administration Information Event Entry	Allows for orders, eRx	Allows provider to record timing, frequency, interval, duration, route,
Medication Information	Coded product name, brand name, drug manufacturer, status of medication, indications, patient instructions, reactions, vehicle, and dose indicator	
Order information	Order number, refills, quantity, expiration date, order date, time, provider, dispense date	
Pregnancy Module		
Information Source Module	Author	Allows practice to see who or what captured information so far, date, time, URL, reference/@value.
Comment Module		
Advanced Directive Module	Effective date, relationship, status	Allows practice to contact Power of Attorney in the event patient is incapacitated.
Immunization Module	Date, Time, Refusal, Medication Series Number, reactions	New in HIPAA, allows schools to access immunizations
Vital Signs Module	Results entry, interpretation, reference range	
Results Module	Result ID, date, time, type	
Encounter Module	Encounter type, free text, date, time, provider	
Procedure Module	Order procedures by ID, track status, organize results,	

Abbreviations: @ indicates at; e-Rx, electronic prescribing; DOB, date of birth; ID, identification; and URL, uniform resource locator.
Source: Adapted from HealthIT.gov. Available at www.healthIT.gov. Accessed January 23, 2013.

Other Uses of Clinical Data

Clinical data can inform clinical advancements. In medical meetings, physicians often present findings from a clinical study to influence a disease-specific protocol or encourage surgeons to adopt a new robotic approach to surgery. Verifiable data provide scientific evidence to help demonstrate the efficacy of one treatment protocol over another.

Practice administrators, billing companies, and coders use data in their constant search for improvements to diagnostic and procedure codes. Coding is critical for payment, to ensure accuracy, and to avoid potential fraud. In an EHR, physicians will document and code encounters. An integrated EHR/practice management (PM) system will push the codes from the EHR into the PM system for coders to review and approve for billing. This will result in decreased billing errors and a more accurate reflection of care provided to the patient during the encounter.

When the Department of Family Medicine in the Quillen College of Medicine at East Tennessee State University studied how physicians used Current Procedural Terminology (CPT®) code set for the same visit or procedure, findings indicated that on any given day, one physician may use the same or different CPT code for the same-level visit or procedure. As a result of the study, Quillen College was able to standardize the use of CPT codes and improve revenue.

Critical Point

Medical necessity is not always factored into an EHR/PM system's coding processes. Often medical necessity is determined by the payer and substantiated by the ordering provider; however, if the physician copies and pastes the last progress note into the current note, a case for medical necessity must also be entered for the visit. For data-gathering purposes, E&M coding calculators embedded in EHRs have not yet streamlined the medical necessity decision processes as this topic is a moving target.

Figure 2-1 shows how physicians and coders varied their coding of procedures.

FIGURE 2-1

Coding Discrepancies Between Physicians and Coders

Note that physicians disagree on which code to use, but coders are often in agreement.

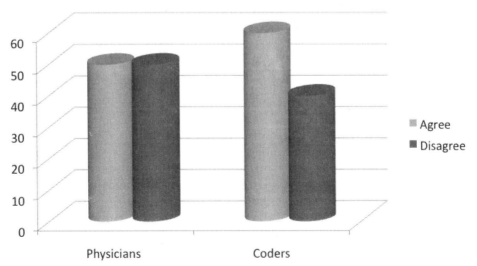

Data Analysis: A Moment of Applause for Data Wonks

Data provide opportunities for physicians, including potential financial revenue, when another organization wants access to the data. Grants, contracted funding opportunities, clinical trials, and business decisions become most valuable when a physician can demonstrate data integrity and credibility. How do you do this?

What to Do: Learn About Your EHR Vendor's Data-Reporting Capabilities

Get involved in state or local EHR workgroups, and develop a list of data-reporting capabilities you'd like. A list built by a group of physicians has a much better chance of getting into the EHR's development cycle than a great idea from one physician, even if it is an idea no one else has considered. A sample list may go from simple to complex and may involve searching the demographics and clinical databases. For example:

■ Where are our patients by zip code and what are the *ICD* codes for their conditions?

■ Has there been a flu outbreak in one or more of those zip codes?

■ Are this year's flu patients coming from a specific region?

■ How much of our business is Medicare and Medicaid?

■ How many patients did we see for a hemoglobin A_{1c} (HbA$_{1c}$) in the last 60 days? Which patients should have come in for this test and have not yet scheduled an appointment?

■ Have we seen many children or adults with Asperger syndrome? What have been our most effective intervention protocols?

■ How effective is this chemotherapy mix on treating a patient with breast cancer?

Submit your list not just to one EHR vendor but to several in your area or specialty.

Review Chapters 6 and 7 to learn what patients would like to know and what outcomes you should be tracking for MU.

Know the Data Your Stakeholders Want

Your stakeholders are those individuals, payers, referring physicians, patients, and public-health agencies that want to participate in sending and receiving data. If you operate a grant-supported clinic, such as a community health center or a not-for-profit clinic, the grant dollars are usually tied to information the grantee wants in exchange for the investment. For example, a state breast cancer awareness organization may provide funding to better learn how frequently women between the ages of 40 and 65 years obtain mammograms. Such data could help the organization determine the public-health messages it should disseminate and also demonstrate the effect the organization has on public health by funding the research. Organizations funding studies such as these generally are required to justify why they allocated dollars for a study. Data help both the physician and the funding organization make that case.

Collaborating *clinicians* in an accountable-care organization or a patient-centered medical home, where all providers have access to the patient's information, want data that demonstrate improved patient outcomes.

Some *patients* actually want to advocate for themselves and become a one-person HIE. More recently, patients have wanted to manage their own laboratory tests and, through DNA tests, learn whether they are candidates for everything from macular degeneration to cancer.

The CMS seeks data that help it provide improved clinical outcomes, define improved measures for quality of care, and effectively manage payments.

The Department of Health and Human Services (HHS) says it needs quality data for more public-health services and to incentivize health care professionals for outcomes.

Hospitals want time-stamped patient data connected to quality data that measures the value of a hospital's services.[14] They also want to discard unused and irrelevant data.

Access to data, however, comes with challenges. Too much data leaves data analytics impossible to manage without a process to connect the dots.[14] Moreover, you have a responsibility to act on data that you collect.

What to Do: Identify What Your Stakeholders Want

Use the chart in Action Item #1 at the end of the chapter to build a list of stakeholders and determine what data they want.

Consider the public-health agencies within the HHS that also leverage data for decision making:

- The Centers for Disease Control and Prevention (CDC) uses data to inform providers of disease-management trends, identify gaps in services, determine where older adults are not getting recommended services, establish motorcycle safety standards, identify causes of birth defects, and much more. For information on data gathered by the CDC, go to www.cdc.gov/datastatistics.

- The Agency for Healthcare Research and Quality (AHRQ) offers robust data sources that typically are of interest to researchers, clinicians, policymakers, and consumers. See www.ahrq.gov/data.

- The Health Resources and Services Administration uses demographic and clinical data to determine how federal dollars can best be distributed and measured to help the underserved and uninsured patients receive medical, dental, and mental-health services.

Pharmaceutical companies want to know whether you are prescribing their medications. They also want to measure adverse events and determine whether the event was a result of patient behavior, medication interaction, or the stage of the disease.

SUMMARY

What's in It for Physicians

- To achieve MU, physicians use EHRs not only for quality reporting purposes, but also to bring relevance and meaning into data. They use EHRs to:
  - Share, print, report, and effect change.
  - Improve medical safety, efficiency, and follow-up.
  - Manage prescriptions, laboratory results, and referrals.
  - Improve quality.
  - Manage costs.
  - Access charts remotely.
  - Reduce potential medication errors.
  - Provide electronic alerts on critical laboratory values.

What's in It for Staff?

- Improved workflow management
- Efficiencies in managing patient information
- Enhanced employee value and employability

What's in It for Payers?

■ Quality services that serve as preventive measures

■ Data that help them make efficient decisions on utilization and care management

What's in It for Public Health?

■ Data to create policy, identify emerging issues and diseases, educate consumers on public-health issues, and establish a safe and healthy environment

ACTION ITEMS

1. Evaluate the stakeholders who are involved in the health of your organization. Complete this chart before or during discussions with other health care providers on sharing or disclosing data to them. Know what you want and what they want, as well.

Stakeholders	What Do They Want?	What Will They Give Up?	Your Risks/Benefits
Employees			
Hospitals			
Payers: public			
Payers: private			
Referring physicians			
Patients			

2. Make a list of decisions or improvements you could make if you had good data. A few suggestions are presented here to get you started.
   • Improve billing and collections or renegotiate contracts with payers
   • Reduce aged receivables
   • Enroll patients in clinical trials
   • Incorporate clinical-trials data capture as part of routine clinical care
   • Decide how much your practice would earn with an in-house laboratory or procedure room
   • Determine where to open a new office
   • Decide whether you need to bring a specialist into your practice or clinic
   • Earn a patient-centered medical home designation
   • Decide whether you want to participate in an HIE and how much data you will make accessible through the HIE

REFERENCES

1. Groopman JE. *How Doctors Think*. Reprint ed. Boston, MA: Houghton Mifflin; 2007:8.
2. The Office of the National Coordinator for Health Information Technology (ONC). What kinds of providers do regional extension centers work with? www.healthit.gov/providers-professionals /faqs/what-kinds-providers-do-regional-extension-centers-work. Accessed January 20, 2013.
3. The Office of the National Coordinator for Health Information Technology (ONC). Certification Progress for EHR Technologies. www.healthit.gov/providers-professionals/certification-process -ehr-technologies. Accessed January 20, 2013.

4. Coffman J, Grumbach K, Fix M, Traister L, Bindman AB. On the road to Meaningful Use of EHR. A survey of California Physicians. University of California, San Francisco; June 2012. www.chcf.org/~/media/MEDIA%20LIBRARY%20Files/PDF/R/PDF%20RoadMeaningfulUseEHRs Physicians.pdf. Accessed January 20, 2013.

5. LinkedIn. EHR Implementation Network (EHRIN). Accessed January 20, 2013.

6. Lewis N. Electronic Health Records Raise Security Risks. *InformationWeek*, March 10, 2011. www.informationweek.com/news/healthcare/security-privacy/229300722. Accessed January 20, 2013.

7. Institute of Medicine. www.iom.edu. Accessed January 20, 2013.

8. Hartley CP, Jones ED. *EHR Implementation: A Step-by-Step Guide for the Medical Practice.* Chicago, IL: AMA; 2011:11–12.

9. Haerian K, Varn D, Vaidya S, Ena L, Chase HS, Friedman C. Detection of pharmacovigilance-related adverse events using electronic health records and automated methods. *Clin Pharmacol Ther.* 2012;92(2):228–234.

10. Behrman RE, Benner JS, Brown JS, McClellan M, Woodcock J, Platt R. Developing the sentinel system: a national resource for evidence development. *N Engl J Med.* 2011; 364(6):498–499.

11. Biomed Central. www.biomedcentral.com/bmcmedinformdecismak/. Accessed March 23, 2013.

12. Hunt JS, Siemienczuk J, Gillanders W, et al. The impact of a physician-directed health information technology system on diabetes outcomes in primary care: a pre- and post-implementation study. *Inform Prim Care.* 2009;17(3):165–174.

13. Bell LM, Grundmeier R, Localio R, et al. Electronic health record–based decision support to improve asthma care: a cluster-randomized trial. *Pediatrics.* April 2010;125(4):e770–777.

14. Richmond R. Why hospitals continue to fail in "connecting the dots" with their data, and what they can do to change. The Health Care Blog. http://thehealthcareblog.com/blog/2012/02/01/why-hospitals-continue-to-fail-in-%E2%80%98connecting-the-dots%E2%80%99-with-their-data-and-what-they-can-do-to-ch/. Accessed March 23, 2013.

Operationalize Meaningful Use

P art II of this book drills down into operationalizing Meaningful Use (MU).

Chapter 3 provides you with details on how to build a Meaningful Use infrastructure that will support a secure environment for networking, data capture and management, and patient-portal decisions. A section on standards is enough to provide highlights on how electronic health records should be built with similar standards that support interoperability, or as it is rapidly becoming known as "data liquidity."

In Chapter 4, we tackle the workflows that often make data entry and management unwieldy. In this chapter, the authors compare MU workflows by measure and by role, and then incorporate the process into a patient visit. Tackling workflows may offer the greatest advantage, as you move into MU Stage 2.

Chapter 5 is your attestation survival guide, providing you with guidance rarely offered until you are at the CMS' attestation work-page, trying to figure out what to do and to come up with the numerators and denominators for a successful attestation. This chapter also identifies documentation strategy so that you can explain how you arrived at the numbers in the event of an audit.

## chapter 3

Building the Meaningful Use IT Infrastructure: What Do You Need to Have in Place?

WHO SHOULD READ THIS CHAPTER?

This chapter, written in plain language, is for the person who oversees the networking, electronic health record (EHR) security processes, compliance activities, and data-management tasks in the practice. A security official may wish to leverage some of the content to assist in risk management.

What you will learn in this chapter:

- Preparedness strategies you won't get from the Centers for Medicare & Medicaid Services or your EHR vendor
- The functions that certified EHR software must be able to achieve
- What health information technology standards are and what they do for you
- Data management and the value of standard operating procedures
- The care and nurturing of data:
  - Privacy, security, breaches
  - Reporting
  - Audits and data validation
- What's in it for
  - Physicians
  - Staff
  - Patients

Key Terms Introduced in This Chapter

Clinical Decision Support

Data Management

Interoperability Standards

Covered Entity

EHR Certification Standards

Unique Patient

Hybrid Chart

MEANINGFUL USE PREPAREDNESS STRATEGIES

One might logically assume that if an electronic health record (EHR) vendor has tested and achieved Office of the National Coordinator for Health Information Technology (ONC) certification status, completing Meaningful Use (MU) attestation should be relatively easy to do. (Under the Temporary Certification Rule, the ONC named approved certification bodies "Accredited Testing and Certification Bodies" [ATCB]. Effective October 4, 2012, the permanent certification program was renamed ONC-HIT Certification Program.) Most practices that have successfully attested to Stage 1 say MU attestation is not a "series-of-mouse-clicks" experience, as once promised by EHR software developers. Stage 1 EHR certification criteria, such as building reports with numerators and denominators, is an exercise in multiple interpretations, an effort that Stage 2 hopes to correct. However, this is an indication that attestation can be successfully completed, and the Centers for Medicare & Medicaid Services (CMS) is making good on paying incentives. In building this chapter, we leverage lessons learned from eligible professionals (EPs) who have already achieved Stage 1 MU. Some of these lessons learned offer substantial guidance for building your MU infrastructure.

Meaningful Use Lessons Learned

- Include in your contract a provision that the EHR vendor's support staff will provide you online and, if needed, onsite consultation through MU attestation.
- Outside of a trained MU project manager, the office staff is the next most critical influencer to successful attestation.
- Clinical policies and procedures help standardize how data are entered into the EHR.
- If physicians collectively agree on the clinical quality measures (CQMs) first, the likelihood that they will meet their numbers increases exponentially while decreasing project-management hours.
- Rushing to meet MU creates gaps in data entry and reporting.
- Protect MU attestation patient lists if you print them.
- Don't attest "yes" to core measure #15 until you have completed or annually updated a Health Insurance Portability and Accountability Act of 1996 (HIPAA) risk analysis and are putting measures in place to manage the risks.
- Conduct a pilot test of the patient portal before using it for attestation.
- Create an MU checklist, and document every decision you make.

To learn more about MU lessons learned, go to www.HealthIT.gov. Select "For Providers and Professionals," and then select "Achieve Meaningful Use." At the bottom of this page, you will find grids for core objectives and menu objectives. For each objective selected, there's a link for "Lessons Learned from the Field" on the right navigation pane.

This chapter not only compiles additional lessons learned posted on HealthIT.gov,[1] but also adds an abundance of our own key findings from years in the field.

FUNCTIONS THAT CERTIFIED EHR SOFTWARE MUST ACHIEVE

On July 28, 2010, the Department of Health and Human Services (HHS) published regulations defining qualified EHR technology and establishing standards and implementation specifications for both complete EHRs and EHR modules.

These standards and certification criteria established by the ONC establish the required capabilities and related standards that certified EHR technology (CEHRT) must include so that, at a minimum, an EP or eligible hospital (EH), defined in Chapter 1, will be able to achieve MU.[2]

When you select a certified EHR system, the system's functions must enable you not only to enter data, but also to analyze, extract, and make clinical decisions from these data. Below, you will find a description of certification criteria in seven areas that EHR vendors are required to demonstrate during testing:

1. Clinical Criteria[3] that include data elements required for clinical decision making, such as demographics, medications, allergies, problem list, and vital signs, many of which CMS now calls the "common MU data set."[4].

2. Transitions of Care[5] defines how a CEHRT electronically receives, displays, and incorporates transition of care and referral summaries. This includes clinical summaries, laboratory orders and results, health information exchanges (HIEs), e-prescribing, and medication reconciliation.

3. CQMs[6] require a CEHRT to capture and export clinical quality measures selected by the EP, but check to be sure your CEHRT can support these CQMs. Often, providers use third-party software to check the status of data entered into the EHR to see if the practice is meeting numerator and denominator, a process that is allowable for Stage 1 because CQMs were not an area of certification focus in the 2011 Edition. As a result, many EPs struggled to calculate and export CQMs data for reporting. However, CQMs will be in the 2014 Edition. Therefore, for each CQM that the EHR technology presents for certification, the CEHRT must be able to electronically record and calculate all data for that CQM. CEHRT must also be able to export all data that it claims it can record and calculate in the certification process [170.204(c) and170.205(h)].

   A list of Stage 1 and Stage 2 CQMs is available at www.healthit.gov. To access each of these CQMs, along with a fact sheet that describes how to capture the numerator and denominator, follow the following steps:

   • On the home page of www.Healthit.gov, select "For Providers and Professionals"
   • On the providers and professionals page, select "Achieve Meaningful Use." On the achieve Meaningful Use page, scroll down to the "Core Objectives" table and select core objective #10, "Clinical Quality Measures (CQMs)"
   • On the CQM page, scroll down to the "National Learning Consortium Resources" table. In the table, scroll down to "Clinical Quality Measure (CQMs) Quick Reference Guide,[7] and select "Download" to obtain a copy of CQMs Quick Reference Guide.

4. Privacy and Security[8] requires a CEHRT to support technical safeguards that the EP must use. In Stage 1, EPs were required to complete or update a risk analysis, an ongoing risk management process, at least annually. In Stage 2, EPs must demonstrate that they use physical safeguards and that the CEHRT's technical safeguards encrypt data both at rest and in an HIE. Reference MU Tables Series 2 110112, which is available at www.healthit .gov/policy-researchers-implementers.

5. Clinical Summaries[9] defines minimum data elements for selection into a clinical summary, including the provider's name and contact office. Other elements included in the Stage 1 clinical summary are[10]:
   • Patient name
   • Provider name
   • Date and location of visit
   • Reason(s) for visit
   • Vitals (temperature, blood pressure, height, weight, BMI [body mass index], exercise status in minutes/week)
   • Problem list/current conditions[a]
   • Medication list[a]
   • Medication allergies[a]
   • Diagnostic test/lab results[a]
   • Patient instructions
   [a]*Required for Stage 1 of MU*

6. Immunization and Disease-Specific Registries[11]

For the 2014 Edition testing, the EHR vendor must be able to electronically create immunization information for electronic transmission to specific registries. If the EP is prohibited from providing immunization data because of state law, the EP may be exempt from this measure.

7. Automated Numerator Recording and Automated Safety Enhanced Design[12]

In the 2014 Edition certification testing, the EHR vendor must be able to create a report or file that measures and calculates whether the patient is eligible for the specific measure's numerator. This applies to Stage 1 and 2 objectives and measures.[13]

The 2014 Edition of the Standards and Certification Criteria (S&CC) also includes the following changes:

■ Redefines the meaning of CEHRT and introduces more efficient means for certification to permit greater innovation and reduce regulatory burden

■ Adopts vocabulary, content exchange, transport, functional, and security standards in certification criteria

■ Adopts certification criteria for transitions of care that will ensure EHR technology supports standards-based electronic HIE

■ Requires that test reports used for EHR technology certification be made publicly available and that EHR technology developers follow certain price transparency practices related to the types of costs (ie, one-time, ongoing, or both) associated with EHR technology implementation for MU

■ Makes available for the first time "gap certification" for certain certification criteria, which will enable more efficient EHR technology certification. "For EHR reporting periods during and after FY/CY [fiscal year/calendar year] 2014, eligible providers will need to have EHR technology certified to the 2014 edition EHR certification criteria that meets a required base amount of functionality and then any other functionality they need to achieve meaningful use. ONC Fact Sheet: 2014 Edition Standards & Certification Criteria (S&CC) Final Rule."[14]

■ Implements a "base EHR" concept. Previously, EHRs for specialists were forced by the CEHRT concept to incorporate functionality that their users would never use and that would be excluded during the incentive attestation process. That requirement is now gone, and only those additional modules that would be used to achieve MU will be required to become certified. This is a critical change for vendors that support chiropractors, diagnostic radiologists, dentists, and other specialists.[15]

■ Implements "gap testing" for EHR vendors, who will not need to retest any unchanged modules that had received 2011 edition certification. Being able to focus on a subset of modules for development and testing is a plus.[15]

■ All EHR technology that is currently in the pipeline must complete 2011 edition testing and certification before achieving the 2014 edition certification. This means that, if you adopt a system that is new to the marketplace, the EHR must have completed both the 2011 edition and 2014 edition certification for you to achieve 2014 MU.

WHICH EHR CERTIFIED EDITION SHOULD A PROVIDER USE?

Prior to 2014, eligible providers will be able to meet the definition of CEHRT in any one of the following three ways:

1. Adopt EHR technology certified to the 2011 edition EHR certification criteria that meets all applicable certification criteria (the original CEHRT definition established in the S&CC July 2010 final rule).
2. Upgrade parts of their 2011 edition EHR technology to the equivalent 2014 edition EHR technology (this is essentially the same as the preceding process but with a mix of EHR technology certified to either the 2011 or equivalent 2014 edition).
3. Adopt EHR technology that meets the CEHRT definition for FY/CY 2014.

After FY/CY 2014, EPs must use CEHRT certified to the 2014 edition certification criteria.[14]

Table 3-1 represents criteria that ambulatory EHR systems must meet so that EPs can meet MU Stages 1 and 2. Column 3 indicates whether there were changes from Stage 1 to Stage 2. Numbers provided in the fourth column reference the location in the final MU Stage 2 rule.[16–18]

T A B L E 3-1

EHR Certification Criteria: Stage 1 and Stage 2 Criteria for Ambulatory Care

Certification Criteria	Stage 1 (45 CFR 170.304) Functional Requirement the System Must Achieve	Changed or Revised in Stage 2?	Stage 2 (45 CFR 170.314)
Clinical Criteria: Common MU [Meaningful Use] Data Set			
Computerized provider order entry (CPOE)	(a)(1) Enable a user to electronically record, store, retrieve, and modify, at a minimum, the following order types: (i) medications; (ii) laboratory; and (iii) radiology/imaging	Yes	(a)(1) Interventions
Conduct drug-to-drug and drug-to-allergy interaction checks	(a)(2) Notifications. Automatically and electronically generate, and indicate in real-time, notifications at the point of care for drug-to-drug and drug-to-allergy contraindications based on medication list, medication allergy list, and computerized provider order entry (CPOE). (2) Adjustments. Provide certain users with the ability to adjust notifications provided for drug-to-drug and drug-to-allergy interaction checks.	Yes.	(a)(2)(i) Interventions. Before a medication order is completed or acted upon during CPOE, interventions must automatically and electronically indicate to a user drug-drug and drug-allergy contraindications based on a patient's medication list and medication allergy list. (ii) Adjustments. (A) Enable the severity level of interventions provided for drug-to-drug interaction checks to be adjusted. (B) Limit the ability to adjust severity levels to an identified set of users, or make this function available as a system administrative–function.

(*continued*)

TABLE 3-1 (continued)

EHR Certification Criteria: Stage 1 and Stage 2 Criteria for Ambulatory Care

Certification Criteria	Stage 1 (45 CFR 170.304) Functional Requirement the System Must Achieve	Changed or Revised in Stage 2?	Stage 2 (45 CFR 170.314)
Demographics	(e) Enable a user to electronically record, change, and access patient demographic data including preferred language, sex, race, ethnicity, and date of birth. (A) Enable race and ethnicity to be recorded.	Yes	(B) Enable preferred language to be recorded as structured data. In the event the patient does not provide preferred language, the system will prompt you to say, "The patient declined to specify."
Record and chart vital signs	(f)(1) Record and chart vital signs. Enable a user to electronically record, modify, and retrieve a patient's vital signs including, at a minimum, height, weight, and blood pressure. (f)(2) Calculate body mass index (BMI). Automatically calculate and display body mass index based on a patient's height and weight. (f)(iii) Optional—Plot and display growth charts. Plot and electronically display, upon request, growth charts for patients 2–20 years old.	Yes	(a)(4) Age restrictions on growth charts and blood pressure
Maintain up-to-date problem list	(c) Enable a user to electronically record, modify, and retrieve a patient's problem list for longitudinal care in accordance with: (1) the standard specified in §170.207(a)(1); or (2) at a minimum, the version of the standard specified in §170.207(a)(2).	Yes. Definition clarity	(a)(5) Maintain problem list over multiple encounters
Maintain active medication list	(d) Enable a user to electronically record, modify, and retrieve a patient's active medication list as well as medication history for longitudinal care.	Yes. Minor revisions for clarity	(a)(6) Over multiple encounters
Maintain active medication allergy list	(e) Enable a user to electronically record, modify, and retrieve a patient's active medication allergy list as well as medication allergy history for longitudinal care.	Yes. Minor revisions for clarity	(a)(7) Over multiple encounters
Clinical decision support	(1) Implement rules. Implement automated, electronic clinical decision support rules (in addition to drug-to-drug and drug-to-allergy contraindication checking) based on the data elements included in: problem list; medication list; demographics; and laboratory test results. (2) Notifications. Automatically and electronically generate, and indicate in real-time, notifications and care suggestions based upon clinical decision support rules.	Yes. Drug-to-drug and drug-to-allergy now consolidated in this measure.	(i) Evidence-based decision support interventions. Enable a limited set of authenticated users to select/activate one or more electronic clinical decision support interventions (in addition to drug-to-drug and drug-to-allergy contraindication checking) based on each one and at least

(continued)

T A B L E   3-1 (continued)

EHR Certification Criteria: Stage 1 and Stage 2 Criteria for Ambulatory Care

Certification Criteria	Stage 1 (45 CFR 170.304) Functional Requirement the System Must Achieve	Changed or Revised in Stage 2?	Stage 2 (45 CFR 170.314)
			one combination of the following data: (A) problem list; (B) medication list; (C) medication allergy list; (D) demographics; (E) laboratory tests and values/results; and (F) vital signs. (ii) Link referential clinical decision support to therapeutic reference information or diagnostic and therapeutic reference information. Technology must enable interventions to be electronically triggered: *Note:* This is not a complete definition. Consult Appendix A of this book.
Electronic notes	Updated: In 2014 Edition testing, the EHR vendor must (1) select the correct patient; (2) record electronic notes; (3) change the electronic notes; (4) access electronic notes; and (5) search the electronic notes.[19]	Updated	(a)(9) Enable a user to electronically record, change, access, and search electronic notes.
Drug formulary checks	(b) Enable a user to electronically check if drugs are in a formulary or if a preferred drug list exists for the patient.	No	(a)(10) Unchanged
Smoking status	(g) Enable a user to electronically record, modify, and retrieve the smoking status of a patient. Smoking status types must include: current every day smoker; current some day smoker; former smoker; never smoker; smoker, current status unknown; and unknown if ever smoked.	No	(a)(11) Unchanged
Image results		New	(a)(12) Electronically indicate to a user the availability of a patient's images and narrative interpretations (relating to radiographic or other diagnostic test(s)) and enable electronic access to such images and narrative interpretations.

(*continued*)

T A B L E   3-1 (continued)

EHR Certification Criteria: Stage 1 and Stage 2 Criteria for Ambulatory Care

Certifica-tion Criteria	Stage 1 (45 CFR 170.304) Functional Requirement the System Must Achieve	Changed or Revised in Stage 2?	Stage 2 (45 CFR 170.314)
Family health history	New	Yes	(a)(14) Enable a user to electronically record, change, and access a patient's family health history
Generate patient lists	Enable a user to electronically select, sort, retrieve, and generate lists of patients according to, at a minimum, the data elements included in: (1) problem list; (2) medication list; (3) demographics; (4) laboratory test results; and (5) care team member.	No	Unchanged
Patient-specific education resources	EHR technology must be able to electronically identify for a user patient-specific education resources based on data included in the patient's problem list, medication list, and laboratory tests and values/results. (Consult Appendix A.)		(a)(15) Note: Not included in CMS' term, Common MU Data Set.
Advance directives	New	Yes	(a)(17) Enable a user to electronically record whether a patient has an advance directive.
(b)(1) Transition of Care: Electronically receive, display, and incorporate transition of care and referral summaries between health care professionals and unrelated systems			
(e)(1) View, download, and transmit to third party; timely access	Enable a user to provide patients with online access to their clinical information, including, at a minimum, correct patient name, laboratory test results, problem list, medication list, medication allergy list, reason for referral, referring or transitioning provider's name and office contact information.	Yes	Timely access added. Transmitted content is encrypted through a secure channel that ensures all content is encrypted and integrity-protected in accordance with the standard for encryption and hashing algorithms. Keep an active history log of transactions when electronic health information is viewed, downloaded, or transmitted to a third party. Consult Appendix A of this book.

(*continued*)

T A B L E   3-1 (continued)

EHR Certification Criteria: Stage 1 and Stage 2 Criteria for Ambulatory Care

Certifica- tion Criteria	Stage 1 (45 CFR 170.304) Functional Requirement the System Must Achieve	Changed or Revised in Stage 2?	Stage 2 (45 CFR 170.314)
Clinical summaries for patients	(h) Enable a user to provide clinical summaries to patients for each office visit that include, at a minimum, diagnostic test results, problem list, medication list, and medication allergy list. If the clinical summary is provided electronically it must be: (1) provided in human readable format; and (2) provided on electronic media or through some other electronic means in accordance with: (i) the standard (and applicable implementation specifications) specified in §170.205(a)(1) or §170.205(a)(2); and (ii) for the following data elements the applicable standard must be used: (A) Problems. The standard specified in §170.207(a)(1) or, at a minimum, the version of the standard specified in §170.207(a)(2); (B) Laboratory test results. At a minimum, the version of the standard specified in §170.207(c); and (C) Medications. The standard specified in §170.207(d).	Yes	(b)(2) and (e)(1) For patients, clinical summary for each office visit
Exchange clinical information and patient summary record	(1) Electronically receive and display. Electronically receive and display a patient's summary record, from other providers and organizations including, at a minimum, diagnostic tests results, problem list, medication list, and medication allergy list. Upon receipt of a patient summary record formatted according to the alternative standard, display it in human readable format. (2) Enable a user to electronically transmit a patient summary record to other providers and organizations including, at a minimum, correct patient, diagnostic test results, laboratory lab results, problem list, medication list, and medication allergy list.	Yes	(b)(2) For referring physician. Also include office contact information. Imaging information included.
Electronic prescribing	(b) Enable a user to electronically generate and transmit prescriptions and prescription-related information in accordance with: (1) the standard specified in §170.205(b)(1) or §170.205(b)(2); and (2) the standard specified in §170.207(d).	Yes	(b)(3) Now included with formulary checking

(*continued*)

T A B L E   3-1 (continued)

EHR Certification Criteria: Stage 1 and Stage 2 Criteria for Ambulatory Care

Certification Criteria	Stage 1 (45 CFR 170.304) Functional Requirement the System Must Achieve	Changed or Revised in Stage 2?	Stage 2 (45 CFR 170.314)
Clinical information reconciliation	Enable a user to electronically reconcile the data that represent a patient's active medication list, problem list, and medication allergy list as follows. For each list type: (i) Electronically and simultaneously display (ie, in a single view) the data from at least two list sources in a manner that allows a user to view the data and its attributes, which must include, at a minimum, the source and last modification date. (ii) Enable a user to create a single reconciled list of medications, medication allergies, or problems. (iii) Enable a user to review and validate the accuracy of a final set of data and, upon a user's confirmation, automatically update the list.	No	(b)(4) Unchanged
Incorporate laboratory tests and values/results	Receive results (ambulatory only)	Yes	(b)(5) Electronically display tests and values/results received in human readable format.
Transmit electronic laboratory tests and values/results to ambulatory physicians	CEHRT must demonstrate it can import lab values into the EHR	Expanded from the 2011 Edition to the 2014 Edition	(b)(6) EHR technology must be able to electronically create laboratory test reports for electronic transmission.
Data portability	Enable a user to electronically create a set of export summaries for all patients in EHR technology according to standards.	No	(b)(7) Unchanged
(C) Clinical Quality Measures			
Calculate and submit clinical quality measures [CQMs]	(1) Calculate. (i) Electronically calculate all of the core clinical measures specified by CMS for eligible professionals. (ii) Electronically calculate, at a minimum, three clinical quality measures specified by CMS for eligible professionals, in addition to those clinical quality measures specified in paragraph (1)(i). (2) Submission. Enable a user to electronically submit calculated clinical quality measures in accordance with the standard and implementation specifications specified in §170.205(f).	Yes. Language is more defined.	(c)(i) Capture. For each and every CQM for which the EHR technology is presented for certification, EHR technology must be able to electronically record all of the data that would be necessary to calculate each CQM. Data required for CQM exclusions or exceptions must be codified entries, which may

(*continued*)

T A B L E 3-1 (continued)

EHR Certification Criteria: Stage 1 and Stage 2 Criteria for Ambulatory Care

Certification Criteria	Stage 1 (45 CFR 170.304) Functional Requirement the System Must Achieve	Changed or Revised in Stage 2?	Stage 2 (45 CFR 170.314)
			include specific terms as defined by each CQM. (ii) Export. EHR technology must be able to electronically export a data file that includes all of the data captured for each and every CQM to which EHR technology was certified.
Clinical quality measures —import and calculate	In 2014 Edition, the CEHRT must electronically capture data elements specified in the data element catalog (170.204(c)).	Yes. Language revised.	(c)(i) Import. EHR technology must be able to electronically import a data file and use such data for certification. (ii) Calculate. EHR technology must be able to electronically calculate each and every clinical quality measure for which it is presented for certification.
Clinical quality measures —electronic submission	CEHRT must export results of the CQM calculation into a report to file. Higher area of focus in 2014.[20]	Yes. Language revised.	(c)(3) Enable a user to electronically create a data file for transmission of clinical quality measurement data that can be electronically accepted by CMS.
(d) HIPAA Privacy and Security **For the 2014 Edition Certification, ONC [Office of the National Coordinator for Health Information Technology] folded in the criteria from HIPAA [Health Insurance Portability and Accountability Act] Privacy and Security that supports Covered Entity requirements 170.314(b)(1) and (2) and 170.314 (d) (1)-(8)**			
User authentication, access control, and authorization	Cross-references HIPAA technical security safeguards, including audit controls, authentication, and user log-off monitoring.	New	(d)(1) Verify against a unique identifier(s) (eg, user name or number) that a person seeking access to electronic health information is the one claimed. (ii) Establish the type of access to electronic health information a user is permitted and the actions the user is permitted to perform with the EHR technology.

(*continued*)

T A B L E 3-1 (continued)

EHR Certification Criteria: Stage 1 and Stage 2 Criteria for Ambulatory Care

Certification Criteria	Stage 1 (45 CFR 170.304) Functional Requirement the System Must Achieve	Changed or Revised in Stage 2?	Stage 2 (45 CFR 170.314)
Auditable events and tamper-resistance	HIPAA Technical Standards added to the 2014 Edition certification.	New	(d)(2)Record actions. (d)(3)Record the audit log status. (C) Record the encryption.
Amendments	HIPAA Technical Standards added to the 2014 Edition certification criteria.	New	(d)(4)Enable user to electronically select the record affected by a patient's request. If amendment is approved, append the amendment or include a link that indicates the amendment's location. For denied amendments, at a minimum, append the request and denial with a link.
Automatic log-off	Prevent a user from gaining further access to an electronic session after a predetermined time of inactivity.	No	(d)(5) Unchanged
Emergency access	Permit an identified set of users to access electronic health information during an emergency.	No	(d)(6) Unchanged
Encrypt data at rest		New	(d)(7) End-user device encryption. Electronic health information that is stored must be encrypted. Default setting: EHR technology must be set by default to perform this capability and, unless this configuration cannot be disabled by any user, the ability to change the configuration must be restricted to a limited set of identified users.
Integrity	Verify that information has not been altered.	No	(d)(8) Unchanged
Accounting of disclosures	Record disclosures made for treatment, payment, and health care operations in accordance with the standard specified.	Feature is optional for EHR vendors.	(d)(9) Optional This puts EPs [eligible professionals] and EHs [eligible hospitals] at some risk in that

(continued)

TABLE 3-1 (continued)

EHR Certification Criteria: Stage 1 and Stage 2 Criteria for Ambulatory Care

Certification Criteria	Stage 1 (45 CFR 170.304) Functional Requirement the System Must Achieve	Changed or Revised in Stage 2?	Stage 2 (45 CFR 170.314)
(continued)			Accounting of Disclosures remains a HIPAA Patient Right but tracking disclosures is not required under 2014 Edition certification.
Encryption when exchanging electronic health information	Encrypt and decrypt electronic health information when exchanged.	ePHI [electronic protected health information] must be exchanged between trusted domains, such as Direct, CONNECT or encrypted delivery system.[21]	170.314(b)(7) Ensure domains for exchange are trusted.
Immunizations and Disease-Specific Registries			
Submission to immunization registries	Submission to immunization registries. Electronically record, modify, retrieve, and submit immunization information.	Yes Revised	(f)(2) "Submit" is included.
Public health surveillance	Electronically record, modify, retrieve, and submit syndrome-based public-health surveillance information in accordance with the standard (and applicable implementation specifications) specified in §170.205(d)(1) or §170.205(d)(2).	Yes Revised Specific disease registries defined.	HL7 Standard Code Set, CVX Vaccines (2009 version); LOINC [Logical Observation Identifiers Names and Codes], v 2.27; Cancer Reporting, SNOMED CT® January 2012 and LOINC v. 2.38
Automated numerator recording	For each MU objective with a percentage-based measure, EHR technology must be able to create a report or file that enables a user to review the patients or actions that would make the patient or action eligible to be included in the measure's numerator. The information in the report or file created must be of sufficient detail to enable a user to match those patients or actions to meet the measure's denominator limitations when necessary to generate an accurate percentage.	No	(g)(1) Unchanged

(continued)

TABLE 3-1 (continued)

EHR Certification Criteria: Stage 1 and Stage 2 Criteria for Ambulatory Care

Certification Criteria	Stage 1 (45 CFR 170.304) Functional Requirement the System Must Achieve	Changed or Revised in Stage 2?	Stage 2 (45 CFR 170.314)
Automated measure calculation	For each MU objective with a percentage-based measure, electronically record the numerator and denominator and generate a report including the numerator, denominator, and resulting percentage associated with each applicable MU measure.	EHR vendors must demonstrate for the 2014 Edition CEHRT	Modified to make calculations more dynamic.
Safety-enhanced design	For 2014, adds focus on "human factors, safety culture, and usability."[a] (170.314 (g)(3))	New	User-centered design processes must be applied to each capability an EHR technology includes.
Quality Measurement System	The 2014 Edition refines data searches as data during early implementation are likely to be entered into the EHR inconsistently into several fields.	New	For each capability that an EHR technology includes and for which that capability's certification is sought, the use of a quality management system (QMS) in the development, testing, implementation, and maintenance of that capability must be identified.

[a] National Research Council. Health IT and Patient Safety: Building Safer Systems for Better Care. Washington, DC: The National Academies Press, 2012.
Copyright © 2013. Physicians EHR, Inc. All rights reserved.

Critical Point

EHR vendors must not only demonstrate clinical data capture, but Stage 2 certification standards require the EHR vendor to enable the provider to meet all HIPAA technical standards. This requirement helps to circumvent some clauses embedded in a few EHR vendors' contracts that they be held harmless if the software does not enable users to meet HIPAA technical safeguards.[22]

HEALTH IT STANDARDS YOU SHOULD KNOW ABOUT FOR MEANINGFUL USE ATTESTATION

Data standards are an agreed-upon, common, and consistent way to record information. When standards are consistently applied, data can be efficiently exchanged among different information systems.[23]

One reason for America's exorbitant health care costs is because of the lack of standards. This has resulted in excessive administrative costs to interpret and re-enter data so that they can be used for patient care, patient communications, and reimbursements. The

Administrative Simplification Rule provisions, embedded in HIPAA, initiated a series of mandates for standardizing and safeguarding health information when used with transactions and code sets. Physicians view HIPAA as primarily promoting patient privacy and data security. Billers, coders, and practice administrators are familiar with HIPAA's Transactions and Code Sets (T&CS) Rule, which allows health care entities to check for a patient's eligibility, assess the payer's preauthorization requirements, conduct a formulary check, and determine if the payer has deposited funds into the physician's account and match those funds to the patient encounter.

To provide oversight and continuity on the development of standards, the ONC, through funding established by the American Recovery and Reimbursement Act (ARRA), established two federal advisory committees (FACs) made up of industry leaders and stakeholders: the Health IT Policy Committee and the Health IT Standards Committee.[24] The Health IT Policy Committee makes recommendations to the ONC on the development and adoption of a nationwide health information infrastructure, including standards for the exchange of patient medical information. The Health IT Standards Committee focuses on policies developed by the Health IT Policy Committee and makes recommendations to the ONC on standards, implementation specifications, and certification criteria for the exchange and use of health information.

Standards Hub[25]

Many organizations contribute to the development and adoption of standards that are included in the 2014 edition EHR certification criteria, which were also included in the final rule. These organizations include the American Dental Association (ADA), AMA, American National Standards Institute (ANSI) ASTM International, Centers for Disease Control and Prevention (CDC), CMS, Health Level Seven (HL7) Internet Engineering Task Force (IETF), National Institute of Standards and Technology (NIST), Office of Management and Budget (OMB), ONC, Regenstrief Institute, Inc, National Library of Medicine (NLM), and the World Wide Web Consortium (W3C)/MIT.

The ONC has provided funding for a number of health IT programs, including the development of CONNECT and the Nationwide Health Information Network (NwHIN) Direct.[26] The NwHIN Direct developed "specifications for a secure, scalable, standards-based way to establish universal health addressing and transport for participants (including providers, laboratories, hospitals, pharmacies and patients) to send encrypted health information directly to known, trusted recipients over the Internet."[27] NwHIN Direct is an open government project that has avenues for a broad range of public participation, while CONNECT is an open-source software used as an HIE portal with governance among users that define how protected health information will be used and disclosed. CONNECT, part of the eHealth Exchange (formerly the NwHIN, is built on Integrating the Healthcare Enterprise (IHE) profiles and managed by Healtheway, Inc, a nonprofit public-private partnership organization.

CONNECT includes one or more open source applications for each of the components, plus some private vendor tools such as IBM/Initiate Systems' master patient index software. CONNECT is real, downloadable software with three components:

- Gateway, which implements nationwide health information network specifications for secure data exchange over the Internet;
- Enterprise Service Platform, which enables an organization to plug practice management and electronic health records systems into a framework to communicate with the Gateway; and

■ Universal Client Framework, a platform to develop end-user applications that support meaningful use if a physician doesn't have an EHR.

While CONNECT was done to meet certain needs of government agencies and large organizations, NwHIN Direct is focused on more modest goals by smaller entities, such as physician-to-physician or physician-to-laboratory connectivity. It builds off CONNECT to offer an additional set of standards and specifications to support point-to-point interactions for meaningful use of health information technology, says Doug Fridsma, MD, acting director of the office of standards and interoperability in the Office of the National Coordinator for Health Information Technology."[28]

Table 3-2 provides an overview of health IT standards, and while most physician practices are expected to reach into the EHR and pull out data, standards make it possible for data analytics and exchange with referral partners. Once standards are agreed upon, often a prolonged process, the NIST tests the standards before they are submitted for adoption.[29]

TABLE 3-2

Health IT Standards, What They Mean, and How They Affect Your Practice

Standard	What It Represents	How It Affects Physicians
Continuity of Care Document (CCD)	Patient health summary standard. Some questions whether the CCD will supplant the Continuity of Care Record (CCR).	Vendors certified by the Authorized Testing and Certification Body (ATCB); or since 2013, the Authorized Certification Bodies (ACB) must demonstrate they can create a patient summary using a CCD. Allows physicians to create a patient summary.
Continuity of Care Record	Patient health summary standard	Vendors certified by the ACB must demonstrate they can create a patient summary using a CCR. As with the CCD, the CCR must gather sections of allergies, medications, problems, and laboratory results and match these to the correct patient.
HIPAA Transactions and Code Sets	In electronic transactions, the billing system must use eight standard formats for health care transactions.	Allows a physician to check for patient eligibility, insurance verification, or preauthorization requirements using standardized medical code sets, such as *International Classification Diseases, Ninth Revision, Clinical Modification* (*ICD-9-CM*), National Drug Codes (NDC), the Code on Dental Procedures and Nomenclature (CDT), Current Procedural Terminology (CPT), and the Health care Common Procedure Coding System (HCPCS).

(continued)

T A B L E 3-2 (continued)

Health IT Standards, What They Mean, and How They Affect Your Practice

Standard	What It Represents	How It Affects Physicians
Logical Observation Identifiers Names and Codes (LOINC® Codes)	Universal code system for identifying laboratory and clinical observations. Enables aggregation of electronic health data from many independent systems.	Translates laboratory results into meaningful terms for physician interpretation.
Systematized Nomenclature of Medicine (SNOMED) Clinical Terms® [CT®])	Standardizes the language of topography (location) with morphology (changes) and many other categories to accurately store and retrieve clinical records. For example, T-28000 references the lung; T-M-40000 references inflammation.	Certified EHRs must demonstrate that structured data are built using SNOMED-CT® technology. This allows one physician to create a record and retrieve data using the same search criteria.
Accredited Standards Committee X12 (ASC X12)	Standardizes the financial/business transactions and HIPAA-related mandated transactions.[30]	These standards are used by the financial industry to process payment and post funds into your account.
Syndromic Surveillance	Allows physicians to report potentially hazardous disease outbreaks to public-health officials.	Supports health care professionals' response to potential emergency situations.
Digital Imaging and Communications in Medicine (DICOM)	Standardizes biomedical diagnostic and therapeutic information.	DICOM standards are most often found in cardiology, dentistry, endoscopy, mammography, ophthalmology, orthopedics, pathology, pediatrics, radiation therapy, and radiology.
Health Level Seven (HL7)	Standardizes the exchange, management, and integration of data that supports clinical patient care and the management, delivery, and evaluation of health care services.[30]	Allows a health care professional to order and obtain results between different systems.
Integrating the Healthcare Enterprise (IHE)	Develops structured document exchange integration profiles.	IHE plays a significant role in helping physicians integrate content from multiple sources accessible by the provider for clinical decision making.
National Council for Prescription Drug Programs (NCPDP)	Creates and promotes interchange standards for the pharmacy sector.	Standardizes the e-prescribing process to pharmacies.
Institute of Electrical and Electronics Engineers (IEEE)	In health care, IEEE standardizes information exchanges for medical devices.	Allows physicians to interface EHR with medical devices.

HEALTH CARE BORROWS STANDARDS FROM OTHER INDUSTRIES

Not only does the health care industry utilize standards from its own sector, it also borrows standards from other industries that today influence how physicians use mobile devices to communicate with each other and practices.

For example, Great Britain brought together its allies during World War II when quality issues in ammunitions plants caused bombs to explode during creation. The request for standardization created the first International Standards Organization, which has evolved into the ISO 9000 series governing the manufacturing sector. ISO standards also are now cross-referenced in the 2014 edition of the EHR certification criteria.

The ITU Telecommunication Standardization Sector (ITU-T) is the organization that built consensus on the technologies and services that form the backbone of core network functionalities from broadband to new technologies.[31] These standards allow physicians to use Wi-Fi networks while traveling so that they can securely access electronic protected health information (ePHI) from smart phones and most mobile devices.

DATA MANAGEMENT AND THE VALUE OF STANDARD CLINICAL OPERATING PROCEDURES

Several years ago, members of the Physicians EHR, Inc, team were called into a 10-physician practice that had gone live about 2 years prior and transitioned from an EHR that probably would not get ONC certification. The eight servers initially recommended by their certified vendor had run out of space. The system ran exceptionally slowly during peak use and occasionally shut down if several physicians were simultaneously e-prescribing.

The practice manager had consulted a local IT company that recommended they purchase and install eight more servers, which they did. This was not simply a matter of installing another rack server, but the practice also needed to enlarge the server room, install a 3.5-ton air conditioning unit that would circulate air throughout the room to manage hot spots, and install a temperature alarm, because no one had time to regularly monitor heat in the server room.

Within another 6 months, back-end bottlenecks slowed the practice down so much that it was ready to abandon the EHR. When we began our workflow and IT study, we observed the following:

- The practice was still running their previous EHR on the first set of servers.
- Physicians were e-prescribing on both the previous and current EHR.
- When communicating with the care team, one doctor would attach a document to an Outlook message and copy all physicians. When responding, all physicians would copy each other and attach a track-changes revision to the original document.

For just a moment, put aside the privacy, security, and patient-safety issues and look at how data monopolized server space. Given the growth of the practice, the expanded server room turned out to be a good investment, but once the practice put data management policies and procedures in place and shut down the previous EHR to "view only," we cleaned up the servers and made them fully functional again.

Implementing standard operating procedures for data resulted in three lessons learned:

1. Physicians should be confident that patient medical and demographic information will be stored and accessible through a single source.

2. Multiple e-mails may not only be insecure, but when sent with attachments, they slow the system and create bottlenecks. Server bottlenecks are interrelated, so improving old data also improves system performance.
3. Data are easier to collect and report on when submitted in a consistent and standardized manner. You can learn more about standardizing clinical workflows in Chapter 4.

Many practices develop or modify policies and procedures not only for compliance with organizations and regulations such as the Joint Commission (formerly the Joint Commission on Accreditation of Healthcare Organizations [JAHCO]), HIPAA, and the Occupational Safety and Health Administration (OSHA), but because data can become voluminous once the clinical team begins entering content.

Critical Point

Data-management operating procedures provide a structure for governing how information is entered into the EHR and who enters it. Clinical standard operating procedures (SOPs) set the stage for a healthier infrastructure as you build the system. When building your SOPs, begin by evaluating current-state workflows (discussed in Chapter 4), and then build future-state policies.

CARE AND NURTURING OF DATA

Earlier in this chapter you learned that privacy and security safeguards have been added to the 2014 edition of the EHR certification standards, ensuring that EHR vendors can support technical standards included in the HIPAA Security Rule. While we do not intend to get into a deep discussion on privacy and security in this chapter, this section is designed to help you meet MU Stage 1 core measure #15: *Attest that you have completed or updated a risk analysis and are in the process of developing policies and procedures to mitigate identified risks.*

For Stage 2, as mentioned previously in this chapter, you are not asked to attest to completing a risk analysis, as you have already attested to completing one in Stage 1. The HIPAA Security Rule requires that you evaluate your risks at least annually and also update and train your staff on corresponding policies and procedures. In Stage 2, however, a CEHRT system must demonstrate that it can meet HIPAA technical safeguards.

To that end, we provide a brief overview of HIPAA privacy and security but recommend you reference one of several HIPAA books published by the AMA, including *HIPAA Plain & Simple,* 2nd edition, by Carolyn P. Hartley, MLA, and Edward D. Jones.

There are three agencies under the HHS that govern the creation, use, and disclosure of health information.

■ The Office for Civil Rights (OCR) is the enforcement agency for both HIPAA's privacy and security rules.
■ The ONC requires EPs and EHs to demonstrate they are managing protected health information in a secure environment.
■ The CMS regulates and enforces the use of HIPAA standard transactions.

Terms defined in the HIPAA privacy and security rules have heightened vulnerabilities and protection concerns in relation to EHRs. Table 3-3 provides an overview of those terms and their complications.

TABLE 3-3

HIPAA Terms and Their Heightened Vulnerabilities

HIPAA Terms	Heightened Vulnerabilities and Complications
Protected Health Information (PHI)	PHI has 18 identifiers—information that nurses, doctors, and other providers put into a patient's paper or electronic medical chart, conversations about the patient, payer, and billing information. **Complication:** In a paper chart, many of these identifiers were accessed on individual pages. In an EHR, these can be more readily accessed.
Use	Create, retrieve, revise, or delete PHI. **Complication:** *Use* now includes access controls, servers, software, and audit trails.
Disclose	Release, transfer, divulge, or allow access to PHI outside the holding entity. **Complication**: PHI is stored in multiple systems; inhibits the ability to pull together record. Source records include images, voice records, and other provider records.
Data at rest	Stored in paper charts, databases, servers, flash drives, etc. **Complication:** Data are now stored in portable notebooks and/or handheld devices, creating new exposures. The 2014 edition certification must provide capabilities to encrypt data at rest.
Data in motion	Data being transmitted. **Complication:** Data-transmission carriers are not business associate. However, both sender and receivers must ensure integrity and confidentiality.
Covered entity	For physicians: a health care provider who transmits any information in an electronic form in connection with a transaction for which the Department of Health and Human Services has adopted a standard.

Embedded in the HIPAA Privacy Rule are HIPAA privacy safeguards. Both these privacy safeguards and the HIPAA Security Rule implementation specifications are divided into three categories:

■ Administrative safeguards
■ Physical safeguards
■ Technical safeguards

The framers of both statutes and associated regulations intentionally designed the overlap. Privacy Rule safeguards, effective April 14, 2003, served as a stopgap measure until Security Rule specifications became effective 2 years later, on April 20, 2005. The Privacy Rule[32] gained widespread recognition when thousands of health-law attorneys, consulting groups, medical societies, and publishers helped spread the word of the rule's compliance standards. The Security Rule, designed to put good security business practices in place, really came of age when Congress approved the HITECH Act's[33] investment of more than $20 billion to build a health IT infrastructure. The HITECH Act also required the HHS to significantly enhance enforcement penalties and corrective action plans for covered entities' privacy breaches and willful neglect of security and privacy safeguards.

As one of three agencies within the HHS assigned to regulate privacy and security, the ONC included a requirement that EPs and EHs demonstrate how they safeguard PHI when they attest to core measure #15 for EPs and core measure #14 for EHs. These core measures are met by attesting that the EP or EH has completed a risk analysis and also put in place measures to mitigate those risks.

PERFORMING A RISK ANALYSIS

A risk analysis, also referred to as a security risk analysis (SRA), is a series of queries designed to help you determine where risks have been, where they might still be, and how to mitigate them. The NIST posits 492 questions you should include in a risk analysis in its toolkit, which is available online.[34] While the questions are directed at larger organizations, some of the administrative requirements applicable to providers include:

- Did you appoint a security official?
- Did you conduct a risk assessment and build your policies and procedures based on risks you identified in that assessment?
- Have you trained your workforce on those policies and procedures?
- Do you monitor reports of persons who access systems and patient files?
- Do you have a disaster recovery plan in place? Have you tested it?
- Do you also comply with other state and federal privacy requirements?

To meet core measure #15 and also comply with HIPAA, you must not only identify your practice's vulnerabilities and threats, but also mitigate those risks with policies and procedures and train staff on those processes. The measure requires that you conduct or review a security risk analysis in accordance with the requirements under 45 CFR 164.308(a)(1), implement security updates as necessary, and correct identified security deficiencies.

What to Do: Complete a Security Risk Analysis to Meet Core Measure #15

Identify a risk assessment that meets the needs of ambulatory practices. The HIPAA Security Rule is scalable, which means that each specification applies to your size, budget, and number of workforce members. If yours is a large multispecialty practice, your risks may be more significant than a small rural practice, but that is not always the case if the practice has retained the services of an IT director. Free risk assessments for a small practice are available at HealthIT.gov.

A good risk assessment should ask you a series of questions that correspond with the administrative, physical, and technical components of the Security Rule. For each question, you want to assign a risk scaled from:

- **Not really a risk** for us. For example, you hire only family members in your practice, so not performing a background check may not be a risk for you.
- **Could be a risk**, since we believe this could happen to us. For example, a workforce member may be reviewing records from patients not on his or her patient panel.
- **Definitely a risk** for us. For example, you live in North Dakota, hurricanes are unlikely to affect you, but tornadoes and floods have been a real threat to accessing EHRs.

Score each risk on a scale of one to six, with one being a low risk and six being a very high risk. Risks that score above four should be assigned to a risk manager or to someone in the office who can provide answers and responses to both workforce members and an auditor, should questions or situations arise when the security official is not easily available.

Identified risks require a policy and procedure to be put in place. Consult AMA's *Policies and Procedures for the Electronic Medical Practice* for templates you can use to develop your policies.

MAJOR TYPES OF RISKS

The following six risks may not apply to all situations, but they do reflect the general state of privacy, security, and patient safety as the health care community transitions into EHRs and interoperability.

Risk #1: Establish Secure Health Information Exchange With Hospitals, Accountable Care Organizations (ACOs), and Super Groups

HIEs must establish a governance board. The governance board then sets policies and procedures that all members of the HIE agree to follow.

As hospitals acquire ambulatory medical practices, establish ACOs, or take leadership roles in state and local HIEs, privacy policies may need to be reviewed and updated, especially as patients transition between primary care and hospitals or between skilled nursing facilities and hospitals.

Risk-Prevention Strategies

- Participate in HIE governance structures. Part of their governance is to determine privacy and security policies between members as well as sanctions if an organization fails to protect privacy.
- Ask for assurance that HIE interoperability standards will meet the consent requirements in 42 CFR, Part 2, for consent and privacy authorization if behavioral health providers are included.
- If part of a hospital system, read the consent forms to ensure that PHI safeguards meet all clinical and behavioral specialty requirements.
- As this is a legal issue, consult a health-law attorney for additional guidance.

Risk #2: Manage Access and Audit Controls

Access control, an implementation specification in HIPAA's Security Rule, is a companion to the minimum necessary requirement in the Privacy Rule. In both rules, the covered entity is required to determine the minimum amount of access to PHI necessary for any given employee to do his or her job effectively. For example, a physician, nurse practitioner, or physician assistant may need access to clinical information, while a registration clerk or scheduler most likely will not require the same access privileges.

Audit controls, a required specification in the Security Rule, allow administrators to see who has had access to PHI, when they had access, and what they created, viewed, modified, or deleted. Risks associated with access control and audit controls come with several issues:

- Some EHR vendors don't train administrators how to run the audit control feature.
- Audit controls take up space on the server and can slow the system.
- Some EHR vendors embed administrative functions, such as scanning driver's licenses and insurance cards into the clinical screens. So when a front-office staff member admits a patient, he or she may immediately compromise role-based policies and procedures to gain access to the patient's insurance information or authenticate the patient's identity by looking at the driver's license.

- The clinic may need to develop a script to run an audit control report.
- Employees may not access another patient's chart if they are not directly involved in the patient's care

---

Critical Point

Access control refers to the people who *may* have access according to their role. *Audit control* refers to who actually *had* access and what they created, changed, modified, deleted, or downloaded and when.

Risk-Prevention Strategies

- If you have yet to implement the audit controls feature of your EHR system, talk to the system's technical support team, as this feature will be invaluable in the event of a breach. Audit controls are a required feature for the 2014 edition EHR certification. Even so, the HITECH Act's Breach Notification Rule requires covered entities to report an impermissible use or disclosure of PHI (a breach, in other words) of 500 individuals or more to the Secretary of HHS and the media within 60 days after the discovery of the breach. Smaller breaches affecting fewer than 500 individuals must be reported to the HHS Secretary on an annual basis.

Risk #3: Manage the Hybrid Record

A hybrid record is one that is part paper and part electronic. Both have essential information for the physician's clinical decision making. During the transition from paper to an EHR, patient safety may be at risk as PHI can now be found in EHRs, interfaces, audit trails, servers, tablets, handheld devices, annotations, data exchanges, e-prescribing systems, faxes, and much more, including paper.

Without a plan to manage the hybrid record, the physician risks making clinical decisions based on an incomplete record. For example, a physician would not logically look for results of a chest X-ray ordered at a hospital unless someone either faxed or e-mailed results, verbally notified the physician of the order, or scanned the order and results into the electronic patient chart that the physician would normally access. The EHR then would enter the results into the physician queue. Maintaining access to medical information is creating a new class of malpractice claims if access is not managed.[37]

During chart abstraction and data migration, the paper record remains the official record until a thorough representation of the paper record has been migrated into the EHR. For this reason, physicians frequently take the paper chart into the exam room for the first two or three visits to maintain as complete a picture as possible. Once the physician team deems the EHR to be a complete record, the electronic chart then becomes the legal health record (LHR). There is no legal one-size-fits-all definition of the LHR because laws and regulations governing the content vary by setting and by state.

However, there are guiding principles that the American Health Information Management Association (AHIMA) provided in a legal brief to help define the legal record.[35] Refer to the AHIMA's "Practice Brief: Definition of the Health Record for Legal Purposes," for some of the more frequently asked questions and responses.

If the patient provides the physician with information from a personal health record (PHR), does it become part of the LHR? Copies of PHRs that are owned by the patient but provided to the physician and that become part of the EHR are now part of the LHR. These might include advance directives, anesthesia records, care plans, consent-for-treatment forms, discharge summaries, immunization records, medication profiles, and orders. For a complete list, go to http://ehim.wikispaces.com/file/view/AHIMA+book+1.htm.[36]

How should we handle paper that comes into the practice after we have declared the EHR the LHR? Nontraditional patient information should now be considered in the LHR definition process. Documents may include patient inquiry forms, such as patient intake questionnaires, clinical protocols/critical pathways, intravenous flow measures, e-mails, expert system rules, physician alerts/reminders, research protocols, and user-specific screen views.[33]

Critical Point

If you have concerns about the definition of your practice's legal health record, consult a health-law attorney for guidance. The American Health Lawyers Association can be a helpful resource. See www.healthlawyers.org.

Privacy and security measures play a significant role in the PHI data migration process. For example, as part of the scanning process, a practice might adopt a policy that paper containing PHI must be placed into a "shred" pile after data are either scanned or entered as discrete data into the EHR. The shred pile then must be shredded at the end of the day. But that doesn't always happen. Over several days, the pile of paper might build to overflow and an employee might use the back of a progress note to create a grocery list.

Until a clinic establishes, trains, and enforces policies and procedures for how it will manage a hybrid record, the chart will remain a combination of paper and EHR, creating both patient safety and privacy issues and missing one of the most significant benefits of an EHR—having a patient's record in one place. Hybrid records also can present unmanageable privacy exposures.

Risk-Prevention Strategies

- Decide upon an event that will prompt the practice to determine when the EHR is the LHR. For example, when all data on a checklist are entered into the EHR, the EHR will become the LHR.[38]
- Put in place policies that require paper to be shredded at the end of each workday. Enforce this policy.
- Build a strategy for managing hybrid medical charts. This is part of your go-live strategy and should be part of your strategic implementation plan.
- Ask your EHR vendor how it plans to help you comply with access and audit controls.

Risk #4: Establish Legal Clarity on Who Owns the Data, Especially in Secondary Use

To meet one of the MU measures, you must agree to participate in an HIE and load either test or real data for Stage 1 and real data for Stage 2. The board of this HIE has to establish policies and procedures that govern how data will be used and disclosed in a secure environment. Offending members are subject to sanctions.

The HIE must also provide policies for secondary use. For example, suppose a laboratory enters laboratory values into an HIE so a provider can access those results. The preparers of a clinical study demonstrate that they will benefit greatly from accessing deidentified data from that HIE's laboratory data. What policies and procedures will the institutional review board present to the HIE? And who should be informed of the study?

Risk-Prevention Strategies

If you are asked to participate in an HIE, ask these questions:

- What PHI can a health care professional put into the HIE and expect that it will be protected?
- Can PHI be leveraged into another covered entity's database, and what would those conditions look like?
- If erroneous information is provided by another caregiver, how will it be corrected?
- Who owns the record and is responsible for its upkeep?

What Is Secondary Use?

The *Journal of American Medical Association* (*JAMA*) has provided a standard description of secondary use as:

> Secondary use includes such activities as analysis, research, quality and safety measurement, public-health reporting, payment, provider certification or accreditation, marketing, and other business applications, including strictly commercial activities. Secondary use of health data can enhance health care experiences for individuals, expand knowledge about disease and appropriate treatments, strengthen understanding about the effectiveness and efficiency of health care systems, support public-health and security goals, and aid businesses in meeting customers' needs. Yet, complex ethical, political, technical, and social issues surround the secondary use of health data. While not new, these issues play increasingly critical and complex roles given current public and private sector activities not only expanding health data volume, but also improving access to data. Lack of coherent policies and standard "good practices" for secondary use of health data impedes efforts to strengthen the US health care system. The nation requires a framework for the secondary use of health data with a robust infrastructure of policies, standards, and best practices. Such a framework could guide and facilitate widespread collection, storage, aggregation, linkage, and transmission of health data. The framework will provide appropriate protections for legitimate secondary use.[37]

Risk #5: Monitor Privacy, Mobility, and Breach Notification

The question about mobility is not whether your organization will embrace handheld devices, but rather how, when, and what secure solutions, including encryption, you will put in place to protect patient confidentiality. Considerable debates have emerged regarding bring your own device (BYOD) policies and how an organization will protect PHI when it resides on a device owned by a provider, not the organization. Organizations may put policies in effect, but the real measure of this policy is how BYOD is enforced with sanctions applied consistently across the organization. Organizations may choose to confiscate a device and wipe out all PHI and relevant and associated applications, if policy dictates.

As physicians join the ranks of iPad® and smartphone users, a HIPAA covered entity must begin to assess and mitigate risks in the rapidly expanding mobile environment. In patient care, providers can access the patient record from home in the event of an episode, hospitalization, or setback to quickly identify medication and behavioral histories.

One of the most frustrating HIPAA questions for an office manager comes from a patient asking, "I'd like to know where my protected health information has been used and disclosed." Yet, this very capability is still optional for 2014 edition of EHR vendor certification standards.

During an onsite HIPAA training course with New York[38] primary-care providers, the providers collectively said they received from one to three requests for an accounting of disclosures each month. In contrast, participants in a May 2012 webinar on privacy and behavioral health in an electronic environment reported they received approximately 30 requests a month. The lesson learned is that behavioral health providers will receive at least 10 times the number of requests for an accounting of disclosures. As a result, they are much more prepared to handle an accounting of disclosures request than their primary-care colleagues.

Lost, stolen, or missing mobile devices are the leading cause of breaches that must be reported to the OCR, either once yearly (fewer than 500 records affected) or within 60 days of the breach (500 or more records). Fines have dramatically escalated, rebuffing the notion that OCR was a sleeper agency. In a recent "war game" with 23 EHR consultants who were enrolled in a course called Breach Communication and Issues Management,[39] the task they struggled with most was how to identify the location of patient records.

Risk-Prevention Strategies

- Conduct a PHI gap analysis, and identify the location of PHI within your facility.
- Encrypt mobile devices.
- Prevent download of patient information onto mobile devices, including USB hard drives, by locking PHI onto the server. Clinicians can still access patient information but through a secure virtual private network (VPN).
- As your organization transitions into EHRs, be sure the EHR software you select not only meets the clinical and functional elements for behavioral health,[40] but also has the technical capacity to electronically provide you with these disclosures.
- Put in place a strategy that will help you identify patient records *before* a breach occurs.

Risk #6: Handle Consumer Complaints

Every organization should put in place a process that encourages patients to file complaints to someone inside the clinic. These complaints are easier to manage than having to work through an OCR audit. Audit controls embedded in an EHR allow the owner/administrator to run an internal report on the EHR system. An OCR audit is an external audit in which an investigator from the HHS is investigating the reasons behind a valid privacy complaint. An audit from any organization is time consuming, but OCR audits are much more investigative in nature. They may begin with a phone and e-mail investigation but can quickly ramp up to onsite visits, deeper investigations into multiple policies, fines and penalties, as well as additional investigation into potential fraud and abuse activities.

If a patient does file a complaint with the OCR, the four consistently asked questions are these:

1. What is your policy for this complaint? For example, a patient says your clinic disclosed information to another clinic without consent. You would provide your written policy for use and disclosure for treatment, payment, and health care operations.

2. What is your training policy and when did you last train on this policy? You would provide a list of attendees at a HIPAA training session, the topic, and the date of training.
3. What is your sanction policy and did you follow it? Be able to report that sanctions are not applied inconsistently.
4. What is your plan to remediate this complaint? Document steps you are taking to repair any damage, if any, to the patient.

On its Web site, the OCR says it has processed 71,849 HIPAA complaints since April 2003, more than 40,000 of which were found to have no basis for enforcement.[41]

Figure 3-1 shows the HHS/OCR enforcement highlights in terms of the numbers of complaints received and the status of these complaints as of January 31, 2012. Note that these figures are nonstatic figures, ie, they change with each OCR report of incidents and resolutions.

FIGURE 3-1

OCR Enforcement Highlights: Status of All Complaints—April 14, 2003–January 31, 2013.

■ Complaints Remaining Open 7,077 (9%)

☐ Complaints Resolved 70,800 (91%)

   Total Complaints Received 77,877*

* Referrals to [Department of Justice] DOJ – 514
Source: Office for Civil Rights. Health Information Privacy. HIPAA Enforcement Highlights.
Available at www.hhs.gov/ocr/privacy/hipaa/enforcement/highlights/indexnumbers.html. Accessed January 20, 2013.

Figure 3-2 shows the HHS/OCR enforcement highlights in terms of the total number of complaints investigated and the results of these investigations as of January 31, 2013. Of the 77,877 complaints, 514 were referred to a state or Department of Justice (DOJ), as the complaint was of a criminal nature.

FIGURE 3-2

OCR Enforcement Highlights: Total Investigated Resolutions—April 14, 2003–January 31, 2013

☐ No Violation (34%) 8,971

■ Corrective Action Obtained
(Change Achieved) (66%) 18,711

   Total Complaints Investigated 27,682

Source: Office for Civil Rights. Health Information Privacy. HIPAA Enforcement Highlights.
Available at www.hhs.gov/ocr/privacy/hipaa/enforcement/highlights/indexnumbers.html. Accessed January 20, 2013.

Figure 3-3 shows the HHS/OCR enforcement highlights in terms of the total number of investigated resolutions from April 14, 2003 through December 31, 2011.

FIGURE   3-3

OCR Enforcement Highlights: Investigated Resolutions—April 14, 2003 through December 31, 2011.

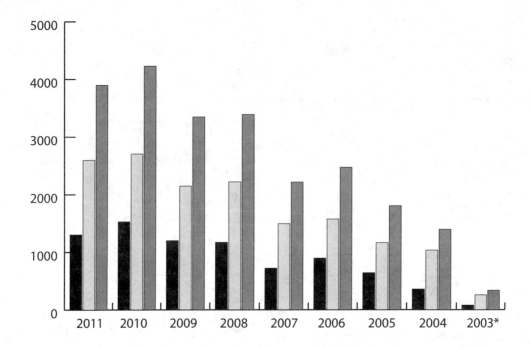

* Partial data for 2003.
Source: Office for Civil Rights. Health Information Privacy. HIPAA Enforcement Highlights. Available at www.hhs.gov/ocr/privacy/hipaa/enforcement/highlights/indexnumbers.html. Accessed January 20, 2013.

The most common types of covered entities that have been required to take corrective action to achieve voluntary compliance are, in order of frequency[42]:

1. Private practices
2. General hospitals
3. Outpatient facilities
4. Health plans (group health plans and health insurance issuers)
5. Pharmacies

Risk-Prevention Strategies

- Train staff on privacy and security policies and procedures on a regular basis.
- Ensure staff knows what is included in your notice of privacy policies.
- Privacy officials should participate in organizational workgroups, such as those aligned with the Workgroup for Electronic Data Interchange (WEDI), to keep up-to-date on privacy and security situations and best practices.
- Consult a health-law attorney if you receive a call from the OCR.
- Train staff on how to respond to a complaint and refer complainants to the privacy official.

SUMMARY

What's in It for Physicians?

■ Physicians need to have access to data to make clinical decisions. An IT infrastructure that is strategically designed, implemented with skill according to plan, and then supported by SOPs means the physicians can trust data will be available to them when needed, irrespective of where they are located.

■ Physicians also want peace of mind that their access will be conducted in a secure environment and that the internal security staff will run audit trails to be sure data are secure.

What's in It for the Staff?

■ Staff want to know what their limits are so that they can perform to the highest level of their licensing credentials. As staff transitions from a paper to an electronic environment, the SOPs, including those for privacy, security, and patient safety, become a comfort zone for all employees to understand the baseline of permissions and requirements.

What's in It for the Patient?

■ The entire medical community—primary-care physicians, specialists, hospitals, laboratories, patients, makers of medical devices—benefits from data when the data are in a secure environment and can be exchanged in a standardized way. Patients/consumers are the greatest beneficiaries of standardized data as they continue to take greater control of their own care.

ACTION ITEMS

1. As a group, play the cyber security game offered at www.healthit.gov/sites/default /files/cybersecure/cybersecure.html. Select "Providers & Professionals," then select the "Privacy & Security" tab.[43] The game requires you to respond to privacy and security challenges by answering a multiple-choice question about security. When you choose the right response, you earn points and can add rooms or features to your virtual office. If you select the wrong response, your virtual office must work through the consequences.
2. Refer to the 2014 edition EHR certification criteria to determine how MU criteria will help your practice be more efficient. For example:
   • Imaging results: By 2014, what server or online capabilities will you need to accommodate imaging?
   • Family health history: Are you currently gathering family history information and where are you entering it into the system?
   • Generate patient lists: How can you use patient lists more effectively to make clinical and business decisions for your practice?
   • Timely access: What should you do now to help your EPs generate a clinical summary within 3 business days or (Stage 2) 24 hours?

REFERENCES

1. HealthIT. How to Implement EHRs. www.healthit.gov/providers-professionals/ehr-implementa tion-steps/step-5-achieve-meaningful-use. Accessed February 4, 2013.

2. 45 CFR Part 170, Health Information Technology: Initial Set of Standards, Implementation Specifications, and Certification Criteria for Electronic Health Record Technology; Final Rule Federal Register, 77(171). September 4, 2012.

3. 45 CRF 170.314 (a)(1) through (a) (17) for Stage 2.

4. 45 CFR Part 170, Federal Register p. 54170, Table 2.

5. 45 CFR, 170.314 (b)(1) through (b)(7).

6. 45 CFR 170.314 (c)(1) through (c)(3).

7. HealthIT. Step 5: Achieve Meaningful Use—Core Measure 10 Clinical Quality Measures (CQMs). www.healthit.gov/providers-professionals/achieve-meaningful-use/core-measures/clinical-quality -measures. Accessed February 4, 2013.

8. 45 CRF 170.314 (d)1 through (d)(9).

9. 45 CFR 170.314 (e)(1) through (e)(3).

10. Health IT. Step 5: Achieve Meaningful Use—Core Measure 13 Clinical Summaries. www.healthit. gov/providers-professionals/achieve-meaningful-use/core-measures/clinical-summaries. Accessed January 29, 2013.

11. Office of the National Coordinator for Health Information Technology. Test Procedure for §170.314(f)(2) Transmission to Immunization Registries. www.healthit.gov/sites/default/files /170.314f2transmissiontoimmunizationregistries_2014_tp_approved_v1.3.pdf. Accessed February 11, 2013.

12. 45 CFR 170.314 (g)(1) through (g)(2).

13. HealthIT. Test Procedure for §170.314(g)(1) Automated Numerator Recording and Test Procedure for §170.314(g)(2) Automated Measure Calculation. www.healthit.gov/sites/default/files/170.314g 12numrec_automeascalc_2014_tp_approved_v1.2_0.pdf. Accessed January 29, 2013.

14. ONC Fact Sheet: 2014 Edition Standards & Certification Criteria (S&CC) Final Rule. www.healthit .gov/sites/default/files/pdf/ONC_FS_EHR_Stage_2_Final_082312.pdf. Accessed February 4, 2013.

15. Tate J. EMR Advocate Newsletter. January 2013. www.emradvocate.com. Accessed January 20, 2013.

16. The Office of the National Coordinator for Health Information Technology (ONC). Certified Health IT Product List. http://oncchpl.force.com/ehrcert?q=CHPL. Accessed January 20, 2013.

17. HealthIT. Final Rules and Regulations. www.healthit.gov/policy-researchers-implementers /standards-certification-rules. Accessed January 20, 2013.

18. The Office of the National Coordinator for Health Information Technology (ONC). Policy Researches and Implementers. www.healthit.gov/policy-researchers-implementers. Accessed January 20, 2013.

19. ———.Test Procedure for §170.314(a)(9) Electronic Notes. www.healthit.gov/sites/default/files /standards-certification/2014-edition-draft-test-procedures/170-314-a-9-electronic-notes-2014-test -procedures-draft-v1.0.pdf. Accessed January 29, 2013.

20. ———. Test Procedure for §170.314(c)(1) – (c)(3) Clinical Quality Measures. www.healthit.gov /sites/default/files/170.314c1-c3cqms_2014_tp_approvedv1.2.pdf. Accessed January 29, 2013.

21. Rules and Regulations. *Fed Regis.* 2013;78(17):5639.

22. Security Standards for the Protection of Electronic Protected Health Information. Technical safeguards. 45 CFR 164.312.

23. Minnesota Department of Health. Public Health Data Standards, Improving How Public Health Collects, Uses and Exchanges Data. www.health.state.mn.us/e-health/standards/pubhstandards 08.pdf. Accessed February 5, 2013.

24. Health IT. HITECH Programs & Advisory Committees. www.healthit.gov/policy-researchers -implementers/hitech-programs-advisory-committees. Accessed February 5, 2013.

25. HealthIT.gov. Standards Hub. www.healthit.gov/policy-researchers-implementers/meaningful-use -stage-2-0/standards-hub. Accessed January 29, 2013.

26. Health IT. Interoperability Portfolio. Nationwide Health Information Network (NwHIN). www .healthit.gov/policy-researchers-implementers/nationwide-health-information-network-nwhin. Accessed February 7, 2013.

27. The Direct Project. http://wiki.directproject.org/. Accessed February 7, 2013.

28. Goedert, J. CONNECT & NHIN Direct: What Are They? Health Data Management. www.health datamanagement.com/news/interoperability-connect-nhin-direct-hie-40313-1.html. Accessed February 7, 2013.

29. International Standards Organization. www.iso.org. Accessed February 4, 2013.

30. Public Health Data Standards Consortium. www.phdsc.org/standards/health-information/IE _Standards.asp#DICOM. Accessed February 4, 2013.

31. ITU-T Telecommunications Standardization Sector. www.itu.int/net/ITU-T/info/Default.aspx. Accessed January 4, 2013.

32. US Department of Health & Human Services. www.hhs.gov/ocr/privacy. Accessed January 4, 2013.

33. American Recovery and Reinvestment Act (ARRA). www.recovery.gov. Accessed January 4, 2013.

34. National Institute of Standards and Technology (NIST). http://scap.nist.gov/hipaa. Accessed January 4, 2013.

35. Quinn AM, Kats AM, Kelinman K, Bates DW, Simon SR. The relationship between electronic health records and malpractice claims. *Arch Intern Med.* 2012;172(15):1187-1189. doi:10.1001/ archinternmed.2012.2371.

36. Amatayakul M, Brandt M, Dennis JC, et al. Definition of the health record for legal purposes (AHIMA Practice Brief). *J AHIMA.* 72(9);2001:88A-H. http://ehim.wikispaces.com/file/view /AHIMA+book+1.htm. Accessed February 5, 2013.

37. Safran C, Bloomrosen M, Hammond WE, et al. Toward a national framework for the secondary use of health data: an American Medical Informatics Association White Paper, *J Am Med Inform Assoc.* 2007;14(1);1-9. Also available at www.ncbi.nlm.nih.gov/pmc/articles/PMC2329823. Accessed January 4, 2013.

38. Hartley C. Presented at New York State Society of Medical Oncologists and Hematologists, Inc; October 2009: Warwick, NY.

39. Physicians EHR Data Breach Response Plan [free breach communication and issues management course]. http://physiciansehr.org/data-breach-response-plan.aspx. Accessed January 4, 2013.

40. Physicians EHR Resource Library. Behavioral Health Clinical Functional Elements. http://physiciansehr.org/ehr-resource-library-2.aspx. Accessed February 4, 2013.

41. Office for Civil Rights. www.hhs.gov/ocr/privacy/hipaa/enforcement/index.html. Accessed November 20, 2012.

42. US Department of Health and Human Services. Health Information Privacy—Enforcement. www.hhs.gov/ocr/privacy/psa/enforcement/index.html. Accessed February 4, 2013.

43. Health IT. Privacy and Security Training Games. www.healthit.gov/providers-professionals /privacy-security-training-games. Accessed February 4, 2013.

Redesigning Your Workflows to Achieve Meaningful Use

WHO SHOULD READ THIS CHAPTER?

This chapter is for physicians, nurse practitioners, and other eligible professionals who would like to understand the "how to" of implementing the Meaningful Use (MU) measures. It is written for staff who would like to know why they are doing what MU requires and how to redesign workflows and facilitate the changes required throughout the medical office to meet MU. It is also written for those staff who is interested in performance improvement and concerned with information being entered correctly into the electronic health record so that they can use the data to make improvements.

What you will learn in this chapter

- The basics of workflow analysis and redesign
- The role of staff in workflow redesign to achieve MU
- The importance of documenting and analyzing the current workflows in your office
- How to transform your paper workflows into efficient electronic workflows
- How consistent data capture is linked with achieving MU
- How to incorporate MU throughout the patient visit
- How to satisfy some MU measures outside of the patient visit

Key Terms Introduced in This Chapter

Workflow
Workflow Redesign
Current State
Future State
Process Mapping

WHAT IS WORKFLOW REDESIGN?

To understand workflow redesign, we must first define the term *workflow*. Workflow is defined as "defining the interaction patterns among a practice's staff as they fulfill tasks and produce outcomes using available resources."[1]

Simply put, in health care, workflow is the processes or steps that move people and information through a medical environment to accomplish a task. Examples of steps in a workflow might include checking in patients or putting them in an examination room.

Other workflows might be ordering medications or laboratory tests. In one office, the workflow might be very efficient when using paper medical records, but the workflow changes when a new paper form, test, or procedure is added to the current practice. On the other hand, the workflows in another office may be understandably inefficient and frustrating, but too often "this is the way we've always done it" prevails.

Small practices are busy, and usually few take the time to examine why things are done the way they are. The standard processes for checking in patients, gathering patient information, and moving patients through the office have, most likely, evolved over time. And if asked, staff members can usually easily state where things get bogged down, lost, or delayed during patient visits.

When a practice implements an electronic health record (EHR), the practice will experience a great deal of change. These changes might include:

- Using an electronic tool instead of a pen and paper chart to document the visit
- Carrying a tablet or laptop from room to room
- Learning to maintain eye contact with a patient while documenting the visit in the computer
- Communicating with staff or signing off on test results electronically

There's very little in a physician practice that is not affected by an EHR implementation. Nevertheless, this is a perfect opportunity for the practice to document and analyze current workflows or to take a look at *how* and *who* currently does *what* in the office and how these activities will change when the practice adopts an EHR.

Paper-based offices often use paper triggers as prompts for the next step in the patient-visit process. For example, the paper chart outside an examination room door alerts the physician that the nurse has completed an initial intake and that the patient is now ready for the physician.

In order to redesign a practice's workflows to accommodate an EHR, all staff members need to look at how they currently perform their tasks before they can change or redesign their workflow. Then they must evaluate how those same tasks are performed using an EHR. In Figure 4-1, we show how workflow may change when an office that currently processes a prescription refill request or uses a stand-alone e-prescribing system adopts an EHR with an integrated e-prescribing module.

Workflow redesign in a physician practice is critical to a successful EHR implementation. If the practice has already implemented an EHR and is planning to meet the specifics of the Meaningful Use (MU) measures, this is another opportunity to examine the current workflows in the office to meet MU goals.

WHO SHOULD DO WORKFLOW REDESIGN AND HOW SHOULD IT GET DONE?

Each member of the staff understands what he or she does every day. Staff also can easily identify what works well and what doesn't. It is essential that all staff members in the office be involved in documenting what they currently do and how and when they do it (the *current-state* workflow), because they know the processes best.

By involving the entire staff in documenting the current-state workflows, you engage in change management, illustrating the following key principles:

1. Many people need to be involved in documenting current workflows.
2. Documentation accuracy becomes a vital part in building the patient's electronic chart.
3. Staff buy-in will be greater by those who have been asked to participate in your practice workflow redesign.

F I G U R E   4-1

Redesigned eRx Workflow Diagram

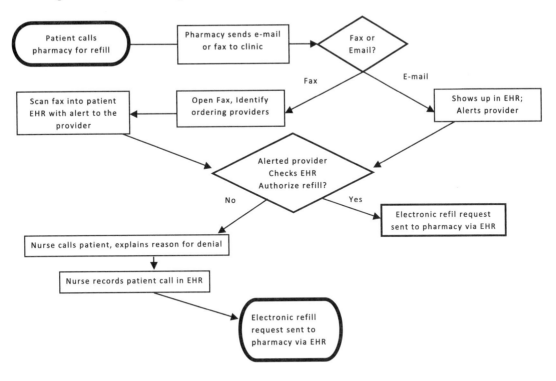

4. The redesign will be seen as an overall practice change effort rather than changes to individual staff members or roles.
5. Staff roles may change, affording staff an opportunity to work at a higher level. When a practice begins to focus on a team approach to care delivery, with staff assuming responsibility for additional tasks, providers can spend more of their time on the medical assessment and decision making that only they can do.
6. Workflow inefficiencies can be identified and addressed, fostering new opportunities for staff to do things differently and to do different things, which may allow for more meaningful patient interactions with the team and greater staff satisfaction.

HOW DO WE START TO DOCUMENT WORKFLOWS?

A team approach to documenting workflows, planning the work, and identifying individual staff roles will facilitate an organized process. Below are suggested steps to consider when planning to document the current workflows in your practice.

Develop a Plan

The best way to accomplish any task is to have a plan. In order to accomplish the task of having your staff document their current-state workflows, define the following:

- The staff member who will lead/oversee the task
- The time when staff will be expected to work on the task—for example, during or beyond the workday, compensated or uncompensated time

- How you will communicate the purpose for documenting workflows—for example, staff meetings, one on one, functional role meetings, written communications, newsletters, Intranet, e-mail
- The target date or timeline for completion
- A list of workflows that are a priority for redesign
- The staff members who will be involved in documenting the current workflows
- The tools/training the staff will need to accomplish the task
- The plan for reviewing the documentation among individuals and as a group

Create a List of Priority Workflows

Some of the most important workflows affected by an EHR implementation and/or to meet MU are as follows:

- Previsit preparation of chart
- Appointment scheduling
- Patient check-in/registration
- Rooming the patient
- Provider-patient visit
- Nurse visit
- Laboratory-only visit
- Patient checkout
- Prescription refill process
- Medication reconciliation
- Laboratory order process for in-house laboratory tests
- Laboratory order process for outside laboratory tests
- Laboratory test results communication
- Laboratory/radiology results management
- Referral process
- Telephone messages
- Paper correspondence processing—mail, fax

Communicate/Train

To help staff through the transition, build a communication and training plan so that they understand why they are being asked to document their tasks and how they are supposed to document them. A team will adjust to documenting (or mapping) the workflow process if provided with some uniform instructions, demonstrations, tools, and resources that focus on the information to be captured.

Suggested actions to facilitate workflow documentation in a practice might be to:

1. Assign specific workflows to individual staff members.
2. Post a document identifying the workflow, staff assigned, and due date.
3. Provide a documentation template with an example.
4. Demonstrate the preferred method for documentation of a common workflow (eg, list of steps, sticky note for each step, Visio diagram, swim-lane diagram [see Figure 4-2]).
5. Provide written and staff resources to assist staff and answer questions.
6. Identify who is to receive the completed documentation, how, and by when.

A swim-lane diagram illustrates a workflow, the different staff roles, and where the process transitions from or to another staff member. In Figure 4-2, you can see how a practice can map, or diagram, its workflow using figures. A swim-lane diagram is one of several process-mapping formats; one is used here to demonstrate the information exchange between eligible professionals (EPs), staff and the patient.

F I G U R E   4-2

Swim-Lane Diagram

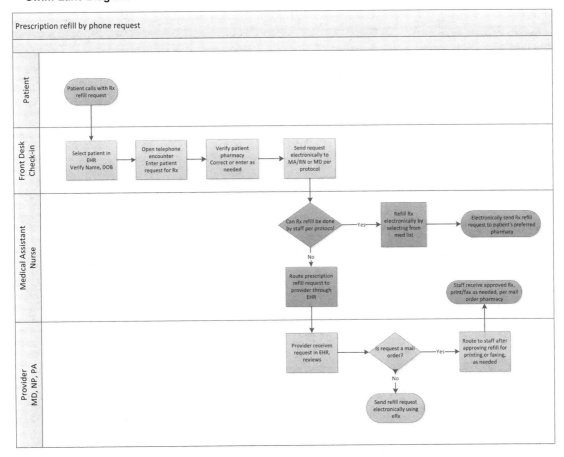

Abbreviations: DOB indicates date of birth; EHR, electronic health record; MA, medical assistant; MD, doctor of medicine; NP, nurse practitioner; PA, physician assistant; and RN, registered nurse.

WHAT WILL WE LEARN FROM AN ANALYSIS OF OUR CURRENT WORKFLOWS?

When practices take the time to document their current workflows and actually look at how they currently do things, many recognize that, for example, several staff members are unnecessarily doing the same task, performing the task in a different way, or documenting the task in a different place—or not at all. Such realizations provide great motivation to change a current process that may not be as efficient or effective as it could be. Analyzing their current workflow allows practices to identify potential areas for improvement, as well as to identify processes that are working well.

> **Critical Point**
>
> A practice must first understand how it currently does things in its office before redesigning workflows, irrespective of whether the redesign is intended to incorporate an EHR into the workflow, meet MU requirements, or achieve particular practice goals. Omitting this step often becomes a point of failure for stabilizing the practice after go-live.

Workflow changes in the clinical setting "first must do no harm" and, second, should aim to improve the following processes that are found to affect the cost, quality, and access to health care:

- Increase efficiency
- Decrease delays, errors, and cost
- Increase quality and safety
- Improve the work environment
- Improve ability to care for patients
- Create a better overall patient experience
- Improve staff and provider satisfaction
- Improve care coordination

Looking for Efficiency

If a practice is looking for efficiency by analyzing current workflows, the goal should be to identify:

- An easier way to accomplish the task.
- A different staff person who may be more appropriate for the task.
- A change in when the task could be done in relation to the patient visit.

Improving Quality

If the focus is on improving quality, analyzing current workflows might identify areas for improvement, such as:

- Staff training to understand the documentation needed to create accurate reports for monitoring quality.
- Cross-training staff to reduce delays in a patient's movement through his or her visit or to curb excessive walking or movement required by the staff or patient, which may affect patient and staff satisfaction.

EHR Implementation

If the focus is an upcoming EHR implementation, analyzing the current workflow provides:

- The starting point for redesigning the current process into the electronic process.
- A focus to create the training script for the EHR vendor.
- Opportunities for the staff to work as a team and brainstorm about how the EHR will change the way they currently work.
- An opportunity to discuss what tasks will change or be eliminated, and how the workload can be redistributed among the staff.

MEETING MEANINGFUL USE

In Chapters 1 through 3, we emphasized that the most significant goal of EHR adoption is to use data in a meaningful way. This also means that health care professionals optimize the EHR to support patient care, quality improvement, clinical decisions, and office efficiency. Because all certified EHR technology (CEHRT) systems feature proprietary designs, practices often find they must also accommodate the system's data entry and reporting structure.

To that end, nearly all of the major EHR companies provide MU workflows that demonstrate how data must be entered into the system. Often, these workflows are different and more complicated than the workflows adopted during the implementation stages.

Part of MU's Stage 1 frustration has been that while health care professionals originally focus on migrating to an EHR, to meet MU they may also need to focus on how the EHR developers built their reports to capture core, menu, and clinical quality measures (CQMs). For example, in some systems, data may only be captured when they are entered using one screen but not another. Or a report may capture the physician's entry on smoking-cessation counseling but not capture smoking-cessation counseling for the second visit if entered in another screen.

By evaluating the CEHRT's MU workflows, the practice can then discuss the following:

■ How workflows will need to be redesigned to achieve MU
■ How information is currently captured in the EHR
■ The need for consistency of documentation among all providers and staff
■ The changes that need to be implemented to meet the requirements

TRANSFORMING PAPER WORKFLOWS INTO EFFICIENT ELECTRONIC WORKFLOWS

A practice that is currently using paper charts and has not been exposed to the use and operational benefits of an EHR in the practice setting often has a hard time envisioning what life will be like when it no longer has paper charts. Unless the practice is already acquainted with EHRs and how they work, it's difficult to know how workflows will be affected and what to expect in the transition process. In Chapter 2, we discussed the value of data. Here, we will build on the value of data entered into the EHR and apply it to various reports the practice may want to generate for incentive programs.

Using Data to Generate Reports

MU reporting often sets the stage for quality-improvement benchmarking, state initiatives, additional incentive or quality-improvement programs, or clinical trials the practice may choose to participate in, such as:

- The Physician Quality and Reporting System (PQRS)
- Patient-centered medical homes (PCMHs)
- Accountable care organizations (ACOs)

Structured data provide the baseline data for these and other studies and incentive programs. To meet data requirements for each program, consider developing reports that might be needed to monitor performance levels on MU measures as well.

We describe the data entry and report planning process using two scenarios: **Scenario 1: Migration in Process.** In this scenario, the practice is preparing for MU while implementing the EHR and has not yet gone live; and **Scenario 2: Go-Live Complete.** In this one, the practice has migrated to an EHR and is stabilizing its workflows so that it can participate in MU and other incentive programs.

SCENARIO 1: MIGRATION IN PROCESS

Let's look at several case studies to see how practices can redesign workflows while they are migrating to an EHR.

Case Study: Mammogram Report

For the CQM "Preventive Care and Screening: Screening Mammography,"[2] the measure focus is the percentage of women aged 40 through 69 years who had a mammogram to screen for breast cancer within the last 24 months. For PCMH recognition, you may be asked to demonstrate when and how you recall female patients for breast cancer screening.

Start by identifying what is needed for this outreach activity.

- Identify the report you would like to generate. For example, how many women between the ages of 40 and 69 years have or have not had a mammogram in the last 2 years. This report would satisfy the Stage 1 menu set measure or Stage 2 core measure regarding patient lists.
- Consider the information needed to generate this report:
  1. Patient date of birth (determine age range of patients to run report on and translate that into dates)
  2. Patient gender
  3. Today's date (month/day/year)
  4. The date 1 year ago (or whatever period you would like to run the report on; month/day/year)
  5. Date of last mammogram
- Identify where the data are stored. The patient's date of birth and gender are usually captured during patient registration and stored in the practice-management system or patient demographic section of the EHR.
- Identify relevant data. The single most important fact needed in order to run this report is the date of the patient's last mammogram.

Scanning a copy of the patient's last mammogram report into your EHR would *not* provide you with this information in a structured or reportable manner. Instead, the date the mammogram was performed must be entered into the correct field in the EHR where health maintenance or preventive information is stored. Saving a scanned copy of a mammogram report that is normal into the patient's EHR may not be necessary. The facility that performed the mammogram will retain a copy of the results. Saving a scanned copy of an abnormal mammogram report is essential to the patient's care plan, but *the date of that mammogram* is the essential data for running reports for follow-up and recall. Identify which staff member is responsible for managing mammogram reports, and include this person in workflow training.

If, however, you are participating in a pay-for-performance program, the payer might require more documentation than the date on which the mammogram was done and ask for the actual mammogram report as proof of the test being done. By saving the normal report into the patient's EHR, if the patient changes insurance carriers, you will have the documentation necessary to satisfy the new payer that did not pay the claim, and won't have to go back to the facility or patient to obtain the full mammogram report as proof to be eligible for your pay-for-performance incentive.

Case Study: Transitioning From Paper to Electronic Laboratory Orders and Results

When transitioning from paper records to an EHR or redesigning an EHR to meet MU, comparing the paper workflow for the communication of laboratory orders and results with the redesigned electronic workflow helps staff to envision the *future-state* workflow. Creating an efficient electronic workflow for laboratory test orders and results can reduce the staff time that is consumed by a paper process. Lost charts, missing orders, missing results, and piles of charts on provider desks awaiting review can all be addressed with a redesigned paper workflow that incorporates the EHR into the process. The timely receipt of results and patient safety improve as a result.

Using the following laboratory order and result communication process, map out the workflow in your practice using the questions presented for each step.

- The provider completes the paper laboratory requisition during a patient visit. (A sample requisition is shown in Figure 4-3.)
    - Where are laboratory requisitions currently stored? In each examination room? Centrally located?
    - Who currently completes the requisition? Doctor, nurse, other staff?
    - How are laboratory tests that are not listed on the requisition ordered?
- The patient takes the requisition to a laboratory.
    - Is the laboratory in-house or outside? Does your office use more than one laboratory? Can the patient use the same paper requisition form at any laboratory selected by the patient or does each laboratory require its own form?
    - Does the practice, either via a payer portal or EHR, consider the patient's insurance coverage prior to writing the requisition?
    - Who gives the requisition to the patient? Does that person also give the patient instructions or directions to the laboratory?
- The phlebotomist draws the specimens for the tests that are indicated on the paper requisition.
- The laboratory sends results to the ordering EP.
    - How are these delivered? Dedicated printer? Fax? US mail?
    - Who is responsible for collecting the results? What do they do with them?
    - Are the results reviewed by someone in the practice before they are placed in the paper chart? Who pulls the charts? Who attaches the results? Are paper results ever delivered to EPs without the chart?
    - Are abnormal results handled differently than normal results? How and by whom?

- If the EP is a specialist, is the primary-care physician (PCP) listed on the requisition? Is a copy of the results routinely sent to the PCP? Who is responsible for sending them? How are they sent?
- The charts are delivered to the EP for review and sign off.
    - How often are they delivered to the EP? Daily? Twice or more daily?
    - Are the results reviewed daily by the ordering EP? If not, how long can the review process take?
    - Who reviews the results if an EP is not scheduled to work for a day or more?
- Instructions/results are communicated.
    - How are additional instructions communicated to the staff? To patients?
    - Who is responsible for communicating the results to the patient? How is this done? By whom?
    - Does your practice send letters to patients regarding the results?
    - Under what circumstances and when are the patients called? Who is responsible for calling the patient with follow-up requests, such as a return office visit or another laboratory order?
    - How long does the process of calling patients take? Is it completed daily?
- Someone follows up on missing laboratory results.
    - Does your practice track tests that were ordered for which there are no results? Who does this? How is it done? Paper log? File system?
    - Are patients called to determine if they followed up on a laboratory order or, if not, to remind them to have the tests done? By whom?
- The paper results are filed in the paper chart.
    - Who does this? When is it done? What happens if a chart cannot be located?

Figure 4-3 is an example of a paper laboratory requisition used to communicate orders to the phlebotomist/laboratory.

After documenting the current process and asking the above questions, very often a practice will realize the inefficiencies and potential issues with its current process. This reinforces the value of staff being involved in the process.

Redesigning to an Electronic Laboratory Workflow

For this example, we turn to Stage 1 MU menu set measure #2, "Clinical Lab Test Results." The objective is to incorporate clinical laboratory test results into the EHR as structured data. The Stage 1 measure is as follows:

> More than 40% of all clinical lab test results ordered by the eligible professional during the EHR reporting period whose results are either in a positive/negative or numerical format are incorporated in certified EHR technology as structured data.

Note: This measure becomes a core measure in Stage 2. See Appendix A for a comparison of Stage 1 and Stage 2 measures.

Saving laboratory results into an EHR, whether manually as structured data or by receiving structured results automatically via an electronic interface between the laboratory and the EHR, improves efficiency and facilitates the discovery of laboratory result trends over time and the sharing of those results with the patient. The ability to outreach to patients who are due for certain tests relies on the availability of structured data within the EHR to be able to run a report query and create a list of patients who are due for tests.

FIGURE 4-3

Sample Paper Order Requisition

Reprinted with permission from Beth Israel Deaconess Medical Center.
Available at: https://intraweb1.bidmc.org/LabManual/lab_manual/images/req1.pdf.

The redesigned laboratory workflow in a practice using an EHR is different from the paper "laboratory order and results communication" workflow just reviewed. Below we will outline an electronic laboratory workflow and questions worthy of consideration as you redesign to an electronic workflow:

- The EP orders the test within the patient's record in the EHR, most often during a patient visit. This is facilitated by training EPs on how to use computerized provider order entry (CPOE), in this case for laboratory orders, utilizing customization that may have been created during your EHR implementation process:
  - Access the short customized list of tests most frequently used by the EP.
  - Double check the orders that may have been renamed to familiar names.
  - Know how to create a new order in the EHR. (The process to enter an order during a patient visit vs outside of a patient visit is usually not the same.)
- Ideally, using the interface between the EHR and the laboratory information system (LIS), the order is sent directly from the EHR to the laboratory.
  - Is there an interface that directly sends orders from your EHR via an electronic interface to the laboratory?
  - Will this happen for all of the laboratories the practice uses? If not, can the order be faxed to the laboratory from the EHR? Or can it be printed for the patient to hand carry to the laboratory?
- The phlebotomist draws specimen, and the specimen is processed.
  - If the order was sent electronically, the phlebotomist will draw specimens for the tests indicated on the electronic order. The results will be electronically linked to the order for delivery back to the ordering EP.
  - If the order was entered into the EHR by the ordering provider but an electronic interface does not exist or the patient was not clear on where he or she would be having the tests done, the ordering provider may print the requisition from the EHR for the patient to hand carry to the laboratory. If the patient takes a paper requisition to the laboratory, the phlebotomist will enter the orders into the laboratory's electronic system. The results of the tests can then be recorded electronically and returned to the provider electronically via the interface, if available, or by fax.
- The results are sent to the ordering EP.
  - Is there an interface to deliver the results from the laboratory back to the practice's EHR? If so, the results are entered into the EHR as structured data and are reportable.
  - Are they delivered to the ordering EP's inbox automatically or does a staff member sort and send to the appropriate EP?
  - Are the results sent by fax? Is it a paper fax? (See below for information about results coming both as paper and electronically.)
  - Does the practice have a fax server? If noninterfaced results are sent to your practice to a fax number for your fax server, the results will be delivered electronically, which allows the results report to be easily saved to the patient's EHR without having to scan and save the results.
  - Who is responsible for routing the results to the EP for review and sign off?
  - If you have a portal, are the results automatically sent to the portal when the provider signs off on them or does the provider need to do something to send the results to the portal?
  - Do the results come by paper or electronically or both? The most efficient delivery method is by interface directly to the ordering EP.

- Are results delivered only to the ordering EP?
- Who will share the results with the PCP or specialist involved in the patient's care? Are they on an EHR? Can the results be shared electronically from the EHR or sent to a fax server with other EPs?

Critical Point

Many laboratory vendors will require the provider to sign a release to stop the dual delivery of results by electronic interface and also by paper. Once comfortable with the electronic delivery of results, eliminating duplicate delivery of results will improve efficiency with the results review and sign off process.

- If the results come both by paper and electronically:
  - How is your practice going to handle that?
  - Who will reconcile the paper results with the electronic results?
  - Who will shred the paper results?
- If the results come only by paper:
  - Who will scan and save the results into the EHR?
  - Has your practice decided on a standard naming convention for filing and saving scanned documents—eg, YrMoDay_Test20120913_CBC?
  - When will the scanning be done?
- The results are communicated.
  - Does your practice have a portal where patients can log in and view their own results?
    - If not, does your practice send the patient a letter as follow-up to the tests?
    - Who is responsible for generating the letters?
    - Who is responsible for preparing the letters for mailing? Is a copy of the letter saved to the patient's record?
  - How will abnormal results be communicated and by whom? When?
  - Are the results saved to the patient's EHR when reviewed and signed off on by the EP?
  - Are results received as structured data from all or most of the laboratories you use?
  - Does the staff know how to save paper results received by mail or fax into the EHR as structured data?

Critical Point

If your laboratory results are still coming in on paper for physician review, ask the staff to scan the result into the patient's EHR and route the result to the appropriate EP for electronic review and sign off. This workflow often results in reduced manual data entry of needed results and dates.

The staff responsible for scanning the results into the EHR should have a clear understanding of which test results and dates need to be manually entered, especially for accurate capture of the data needed for CQM reports.

Many EPs need further training on how to efficiently document and communicate further instructions to the nursing staff through internal electronic communication. These instructions may include: "Ask the patient to schedule an appointment in the next 24 hours." Or, "No further action needed. Schedule next appointment in 1 year." If the results are initially scanned into the EHR, orders such as these are easier to find and fulfill.

For example, patients with diabetes have hemoglobin (Hb) A_{1c} laboratory tests drawn frequently. If their results come into the EHR electronically, then a report can be generated that lists the patients who have HbA_{1c} levels of more than 9% in the current month. If, however, a few patients' results are more than 9% and are delivered to the practice by fax and then scanned and saved into their record in the EHR, the HbA_{1c} results on the scanned reports will not show up on the report previously run of patients with an HbA_{1c} level of more than 9%. Scanned data are not saved as structured data and are not reportable.

If the staff wanted to use the list to reach out to the patients with high HbA_{1c} levels, the patients with only scanned reports would not appear on the list. If someone had scanned the report and known that HbA_{1c} is an important result to monitor, he or she would have known to manually enter the date of the HbA_{1c} test and the result into the reportable field in the EHR, so that the patient's data would be reportable.

Critical Point

The percentage of laboratory results that need to be entered into the EHR as structured data to meet this MU measure is challenging to attain without an electronic laboratory interface and a workflow that will ensure that noninterfaced results are manually entered as structured data.

The redesigned electronic laboratory order and results workflow is illustrated in Figure 4-4.

FIGURE 4-4

Redesigned Electronic Laboratory Order and Result Workflow

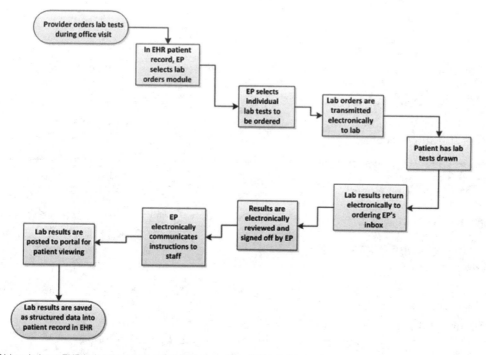

Abbreviations: EHR indecates electronic health record; and EP, eligible professional.

The laboratory workflow is just one example of a very time-consuming risk management, patient safety, and staff satisfaction issue that should be redesigned to optimize the use of an EHR in your practice and to be able to use the data to improve the quality, efficiency, and safety of care and to achieve MU.

MEANINGFUL USE AND CONSISTENCY OF DATA CAPTURE

Stage 1 MU focuses primarily on capturing data in the EHR in a way that is reportable and to prepare for the electronic sharing of information. Many of the Stage 1 MU core measures require the entry of structured data to a certain percentage threshold in order to meet the measure. Structured data, as well as coded data, are also needed to produce the numerators and denominators that will be generated by the EHR to report CQMs for MU.

Because documentation in the EHR during a patient visit is done by various staff members, all staff must understand what needs to be documented, and where it needs to be documented, to meet the MU thresholds.

Case Study: Smoking Status Core Measure

The core measure on smoking status requires that all patients 13 years old or older who are seen during the reporting period have their smoking status documented in the EHR. Consider these documentation questions as you evaluate how to capture patient smoking status.

- Does someone in the office currently and routinely document a patient's smoking status?
- What age patients are routinely asked about smoking and tobacco use?
- What is documented? Where is it documented? Do different staff members document differently?
- When is smoking status documented? Is it documented once or is it a question that is asked at every visit or only at annual examination visits?
- Which staff member usually asks the question and documents the answer? EP? Nurse? Medical assistant?

In a paper medical record, this information may be gathered on the patient registration form. Consider who currently discusses this with your patients and who enters this information into the record. Very often, it is the EP who documents the smoking status, including how many packs per day the patient smokes.

Smoking status is most often documented in the social history section of an EHR. With an EHR and the focus on MU, the medical assistant or nurse could be trained to capture this information when "rooming" the patient. When recording a patient's smoking status in your EHR, how and where it is documented will determine the ease or complexity of gathering data. For example:

1. Data must be entered in a structured field in order for the EHR to pull the information into a report.
2. There is probably more than one place that smoking status could be documented, but there is most likely only one place that will populate reports.
3. If smoking status is documented in the social history as free text, it will not show up in reports.

So who is the most appropriate-level staff person to document smoking status, and when during the patient visit should it be documented?

In one office, there may be multiple workflows for capturing smoking status.

Workflow 1
- Patient documents smoking status on the registration form.
- Patient's form is then scanned and saved into the EHR.

Workflow 2, same office
- Provider documents smoking status as free text in the social history part of his or her notes.

Workflow 3, same office
- Medical assistant asks smoking status while taking the patient's vital signs and documents smoking status in the social history section of the EHR by checking off the appropriate choice of smoking status.

Workflow 4, same office
- Nurse documents smoking status as historical information when abstracting the information from the paper record, if the information was available.

For MU, a report has to be generated listing the smoking status of all unique patients seen by an individual EP during the reporting period who were 13 years old or older. The only patients whose smoking status from the previous scenarios would appear on the report generated by the EHR would be those patients whom the medical assistant documented by selecting and checking off the appropriate choice of smoking status directly in the EHR, because in this way the information was captured as structured data. In all of the other cases, the smoking status is recorded, but the data are not captured in such a way that the EHR can query the database and generate a report that accurately reflects how many patients seen during the reporting period actually have their smoking status documented.

EHR vendors/trainers should be asked to provide training to staff on how and where to document reporting elements, such as smoking status, in a particular EHR, so that they will be accurately reflected in the report generated by that EHR. Include this in an internal user's manual so that all staff members can check to make sure they are documenting correctly. Consistency becomes your ally as you think about redesigning your workflows to satisfy MU measures.

Critical Point

Aim to redesign your paper workflow into an efficient electronic workflow that will accomplish having a patient's smoking status documented 100% of the time in the EHR as structured data. This is a worthwhile goal.

Once the new workflow to capture smoking status is understood, documented, and implemented in a practice, periodic monitoring should be done for the percentage of patients whose smoking status is being recorded as structured data in the EHR. While a worthwhile goal is 100%, the Stage 1 MU threshold is greater than 50%, which increases to greater than 80% in Stage 2. By checking periodically, there will be time to address a low completion rate, whether due to a workflow issue or inadequate staff training, before it is too late to improve documentation enough to meet the threshold for attestation at the end of the reporting period.

SCENARIO 2: GO-LIVE COMPLETE

Gathering data for Year 1, Stage 1 MU can be stressful because the practice staff is not only learning how to use CEHRT, but also balancing MU workflows with patient care. To minimize the stress, aim to complete go-live for all EPs at least 60 days prior to beginning the 90-day reporting period. In this scenario, we discuss how to incorporate MU measures into the patient visit once the practice has transitioned to the CEHRT.

Incorporate Meaningful Use into the Patient Visit

One of the broader MU objectives is to improve quality, safety, and efficiency and to reduce disparities of care. The MU measures that apply to this objective require that data be captured in a way that will result in useful, reportable data. Workflows necessary to capture a majority of the documentation take place during the patient visit.

To retrieve useful information from your EHR, you need to work backward. Rather than beginning with the MU measure, start with the attestation worksheet and know the data you need to gather.

For example, to extract CQM data for diabetes mellitus, you want to first run a report on how many of your patients have a diagnostic code for diabetes mellitus.[a] Then, to understand your performance on a diabetic CQM, it may be necessary to frame the question as, for example, "How many of my patients with diabetes have an HbA_{1c} level of 9% or greater?"

With your chosen diabetes CQM in mind, you can then begin to better analyze and design your EHR workflow.

- Identify the question you want answered.
- Understand where the information required to answer your question needs to be entered into your EHR for it to be displayed in the report.
- Consider your office workflow and which staff members are the most appropriate staff members to document or capture the information.
- Identify during which part of the patient visit this information most efficiently gets captured based on the flow of documentation screens in your EHR.

While the EHR vendor's project manager is available during implementation, ask questions regarding CQMs, such as, "How do I generate a report that allows me to know how many of my patients with diabetes have an HbA_{1c} level of 9% or greater?"

Based on the vendor's response, the second round of questions then becomes:

- Where in your EHR does that information get entered?
- Who in your office enters patient diagnoses into the EHR? During what part of the patient visit is this information captured?
- Where in the EHR does this information need to be entered to show up in the report?
- Does the database query pull the diagnosis from the problem list?
- Is the problem list structured (reportable) data or is it entered as free text?
- Does the database query look to your practice management system for certain *International Classification of Diseases* (*ICD*)-9 codes?
- Do all staff and providers know where and how to enter the information into the fields that feed the reports?

---

[a]Diabetes Mellitus CQMs may include: NQF 0055/PQRI 117 (Diabetes Mellitus: Dilated Eye Exam in Diabetic Patient); NQF 0062/PQRI 119 (Diabetes Mellitus: Urine Screening for Microalbumin or Medical Attention for Nephropathy in Diabetic Patients); or NQF 0056/PQRI 163 (Diabetes Mellitus: Foot Exam).

The internal workflow questions to ask your staff, then, are:

- How is a laboratory test ordered in your EHR? By whom?
- How would you identify patients who have had an HbA_{1c} test done?
- Is there an orders module where you select the particular laboratory test?
- Is your EHR interfaced with all of the laboratories your office uses or only some of them?

Critical Point

There needs to be a clear understanding of where your particular EHR pulls the documented information from and where you need to document to capture the information. This is crucial to generating reports that answer the questions you'd like answered.

Once the information that is needed to answer your question is entered correctly into the EHR and all staff responsible for entering results clearly understand why consistency in the process is necessary for all HbA_{1c} results, the data in the report should reflect the information that is in your EHR and answer the question you posed: "How many of my patients with diabetes have an HbA_{1c} level of 9% or greater this year?" (or whatever timeframe you are interested in viewing).

To improve quality of care, this report could then be used by staff to outreach to patients with an elevated HbA_{1c}. The provider may communicate the desired patient outreach to the staff. Perhaps patients should be encouraged to return for a visit or have another level done to determine any change in their HbA1c level, particularly if they have started a new dose of medication or have recently lost weight. Having the data opens the door to new opportunities to understand and help manage your patients' conditions.

In the following sections, workflow considerations to facilitate consistent data capture 100% of the time will be discussed. This will facilitate your success on many measures as you move through the future stages of MU.

MEANINGFUL USE WORKFLOWS FROM CHECK-IN TO CHECKOUT

In this section, we will examine the MU measures that common staff roles within a practice should be responsible for. Unlike the MU objectives and measures published on the Centers for Medicare & Medicaid Services' (CMS') Web site, this section presents work-by-role responsibilities using the following format:

- Part of patient visit
- Staff role
- MU objective and measure
- Why the measure is relevant
- What to do
- Other measures for this role/staff member to capture

MU is a team effort. Using the EHR in a consistent manner is the responsibility of everyone in your office. Redesigning your workflows to ensure accurate data capture to meet the MU measures will include deciding the role each member of your staff will have for entering documentation correctly into the EHR and on a consistent basis.

A team approach to satisfying the MU measures will improve the use of your EHR by everyone, reduce the perceived burden on any single person, and also prepare your practice for the teamwork and goal setting that will be necessary to improve quality. Let's look at the patient visit and the roles everyone on your team can play in meeting the MU measures during the patient visit. The measures are listed according to the primary staff role with responsibility for the documentation to meet the MU measure. Secondary roles in meeting MU measures will also be mentioned. Figure 4-5 provides an at-a-glance view of how to achieve all of the MU measures according to staff role.

FIGURE 4-5

Meaningful Use Measures for Patient Visit

Meaningful Use Measures for Patient Visit (by Staff Role)
(Items in gray may be new or indicate a different role/duty/task for staff)

Patient Checkin
(Administrative staff/front-desk/cross-trained staff)

Data to capture in EHR:

Core Measures	Menu Set Measures
• Demographics—add new fields to registration form: race, ethnicity, and preferred language to begin capture.	• Document patient preference for reminders/communications from practice.
• Document preferred pharmacy for prescriptions to be sent by e-Rx.	• Document e-mail address (for portal use/secure messaging).

- Collect copay at check-in
- Scanning of forms, insurance cards
- Answer phones
- Send electronic messages to staff
- Schedule appointments
- Have patients sign HIPAA Privacy Notice/ Consent to treat/RxHub consent/ Portal registration/consent (Signature pad will help eliminate need to scan consents.)

Add waiver to practice form stating patients' responsibility to maintain privacy when they are provided with paper or electronic copies of their health information.

 Workflow Pearl — Scanner should be near where the front-desk person sits, and ideally it scans both sides of the insurance card at once and saves to the patient's EHR.

Outside of Patient Visit
(Administrative/front-desk staff)

Core Measures	Menu Set Measures
• Medication renewal requests: send requests electronically to appropriate staff for e-Rx preparation.	• Patient reminders sent via patient preference (based on structured data and alerts for follow-up, immunizations, etc). Usually sent according to practice preference.
• Document requests for electronic copies of electronic health information and medical record requests. Keep track of date of request.	

- Eligibility checking/Prior authorizations (referrals)
- Preload/Registration of patients in EHR
- Scanning role

F I G U R E   4-5 (continued)

Meaningful Use Measures for Patient Visit

Patient Intake/Rooming the Patient
(MA/Nurse)

Data to capture in EHR:

Core Measures	Menu Set Measures
• Vitals: height, weight, and blood pressure	• Patient education: may take place before and/or after provider visit
• Smoking status/tobacco use	
• Medication list/reconciliation: prescription meds and OTC/herbals	
• Allergies: medication, environmental, food, insect bites, etc	
• Problem list updates (per patient)	
• CPOE/e-Rx (Rx renewals with protocols from within EHR)	

• Document chief complaint/reason for visit (may document some history of present illness).

Outside of Patient Visit
(MA/Nurse/Provider)

Core Measures	Menu Set Measures

• Electronic Exchange of Clinical Data	• Public-health reporting (Stage 1, choose 1)
	  o Syndromic surveillance reporting, electronic
	  o Immunization registry reporting, electronic

• Prepare electronic copy of electronic health information.	• Enter laboratory results as structured data: manual entry of results, closing loop on lab orders

• Preload patient records in EHR
• Prior authorizations (medications) /ABNs
• Tracking outstanding laboratory results, referrals
• Care coordination/care management
• Scanning role

F I G U R E   4-5 (continued)

Meaningful Use Measures for Patient Visit

Provider Visit

Data to capture in EHR

Core Measures	Menu Set Measures
• Problem list	• Medication reconciliation from hospital discharge, specialist referral, other physicians caring for patient
• ePrescribing from EHR	• Drug formulary
• CPOE: medications, laboratory tests, and referrals (needed to begin electronic tracking process)	• Patient education: patient specific selected from EHR
• CDS: Point of care documentation necessary	• Referral summary/summary of care for transitions in care
• Drug-drug, drug-allergy	
• Additional clinical decision support rule	
• CQM documentation/orders Follow-up, counseling, orders: whatever CQM measures require	
• Electronic exchange of clinical data with other providers (One test required for Stage 1)	
• Clinical summary from EHR. Requires POC documentation by provider of plan/orders – medication list, medication allergies, problem list, diagnostic tests (To be valuable resource for patients: referrals, follow-up appointments, instructions, current vital signs, reason for visit, etc should also be on clinical summary; must be in EHR as structured data to appear on clinical summary)	
Best practice to have provider select to print (paper) clinical (visit) summary with every visit and for it to print out at checkout desk or have checkout desk staff print (unless patient is seen multiple days in a row; rule says one clinical summary at the end is OK) Challenges: Provider may not have documented in EHR by end of visit, laboratory results may not be back, portal is an option	Patient electronic access: Ideally, the clinical summary will be uploaded to the portal and the patient will access it electronically.

• Coding for billable charges associated with office visit (*huge* learning curve for providers).

Meaningful Use Measures for Patient Visit

Patient Checkout
(Checkout-Desk Staff)

Core Measures	Menu Set Measures
• Deliver clinical summary as part of checkout	• Deliver patient education materials
• Deliver paper prescriptions to patient (if printed)	
• Deliver electronic copy of electronic health information (if patient requests) o Keep track of when electronic copy was delivered/sent	

- Collect superbill/payment, reconcile with daily schedule, send to biller (it is hoped, workflow will eliminate superbill)
- Arrange appointments, tests, follow-up, referrals
- Prior authorizations
- Scanning role

Practice Capabilities/Requirements

Core Measures	Menu Set Measures
• Security risk analysis	• Portal: patient electronic access
• Exchange clinical data: HIE capability	

Abbreviations: ABN, indicates advanced beneficiary notice; CPOE, computerized provider order entry; CQM, clinical quality measure; EHR, electronic health record; E-Rx, electronic prescription; HIE, health information exchange; HIPAA, Health Insurance Portability and Accountability Act; MA, medical assistant; and OTC, over the counter.

Patient Check-in: Front-Desk Staff

The beginning of the patient's visit to see his or her provider usually starts at the check-in desk. The following section will explain the potential role for the front-desk staff in your office in helping to meet the MU requirements. Table 4-1 identifies the objective and thresholds to meet the MU measure for recording demographics.

MU Measure: Record Demographics

Objective	Stage 1 Core Measure	Stage 2 Core Measure
Record preferred language, race, ethnicity, gender, and date of birth as structured data.	More than 50% of all unique patients seen during the reporting period have demographics recorded as structured data.	The threshold increases to more than 80%.

Why Is This Measure Relevant?

In order to run reports and look at a patient population in a variety of ways, certain demographic information needs to be entered into the EHR as structured data. Patient name, address, zip code, and insurance are usually entered into the practice management and/or appointment scheduling module of an EHR. Patient date of birth and gender are also routinely entered as structured data and are necessary to identify patients of a certain age or gender for outreach.

Preferred language is another demographic field required for MU. Knowing in which language your patients prefer to communicate will facilitate having appropriate interpreter services, family members, or educational materials available as needed.

Race and ethnicity are also required for MU. These data can be useful to determine a prevalence of disease in patients of a particular race or ethnicity. The deidentified data could also be used on a larger scale to determine if there are any disparities in care depending on race, ethnicity, or geographic area of the state or country. Therefore, capturing race and ethnicity as structured, reportable data opens the door to many possibilities.

As race and ethnicity can be very sensitive topics, consider the following:

■ Request the sensitive demographic information on a paper form a patient can write on or a laminated form that a patient can point to rather than verbally asking for this information at check-in within hearing distance of others.

■ Offer the patient the option of not providing the information by checking off an option to decline, which can then be recorded in the EHR.

Staff

Demographic information is usually captured on a patient registration form or verified at check-in. The front-desk staff in a physician office is the most appropriate staff to be responsible for capturing this information on a consistent basis.

What to Do

■ Train the front-desk and registration staff how to capture demographic data.

■ Remind registration, scheduling, and check-in staff of the importance of demographics. Demographic information is usually captured on a patient registration form or verified at check-in.

■ Explain how and where to correctly enter the demographic information into your EHR system. Any staff member or provider can capture this information in your EHR if the patient provides it; therefore, everyone in the practice needs to know how and where to document the demographic information in the system.

■ Explain why this information needs to be entered on a consistent basis to improve efficiency, meet MU, and qualify for additional incentive programs.

■ Role-play patient Q&A. Patients may not appreciate being asked to provide personal information and they may ask staff why it is needed. One answer is that your practice is participating in quality-improvement programs for multiple populations. If the patients decline to answer, documenting their refusal in the EHR is accepted documentation for the purpose of meeting this MU measure.

■ Explain the importance of consistent answers and explanations to patients by all staff members.

Please refer to the CMS Stage 1 vs Stage 2 Comparison Table for Eligible Professionals in Appendix A for further specifications.

Front-Desk Role in Other Meaningful Use Measures

Front-desk staff can also contribute toward some of the documentation important to satisfy other MU measures.

Prescriptions.   On a routine basis, as patients check in, the front-desk staff should verify with them which pharmacy they prefer their prescriptions be sent. This will help other staff and EPs who are more directly responsible for e-prescribing and CPOE.

Very often, it is the front-desk staff or receptionists who answer the telephones. Many patients call the physician office to ask for prescription refills. The front-desk staff may electronically enter the refill request into the EHR and then forward the message to the appropriate EP or staff member for decision making and action.

Patient Communication.   The front-desk staff could also offer information about the portal to patients as they check in, obtain a signed consent if they would like a portal account, and document their e-mail address in their record. They also could document the patients' preferences for how they would receive communications and reminders from the practice, whether by phone, mail, e-mail, portal, or text. They may also be assigned the task of preparing and sending patient reminders via mail, phone, or portal to remind patients of upcoming appointments.

Electronic Copy of Health Record.   The front-desk staff may receive requests from patients by phone, mail, or in person for an electronic copy of their health record. As Stage 1 MU requires an e-copy of the clinical summary to be delivered within 3 business days of the patient request, determining where the front-desk staff will document the date of the request and when it was sent or provided to the patient is very important to satisfy the requirements of the MU measure.

To accommodate these patient requests, also be certain that the front-desk staff is included in your Health Insurance Portability and Accountability Act (HIPAA) privacy and security training and is aware of the content in your practice's notice of privacy practices.

Now let's look at the medical assistant's and/or nurse's role in helping to satisfy MU measures during the patient visit, particularly while rooming the patient. The following MU measures are those for which the medical assistant or nurse usually has the primary role in completing the documentation.

Rooming the Patient in the Exam Room: Medical Assistant, Nurse, Cross-Trained Staff

The next part of the patient visit involves "rooming" the patient in the exam room. The following four measures are addressed by the medical assistant or nurse when "rooming" the patient in the exam room before seeing their provider.

Table 4-2 identifies the objective and thresholds to meet the MU measure for recording vital signs as structured data.

TABLE 4-2

MU Measure: Record Vital Signs

Objective	Stage 1 Core Measure	Stage 2 Core Measure
Record and chart changes in vital signs, including height, weight, and blood pressure. The BMI is also calculated and displayed. Vital signs and BMI [body mass index] are plotted and displayed on a growth chart for patients 2 to 20 years of age.	More than 50% of all unique patients seen during the reporting period have vital signs recorded as structured data.	Threshold increases to more than 80% and the age for blood pressure rises to 3 years of age and older. No age limit on height and weight. For exclusion, the vital signs requirement separates the requirement for blood pressure from documentation of height and weight. These changes are optional in 2013 and required in 2014.

Why Is This Measure Relevant?

When documented as structured data, information on vital signs (Table 4-2) can be used to display trends in vital signs over time, as well as to calculate the BMI and populate growth charts in the EHR. Identifying patients with an elevated BMI is important for targeted interventions to promote weight loss. The National Heart, Blood, and Lung Institute clinical guideline for obesity recommends an assessment of BMI at each patient encounter. With the rates of hypertension and diabetes rising, monitoring patient vital signs and managing these conditions is a high priority to improve population and public health and to reduce costs.

Staff

Medical assistants and nurses in a small physician practice are important team members who play a role in documenting information in the EHR that is needed to meet many measures for MU. Recording and charting changes in vital signs is very often the responsibility of the staff rooming a patient. To satisfy this measure, the providers and staff in your office should discuss whose responsibility it is to document the vital signs consistently and discuss any circumstances where you may not agree that all three vital signs are necessary.

What to Do

Remember, more than 50% of unique patients older than 2 years seen during the reporting period need to have vital signs recorded in the EHR to satisfy this core measure. To accomplish this:

- For all patients older than 2 years, and if appropriate to the EP's scope of work, the blood pressure, height, and weight need to be documented as structured data in the EHR. This measure does not stipulate how often the vital signs need to be documented. The presence of height, weight, and blood pressure documented at least once as structured data in your patient's record in the EHR will meet this measure.
- Height and weight can be self-reported by the patient and entered into the EHR as structured data.
- When the height and weight are entered, most EHRs automatically calculate and record the patient's BMI.

■ If the patient is between 2 and 20 years old, the height, weight, and BMI are to be plotted and displayed on a growth chart in the EHR. (In 2013, it is optional to raise the minimum age for blood pressure to be recorded from 2 to 3 years of age. In 2014, the requirement changes to 3 to 20 years of age.)

The staff and providers need to be trained on where to correctly document vital signs in the EHR so that the information will be available as reportable data.

An exclusion is available for providers who believe it is outside their scope of practice to record all three vital signs for their patient population. The exclusion criteria change in Stage 2, separating the blood pressure requirement from the height and weight requirement. Please refer to the CMS Stage 1 vs Stage 2 Comparison Table for Eligible Professionals in Appendix A for further specifications.

Maintaining Active Medication List: Medical Assistant, Nurse, Cross-Trained Staff

Table 4-3 identifies the objective and thresholds to meet the MU measure for maintaining an active medication list.

TABLE 4-3

MU Measure: Maintain Active Medication List

Objective	Stage 1 Core Measure	Stage 2 Core Measure
Maintain active medication list.	More than 80% of all patients have at least one medication entry (or an indication that the patient is not currently prescribed any medications) recorded as structured data.	Medication list is incorporated into the summary-of-care record core measure for transitions in care and referrals.

Why Is This Measure Relevant?

Early EHRs were created to store medical information that had previously been stored in paper medical records. Industry standards and common languages described in Chapter 3 were not currently available or agreed upon before early development of EHRs, so various health care technologies could not interoperate. Therefore, clinical dictionaries, such as SNOMED and Logical Observation Identifiers Names and codes (LOINC), were not on vendor development lists. With health care reimbursement shifting to a focus on *quality* from a *quantity* (fee-for-service) delivery model, access to information in EHRs quickly became necessary.

The EHR Incentive Program, and the use of certified EHRs to be eligible for MU incentives, motivated all EHR vendors who sought certification to provide the structured, reportable data that would be necessary to monitor health care quality. By entering medications into the EHR as structured, reportable data, the information on the medication list is available for e-prescribing/CPOE and for the clinical decision support (CDS) functions to work in the EHR. These functions can alert EPs to potential patient safety issues involving medications. The medication list can also be used to identify patients taking certain medications if there is a recall.

Medication lists, entered into the EHR as structured data, will be displayed on clinical visit summaries shared with patients and on transition-in-care documents shared with medical providers outside of the primary-care office. Medication lists are also important information to be shared via health information exchanges (HIEs), as patient information begins to be shared electronically between many providers of care to improve the coordination of care.

Staff

Medical assistants or nurses often review the patient's medication list when rooming the patient. EPs may ask their patients to bring all of their prescription bottles with them to their appointment, which helps to verify what medications the patient is currently taking on a daily basis.

What to Do

- Ensure designated staff is capturing current medications along with other relevant information according to the practice's clinical standard operating procedures.
- Train designated staff and EPs on how and where to enter medications into the patient record in the EHR.
- Train designated staff and EPs on how and where to enter if the patient is *not* currently taking any medications into the patient record in the EHR.
- Share the importance of consistently entering the medication information into the appropriate fields as structured data, so that the patient medication list is accurate and available for reporting and sharing with patients and other providers of care.
- Identify who will be responsible for verifying the active medication list with patients when they are in the office for an encounter.
- Determine who will be responsible for updating any changes to the patient's active medication list.

Please refer to the CMS Stage 1 vs Stage 2 Comparison Table for Eligible Professionals in Appendix A for further specifications.

Maintaining Medication Allergy List: Medical Assistant, Nurse, Cross-Trained Staff

Table 4-4 identifies the objective and thresholds to meet the MU measure for maintaining a medication allergy list.

TABLE 4-4

MU Measure: Maintain Medication Allergy List

Objective	Stage 1 Core Measure	Stage 2 Core Measure
Maintain active medication allergy list.	More than 80% of all patients have at least one medication allergy entry (or an indication that the patient has no known medication allergies) recorded as structured data.	Medication allergy list is incorporated into the summary-of-care record core measure for transitions in care and referrals.

Why Is This Measure Relevant?

By entering medication allergies into the EHR as structured, reportable data, the information on the medication allergy list is available for the CDS feature in the EHR, which is functionality that can alert EPs to potential patient safety issues involving medications to which the patient may be allergic.

Medication allergy lists entered into the EHR as structured data will be displayed on clinical visit summaries shared with patients and on transition-in-care documents shared with medical providers outside of the primary-care office. Medication allergy lists are another type of information that is important to be shared via HIEs.

Staff

Medical assistants or nurses often review patients medication allergy lists with them when rooming the patients. Staff or EPs may also enter into the EHR the type of allergic reaction the patients had when they took the medication.

What to Do

- Standardize clinical office procedures, such as who enters medications and allergies, by putting those procedures in writing and training the staff on those procedures.
- Train designated staff and EPs on how and where to enter medication allergies into the patient record in the EHR.
- Train designated staff and EPs on how and where to enter if the patient does *not* have any known medication allergies into the patient record in the EHR.
- Share the importance of consistently entering the medication allergy information into the appropriate fields as structured data so that the patient's medication allergy list is accurate and available for reporting and sharing with patients and other providers of care.
- Identify who will be responsible for verifying the medication allergy list with patients when they are in the office for an encounter.
- Determine who will be responsible for updating any changes to the patient's medication allergy list.

Please refer to the CMS Stage 1 vs Stage 2 Comparison Table for Eligible Professionals in Appendix A for further specifications.

Recording Smoking Status: Medical Assistant, Nurse, Cross-Trained Staff

Table 4-5 identifies the objective and thresholds to meet the MU measure for recording smoking status.

TABLE 4-5

MU Measure: Record Smoking Status

Objective	Stage 1 Core Measure	Stage 2 Core Measure
Record smoking status for patients 13 years old or older.	More than 50% of all unique patients 13 years old or older seen by the EP have smoking status recorded as structured data.	Threshold increases to more than 80%.

Why Is This Measure Relevant?

According to the Centers for Disease Control and Prevention (CDC), "All Americans—smokers and nonsmokers—pay the price for smoking. Smoking is still the leading preventable cause of death in the United States, causing 443,000—or nearly 1 of every 5—deaths annually. These include 46,000 heart attack deaths and 3,400 lung cancer deaths among nonsmokers who are exposed to secondhand smoke.

> Smoking is also a major contributor to many chronic diseases that are driving up the nation's health care costs. Each year, diseases caused by cigarette smoking result in $96 billion in health care costs, much of which is paid by taxpayers through publicly funded health programs.[3]

Staff

Medical assistants or nurses verify information with patients while rooming them. Asking questions to determine the smoking status of their patients may or may not be a new task or role for them. Verifying and documenting the smoking status of young patients, age 13 years old and older, may pose some new and different challenges to obtaining accurate information, especially when some young patients are accompanied by their parents to the examination room. Medical assistants and nurses in a physician office are the most appropriate staff to be responsible for capturing this information in the EHR on a consistent basis. The EP should also capture smoking or tobacco use on the patient's problem list.

What to Do

- Ensure smoking status is captured according to the EHR's access rules. For example, smoking status may be available only under the physician's user access.
- Determine if any patient registration forms or health history forms need to be changed to capture the patient's smoking status or any other tobacco use.
- Train designated staff and EPs on how and where to enter smoking status into the patient record in the EHR.
- Train EPs to enter *ICD-9* code 305.1 or 305.10 (Tobacco disorder) into the problem list, as this code will be needed for the CQM on smoking. This option could be built into a template to facilitate accurate documentation by the EP.
- Share the importance of consistently entering the smoking status information into the appropriate fields as structured data, so that the patient's smoking status is accurate and available for reporting and sharing with other providers of care.
- Identify who will be responsible for updating any changes to the patient's smoking status when patients are in the office for an encounter.
- Consider a future workflow that may include a portal. Patients may sign into the portal, complete a patient registration form or health history form, including questions about smoking, and send the form to the practice securely through the portal.

Please refer to the CMS Stage 1 vs Stage 2 Comparison Table for Eligible Professionals in Appendix A for further specifications.

Medical Assistant/Nurse/Cross-Trained Staff Role in Other MU Measures

Medical assistants, nurses, or cross-trained staff in the practice can also contribute some of the documentation important to satisfy other MU measures.

Problem List.   When rooming the patient, very often the medical assistant or nurse discusses with the patient the reason for his or her visit. This conversation often leads to the patient sharing other health problems and health information with the medical assistant. The medical assistant may enter some of the mentioned health issues into the problem list.

EP review of those entries is preferable in consultation with the patient, so that the problem list accurately reflects confirmed diagnoses that the EP agrees should appear on the individual patient's problem list. With the problem list available in the EHR as structured data, the staff will be able to run reports listing all patients with a certain diagnosis for targeted outreach, such as patients on a preferred list for flu vaccine. This measure will be discussed in more detail later when we discuss the provider-patient visit.

Prescriptions.   Many patients call their physician's office to ask for prescription refills. The nursing staff receives some of those calls and electronically enters the refill request into the EHR and then forwards the message to the appropriate EP or staff member for decision making and action. In practices with written medication protocols, nursing staff is authorized to renew certain prescription refill requests per protocol, which can have a measurable effect on efficiency in processing prescription refills. The e-prescribing measure will be discussed in more detail when we discuss the provider-patient visit.

Patient Education.   The medical assistant or nurse may have the responsibility to review the patient-specific educational resources with patients prior to the end of their visit. The EP selects which patient-specific education in the EHR is appropriate for the individual patient during the patient visit and then communicates to the staff for further discussion with the patient. Awareness of how and where to document in the EHR which specific educational resources were provided to the patient is important to satisfy this MU measure. This measure will be discussed in more detail when we discuss the provider-patient visit.

Laboratory Results.   For those laboratory results that are sent to the practice as paper fax, printed, or mailed results, the medical assistant or nurse may have an important role in entering clinical test results as structured data. The laboratory results workflow is an important workflow to redesign to accommodate the variety of ways the results may be communicated to the practice and was previously discussed in detail in this chapter.

Ideally, all laboratory orders originate within the EHR whether or not they are sent to the laboratory by interface, printed and/or faxed, or hand carried. The medical assistant or nurse, in the process of entering the noninterfaced results as structured data, should also be trained in how to "close the loop" on the laboratory order connected with those results. By closing the loop on all orders, only those pending or outstanding orders will be reflected in the electronic queue, which is useful for tracking missing results or tests that have not been done.

Quality outcome measures are very reliant on laboratory results being entered as structured data, such that your practice can monitor its performance and incorporate changes into your workflow, documentation, orders, or outreach to improve patient outcomes.

Sharing Electronic Information.   The medical assistant or nurse may receive requests for electronic copies of health information from patients and assist in preparing the electronic copies if requested. Documenting the date of the request and date of delivery is important to meet the MU requirements for this measure and to deliver within 3 business days of the request. The medical assistant or nurse may also have a role in electronically sending immunization information to the local public-health agency.

The Provider-Patient Visit: Eligible Professionals

Now let's take a look at the patient visit while he or she is with the EP. There are many MU measures that are best addressed during the visit between the EP and the patient.

Table 4-6 identifies the objective and thresholds to meet the MU measure for maintaining problem lists.

T A B L E   4-6

MU Measure: Maintain Problem List

Objective	Stage 1 Core Measure	Stage 2 Core Measure
Maintain up-to-date problem list of current and active diagnoses.	More than 80% of all unique patients seen by the EP have at least one entry, or an indication that no problems are known for the patient, recorded as structured data.	Problem list is incorporated into the summary-of-care record core measure for transitions in care and referrals.

Why Is This Measure Relevant?

The problem list should be an accurate, up-to-date list of current diagnoses or health issues for a patient (Table 4-6). Problems may be an acute or chronic condition or may be historical information about the patient's health. The problem list is one example of structured data that will be shared between providers to guide and inform them about the patients who are referred to them for care. Providers often complain that they do not receive the information they need in order to care for the patients that have been referred to them. Patients are often frustrated, when seeing a provider whom they have been referred to and the provider knows little to nothing about them and then seeks the information from the patient. An up-to-date, accurate problem list documented as structured data is important for quality clinical care and also to improve the sharing of information electronically between providers of care and the coordination of care between providers and facilities.

Staff

Keeping the problem list accurate and up-to-date concerning current active health issues should be the responsibility of the PCP. In the paper chart, unless a centralized problem list was required, the patient's active and past diagnoses were often found within the written documentation for each individual patient encounter. In the EHR, diagnoses are selected by the EP during each visit for the purposes of billing for the encounter. In many EHRs, problems can be designated in the EHR as historical problems, chronic problems, or acute problems. In a shared system, there may be diagnoses made by the PCP and/or specialists using the same EHR system. If some problems have been resolved, an EP may be able to designate the date the problem is resolved in the EHR. The insurance carrier has its own problem list, based on the diagnoses submitted on claims by all of the patient's providers of care.

Patients may also offer information regarding their health that should be included on the problem list. As mentioned earlier, when rooming the patient, the medical assistant or nurse may be told of additional health problems by the patient. Agreeing on the most efficient workflow for how this information will be communicated to the EP is an important consideration.

Given all of these different sources for information that could appear on a patient's problem list, it is important for the patient's PCP to maintain an active current problem list in the EHR.

What to Do

- Ensure data are consistently entered into the EHR for the EP's use and also for MU reporting.
- Train staff who are responsible for entering historical information from the paper chart into the EHR on where and how to enter the information as historical or as current problems. When transferring data from a paper record to the EHR, a review and sign off by the EP, verifying the list as accurate, is required.
- Train designated staff and EPs on how and where to enter problems into the problem list in the EHR.
- If new diagnoses or problems are provided by the patient, or received on a consult report from a specialist, determine whether the staff or the EP will decide if the diagnoses should be entered into the problem list.
- If the patient does not have any problems or diagnoses, the MU measure requires that an entry be made on the problem list indicating that the patient does not have any problems.
- Train EPs to enter appropriate *ICD-9* codes to support the required documentation for quality measures, such as *ICD-9* 305.1 or 305.10 (Tobacco disorder), as this code will be needed for the quality measure on smoking. This option could be built into a template to facilitate accurate documentation by the EP.
- Make sure the staff and EPs responsible for entering problems into your individual EHR are trained in the proper documentation to satisfy this MU measure. Some EHRs require additional clicks or steps after selecting a diagnosis in order for it to actually appear on the problem list itself.
- Identify who will be responsible for updating any changes to the patient's problem list when patients are in the office for an encounter.

Please refer to the CMS Stage 1 vs Stage 2 Comparison Table for Eligible Professionals in Appendix A for further specifications.

E-Prescribing: Eligible Professionals

Table 4-7 displays the objective and thresholds to meet the MU measure for e-prescribing.

TABLE   4-7

MU Measure: E-Prescribing (E-Rx)

Objective	Stage 1 Core Measure	Stage 2 Core Measure
Generate and transmit permissible prescriptions electronically (e-Rx).	More than 40% of all permissible prescriptions written by the EP are transmitted electronically using certified EHR technology.	Threshold increases to more than 50% and includes one formulary check.

Why Is This Measure Relevant?

The MU measure about e-prescribing recognizes that e-prescribing provides benefits to patients and EPs by providing safeguards within the electronic system.

Many medication-related instances of patient harm were noted in the 1999 Institute of Medicine report, *To Err Is Human.*[4] Although paper prescriptions for new medications were most often written and signed by medically licensed professionals, many medication errors occurred because of illegibility or misinterpretation of what was written.

E-prescribing eliminates the illegibility issue, offers electronic tracking of all prescriptions generated within the EHR, and provides CDS to reduce prescription errors related to drug allergies, interactions with other prescribed drugs, and dosing. Prescriptions that are generated and transmitted by the same person also result in fewer errors. Sending prescriptions electronically vs by fax also allows renewal requests to be sent electronically directly to the ordering EP by the pharmacy.

Staff

Prescribing medications, whether by paper or electronically, is the responsibility of professionals whose licensure permits them to authorize the use of certain medications. This privilege may be controlled by state, federal, or local laws, as well as licensure.

The EP is the most appropriate person to be using the electronic prescribing functionality of an EHR during the patient visit owing to the medical decision making taking place during the visit. Many of the benefits of e-prescribing are lost if e-prescribing is allowed to be done by nonlicensed staff. With approved, written protocols, designated staff can renew prescriptions using e-prescribing, if allowed by law. Protocols should not be written to authorize the staff to generate and transmit new prescriptions for patients to the pharmacy without the review and approval of a licensed provider.

What to Do

Many stand-alone e-prescribing systems were introduced prior to widespread use of EHRs in physician practices. Individual prescription orders were entered into the system and then electronically transmitted to those pharmacies equipped to handle electronic prescriptions. This required the EP to document the medications ordered in the paper record, as well as in the e-prescribing system. Many of these systems needed to be certified by insurance carriers for the EP to receive "credit" for e-prescribing. Most of these systems required WiFi and were available at minimal cost or no cost to the EP. As EPs transitioned to the EHR, many found it to be difficult and/or expensive to transfer the history of medications prescribed from the stand-alone system to the EHR. The loss of access to this information was disappointing for many EPs.

In order for a complete EHR system to be Office of the National Coordinator for Health Information Technology (ONC) for the EHR Incentive Program, the system must have integrated e-prescribing within the EHR, including the functionality to offer drug-to-drug and drug-to-allergy interaction checking. The e-prescribing MU measure relies on structured data in the EHR to function accurately, such as accurate medication and medication allergy lists entered into the EHR as structured data. The CEHRT also needs to be able to calculate those prescriptions considered "permissible," which does not include durable medical equipment prescriptions or Schedule II through V controlled substance prescriptions written using e-prescribing except in specific circumstances. For all permissible prescriptions written during the EHR reporting period in Stage 1, more than 40% must be generated and transmitted using e-prescribing through a CEHRT system. The threshold increases to more than 50% in Stage 2 and includes the stipulation that one internal or external drug formulary check is required.

With true e-prescribing, the pharmacy can send electronic refill requests directly to the ordering EP's EHR. When the refill is approved and transmitted electronically back to the pharmacy, this is calculated as a prescription sent by e-prescribing. A history of all medications prescribed by the EP is maintained by the EHR system, as well as a history of when medications were discontinued, if updated documentation is entered into the EHR.

Facilitating regular use of e-prescribing by EPs with prescriptive privileges and discouraging the use of e-prescribing by unauthorized staff are two of the challenges faced when trying to operationalize e-prescribing in medical practices.

Consider the following when promoting the use of the EHR for e-prescribing:

- Train EPs on the proper use of e-prescribing in their particular EHR. Facilitate adoption and regular use; make the process as painless and efficient for the EP as possible.

- Limit the availability of paper prescription pads. Most prescriptions can be entered into the e-prescribing system and sent to the pharmacy, or printed as needed, from the EHR. According to federal law, prescriptions for controlled substances must be manual (paper) unless detailed specifications are met (www.deadiversion.usdoj.gov/fed_regs /rules/2010/fr0331.htm), but most EHRs can calculate how many prescriptions were ordered and sent and how many were ordered and also faxed or printed. Understand what can legally be done in your practice and then facilitate the use of e-prescribing as much as possible. Ideally, paper prescription pads are locked and accounted for and distributed on a limited basis.

- Create customized "favorites" lists to allow access to a shortened list of medications and dosages used most frequently by individual EPs, reducing the time it takes to find and order the medications.

- Minimize the urge to create your own "customized" medications and dosages in your EHR, especially if they are not linked to National Drug Codes (NDCs). The NDCs enable the CDS system to generate drug-to-drug and drug-to-allergy alerts, a major benefit for patient safety in an EHR.

- Consider implementing written protocols for certain long-term medications that can be refilled by staff under specific conditions when authorized by a provider licensed to prescribe (in accordance with Federal and state law and medical board requirements).

Critical Point

Prescription refills will be counted in the denominator of total permissible prescriptions ordered during the reporting period, but if not generated and transmitted via true e-prescribing, those refills that are phoned and faxed will affect the numerator for this measure calculation.

- Work with the EHR vendor to understand how to assign appropriate access privileges for different categories of staff.

- Many staff can facilitate prescription renewals by forwarding the request to the EP using the prescription refill functionality within the electronic messaging in the EHR. This functionality allows the staff to generate the request from the current medication list present in the patient record.

- If the request for a refill comes to the EP/practice via a fax, whether paper or electronic, and the refill is ordered by phone or by returning a fax, even if the fax is generated out of the EHR, this is not considered true e-prescribing for the purposes of this measure. Therefore, if staff is involved in medication refill processing, the EP needs to understand how the percentage of prescriptions sent by e-prescribing is calculated in order to meet the more than 40% threshold (more than 50% in Stage 2) for this measure.

Please refer to the CMS Stage 1 vs Stage 2 Comparison Table for Eligible Professionals in Appendix A for further specifications.

Critical Point

EPs who generate prescriptions in the EHR when in their office may also see patients outside of their office, such as in a nursing home or other facility. The total number of permissible prescriptions written by the individual EP during the reporting period constitutes the denominator for this measure. If prescriptions are written outside of the office and not generated and transmitted using CEHRT, they will not be included in the numerator. This is true even if the total is calculated and recorded manually by the EP who will be attesting to this measure.

Should the patient request a paper prescription, this prescription will be included in the denominator—or the total number of permissible prescriptions written—and will affect the numerator for this measure by being counted as not being sent by e-prescribing. Some EHRs will calculate if the prescription was sent via e-prescribing and will generate a paper copy for the same order. It is important to understand how your individual EHR calculates this measure.

Note: As we have indicated, to meet the e-prescribing MU measure, more than 40% of all permissible prescriptions in Stage 1 (50% in Stage 2) written by an EP during the reporting period must be transmitted electronically using CEHRT. Besides meeting the prescribing thresholds that are part of this MU measure, an EP must attest that the thresholds have been achieved.

Using CPOE for Medication Orders: Eligible Professionals

Table 4-8 identifies the objective and thresholds to meet the MU measure for using CPOE.

T A B L E 4-8

MU Measure: CPOE for Medication Orders

Objective	Stage 1 Core Measure	Stage 2 Core Measure
Use computerized provider order entry (CPOE) for medication orders directly entered by any licensed health care professional who can enter orders into the medical record per state, local, and professional guidelines.	More than 30% of all unique patients with at least one medication in their medication list seen by the EP have at least one medication order entered using CPOE. **New Stage 1 option in 2013:** EPs may choose the number of medication orders during the EHR reporting period as their denominator for the Stage 1 measure.	Threshold increases to more than 60% of medications ordered. Adds requirement for CPOE to be used for more than 30% of laboratory orders and more than 30% of radiology orders.

Why Is This Measure Relevant?

For the purposes of Stage 1 MU, CPOE applies to ordering medications using e-prescribing. The relevance includes what was stated in the previous e-prescribing measure. In Stage 2, the threshold for using CPOE for medications increases to more than 60% of medications ordered, and CPOE use expands to include more than 30% of laboratory orders and more than 30% of radiology orders.

When orders are entered electronically by physicians or other authorized professionals using CPOE, a variety of benefits are realized. In a 2011 study, Baron and Dighe[5] noted, "Adoption of laboratory CPOE systems may offer institutions many benefits, including reduced test turnaround time, improved test utilization, and better adherence to practice guidelines. . . . Clinicians face several challenges, perhaps the most significant of which is that the menu of available tests has expanded, in both number and complexity. . . . Clinicians may compensate for not knowing which test to order by ordering many tests, some of which are unneeded, putting patients at risk for wasteful or even harmful follow-up care. . . . Alternatively, clinicians may fail to order needed tests, leading to delayed or incorrect diagnoses."

In that same study, the authors found the following reported benefits of laboratory CPOE[5]:

- Reduced test turnaround time
- Decreased transcription errors
- Reduced nursing manual steps (paper requisitions, transcription)
- Reduced laboratory manual steps (requisition handling, accessioning)
- Elimination of preprinted requisitions
- Reduced ambiguous orders and missed tests
- Reduced redundant test orders
- Improved test utilization
- Improved compliance with laboratory testing guidelines
- Improved ability to create and modify clinical templates

For those EPs choosing to meet MU, CPOE adoption will expand with the additional requirements to meet Stage 2 MU.

Computerized Provider Order Entry vs E-Prescribing

The e-prescribing MU core measure involves counting the number of permissible prescriptions written and how they are electronically transmitted to the pharmacy. The CPOE measure involves counting unique patients seen by the provider during the reporting period with at least one medication on their medication list in the EHR and how the medication order is entered into the CEHRT.

For the purposes of Stage 1 MU reporting, CPOE refers only to medication orders, not laboratory or diagnostic imaging orders. Essentially, e-prescribing is CPOE for medications for Stage 1 MU, and more than 30% of medication orders must be entered using CPOE. The Stage 2 core CPOE measure increases the threshold for medication orders to more than 60% and also requires that more than 30% of laboratory orders and more than 30% of radiology orders be ordered using CPOE.

If there is a clear understanding by the EP and staff as to what constitutes a medication order generated and transmitted by true e-prescribing and a workflow is in place that minimizes the number of refills that are sent by a method other than true e-prescribing, the EP should be able to meet the measure threshold for MU Stage 1 without difficulty.

Critical Point

The CPOE measure involves calculating the total number of prescriptions ordered through CPOE, not the total number of permissible prescriptions written during the reporting period, as in the e-prescribing measure. Therefore, a workflow that requires all prescriptions to be entered electronically into the EHR and that limits the use of paper prescriptions should make the Stage 1 and Stage 2 thresholds more attainable.

Staff

Entering medication orders into the EHR is usually done through the e-prescribing module or screen. Of particular focus for the CPOE measure is the CDS that may be triggered by a medication order and the EP or staff entering the orders using CPOE.

Which staff is licensed, qualified, or certified to enter medication orders may vary by state, local, or professional guidelines and may vary from one practice to another. The *electronic transmission* of the order is not a requirement of this measure but is a requirement to meet the e-prescribing measure.

The CDS available in the EHR, particularly when using the CPOE feature, if used by an appropriately licensed clinician, can significantly reduce the number of medication errors and the related patient harm. The CPOE measure focuses specifically on medications being ordered for the first time for an individual patient. Examples of the CDS that may be triggered include drug-to-allergy alerts, drug-to-drug interactions, alternative medication choices according to the formulary for the patient's insurance, and appropriate drug dosage information.

Although the technology may facilitate order entry by anyone with permission to access the functionality, the true patient safety benefit is not realized unless a qualified provider is using the system to enter the order and is able to react appropriately to the CDS for that individual patient and circumstance. Assigning appropriate role responsibility, particularly with CPOE, is important for patient safety and for staff to work within the scope of their licensure.

Medication orders are the source of many patient safety issues, as noted below in a press release by the National Academies.

Medication errors encompass all mistakes involving prescription drugs, over-the-counter products, vitamins, minerals, or herbal supplements. . . . Studies indicate that 400,000 preventable drug-related injuries occur each year in hospitals. Another 800,000 occur in long-term care settings, and roughly 530,000 occur just among Medicare recipients in outpatient clinics. The committee noted that these are likely underestimates. . . . A study of outpatient clinics found that medication-related injuries there resulted in roughly $887 million in extra medical costs in 2000—and the study looked only at injuries experienced by Medicare recipients, a subset of clinic visitors. None of these figures take into account lost wages and productivity or other costs.[6]

Critical Point

The CPOE measure stipulates that the person entering medication orders into the EHR be a licensed health care professional and be qualified to exercise clinical judgment should the order entry generate any alerts concerning potential drug interactions or other CDS aids. This also necessitates that CPOE occur when the order is initiated in the patient record and before any action or transmission of the order takes place.

What to Do

- Ensure that all providers licensed to prescribe are trained in using the e-prescribing functionality in the CEHRT in your practice.

- Work with your EHR vendor or EHR administrator to assign appropriate-level access rights to staff for e-prescribing.

- If you are using a shared EHR, where multiple providers can enter medications onto your patient's medication list, understand the ability of your EHR to display the medications that you have ordered separately from the medications other providers have ordered. Specialists, in particular, may have difficulty satisfying this measure if the medications on the medication list ordered by the PCP are attributed to them, especially if they do not routinely order prescriptions for their patients.

- Use CPOE at least once for every patient who has a medication on his or her medication list. Alternatively, you may choose the number of medication orders during the EHR reporting period as your denominator, which is a new Stage 1 reporting option in 2013.

- Understand that if the prescription is entered into the EHR using the e-prescribing function, is entered by a person qualified to react to any CDS, and is then electronically faxed by the system instead of sent via true e-prescribing, the mode of transmission is not part of this measure and will not affect your ability to satisfy this measure. (Electronic faxing does affect your ability to satisfy the e-prescribing measure.)

- Remember that if you write fewer than 100 prescriptions during the reporting period, you can claim exclusion from this measure in Stage 1. The total number of prescriptions written must be entered when attesting.

Please refer to the CMS Stage 1 vs Stage 2 Comparison Table for Eligible Professionals in Appendix A for further specifications.

Drug Interaction Checks: Eligible Professionals

Table 4-9 identifies the objective and thresholds to meet the MU measure for drug interaction.

TABLE 4-9

MU Measure: Drug Interaction Checks

Objective	Stage 1 Core Measure	Stage 2 Core Measure
Implement drug-to-drug and drug-to-allergy interaction checks.	The EP has enabled this EHR functionality for the entire reporting period.	Drug-to-drug and drug-to-allergy checking is incorporated into the clinical decision interventions (CDI) core measure. (CDS is renamed CDI in Stage 2.)

Why Is This Measure Relevant?

The drug-to-drug and drug-to-allergy alerts are CDS tools available in CEHRT that play an important role in helping to improve patient safety. This functionality alerts the provider at the time of writing a prescription that the patient is allergic to the medication and/or that the new medication ordered may interact with another medication the patient is already taking.

With medication errors being a recognized source of patient harm in the health care system, electronic systems, such as interaction alerts, are important tools to reduce patient harm. Although CDS in EHRs is in its infancy, drug-to-drug and drug-to-allergy interaction alerts offer a level of support that is one of the benefits of using technology during patient care. This measure is a Stage 1 core measure and is incorporated into the clinical decision intervention core measure in Stage 2.

Staff

The EHR system administrator in your practice should be one of the few people, if not the only person, in your office who has access to turn the drug-to-drug/drug-to-allergy checking functionality on or off in your EHR.

What to Do

Alerts that appear too often frustrate EPs, and, as with the boy who cried "wolf," alert fatigue can occur. The alerts themselves can become more frustrating than helpful to EPs, especially when adversely affecting their level of productivity.

Many vendors fail to inform the EPs using their EHR product that these alerts usually have an adjustment capability that allows EPs to increase or decrease the sensitivity or frequency with which the alerts will appear. Unaware of this feature, EPs often ask for the alerts to be turned off.

There are two important things to remember about operationalizing this measure.

■ Remember that, in order to meet this measure, the functionality must be turned on for the entire reporting period.

■ Learn how to adjust the sensitivity, and then find a level of sensitivity that alerts the EP to pertinent interaction possibilities and at a frequency that is tolerable.

Please refer to the CMS Stage 1 vs Stage 2 Comparison Table for Eligible Professionals in Appendix A for further specifications.

Drug-Formulary Checks: Eligible Professionals

Table 4-10 identifies the objective and thresholds to meet the MU measure for drug formulary checks.

T A B L E 4-10

MU Measure: Drug Formulary Checks

Objective	Stage 1 Core Measure	Stage 2 Core Measure
Implement drug formulary checks.	The EP has enabled this functionality and has access to at least one internal or one external formulary for the entire EHR reporting period.	Performing at least one internal or one external drug formulary check has been incorporated into the e-Rx core measure.

Why Is This Measure Relevant?

When the EP is e-prescribing, the drug-to-drug and drug-to-allergy CDS or alerts provide information to the EP at the point of care regarding possible interactions. The EHR functions in a similar way for the drug formulary checks menu set measure. Querying the drug formulary when prescribing provides the EP with information regarding the patient's health insurance coverage for medications, the availability of a generic alternative, and the patient copay or cost for the particular medication.

Using the drug formulary functionality while the patient is in the office informs the EP and the patient of valuable information at the point of care. Having access to this information might influence a patient's medication preference, especially if the cost difference is considerable or if the medication is not covered by the patient's insurance. Payers prefer that EPs prescribe medications on their plan's formulary.

Staff

Using e-prescribing to order a new medication is usually a role for the licensed providers with prescriptive privileges in a practice. EPs are responsible for doing drug formulary checks when e-prescribing. The staff with administrative rights to settings in the EHR will need to turn the drug formulary functionality on for the entire reporting period to meet MU.

What to Do

If your EHR has access to a drug formulary, this is one measure you should consider selecting as one of your five menu set measures, as it would be very easily met.

The EP should be aware of who has access privileges to turn on or off the drug formulary functionality and ensure that the functionality is turned on in the CEHRT for the entire reporting period.

There needs to be access to at least one internal or one external drug formulary for the entire reporting period. Verify with your EHR vendor that this access is available.

Drug formularies require occasional updates. Remembering to schedule the formulary updates and having access to many payers' formularies are two of the challenges encountered when sustaining this measure.

For Stage 2, this measure has been incorporated into the e-Rx measure.

Providers are required to check one internal or one external drug formulary when e-prescribing to meet the Stage 2 core measure.

Please refer to the CMS Stage 1 vs Stage 2 Comparison Table for Eligible Professionals in Appendix A for further specifications.

Implement a Clinical Decision Support Rule: Eligible Professionals

Table 4-11 identifies the objective and thresholds to meet the MU measure for implementing a CDS rule and to track compliance with the rule.

TABLE   4-11

MU Measure: Clinical Decision Support Rule (Renamed Clinical Decision Interventions in Stage 2)

Objective	Stage 1 Core Measure	Stage 2 Core Measure
Implement one clinical decision support rule relevant to specialty or high clinical priority along with the ability to track compliance with that rule.	Implement one clinical decision support rule.	Increases to implementation of five clinical decision interventions related to CQMs (high-priority health conditions). This measure also includes enabling drug-to-drug/drug-to-allergy alerts for the entire reporting period.

Why Is This Measure Relevant?

CDS is a key benefit of using an EHR. Built-in electronic alerts and reminders specific to individual patients assist providers and staff to provide the right care at the right time for each patient by alerting the team to the individual needs of each patient, whether for chronic-disease management or preventive care. The alerts and reminders are most beneficial when the electronic support is provided during the patient visit.

Staff

CDS is an important tool available in EHRs. CDS when prescribing is intended to alert those EPs who have the clinical judgment to respond to the drug-related alerts. For Stage 1 MU, the CDS rule must provide a reminder or alert to something other than drug-to-drug or drug-to-allergy interactions. The EP or practice should select and implement a rule that will facilitate patient care, such as one that may address patients with a certain disease or a preventive care need. This rule may be an alert or reminder that appears during any part of the patient encounter, but most likely will occur during the clinical part of the visit, when the medical assistant, nurse, or EP is documenting in the EHR.

What to Do

CDS is most beneficial when the EP or staff is using the technology at the point of care—that is, when the patient is in front of them. Receiving the alert or reminder when documenting in the CEHRT after the patient has left the office or after ordering a contraindicated test or medication negates the value of this supportive feature of EHR technology.

This measure allows the provider to activate a CDS rule that supports the appropriate care of his or her patients. As many payers are incorporating quality measures into their contracts, a rule reminding the EP that a patient with diabetes needs an eye examination or HbA$_{1c}$ test could be a CDS rule activated to meet this measure. Another rule could be an alert for any patients who are due for preventive screening, such as a mammogram or a colonoscopy.

Keep the following in mind as you implement a CDS rule:

- Setting up the CDS rule in your particular EHR may require technology support or training. All CEHRT systems have the functionality for CDS.
- Ensure that appropriate training and support are provided for the EPs and staff to encourage use of the CEHRT at the point of care in the examination room.
- System administrator rights, with the ability to turn on/off such features as CDS, should be available to a limited number of people in the practice.
- The rule must be activated for the entire reporting period to meet MU.
- Work with your EHR vendor/trainer to understand the feature that allows the frequency and sensitivity of the CDS to be adjusted to a level that will appropriately alert the EPs and staff.

Please refer to the CMS Stage 1 vs Stage 2 Comparison Table for Eligible Professionals in Appendix A for further specifications.

Report Clinical Quality Measures: Eligible Professionals

Table 4-12 identifies objectives and thresholds to meet the MU measure for reporting CQMs.

T A B L E   4-12

MU Measure: Clinical Quality Measures (CQMs)

Objective	Stage 1 Core Measure	Stage 2
Report ambulatory clinical quality measures to CMS.	Successfully report ambulatory clinical quality measures selected by CMS to CMS in the manner specified by CMS.	CQM reporting will be directly with CMS, not through MU attestation.

Why Is This Measure Relevant?

As health care begins its transformation from a reimbursement incentive based on volume to reimbursement designed to incentivize quality, cost savings, and managing population health, the importance of CQMs in this transformation is gaining traction. MU builds the foundation for future quality reporting, first by understanding the importance of capturing information in the EHR as structured data so that reporting from the EHR is possible, and second, by focusing the early CQMs to be reported to CMS on those health-related conditions that contribute to high health care costs and poor population health—smoking and obesity. (The Markle Foundation, World Health Organization, and Robert Wood Johnson Foundation are examples of agencies and organizations that study population health measures.)

Staff

For this Stage 1 core measure, the EP will attest that he or she intends to submit at least six CQMs to the CMS. As practices begin to focus on improving the quality of care they deliver, the care will be delivered by a patient-centered team approach, and everyone will play a role on the team to deliver high-quality care.

What to Do

The CQM Stage 1 core MU measure requires only that the EP attest either "yes" or "no" that he or she will report the six CQMs to CMS. The submission of individual numerators and denominators for the CQMs is reported on the CMS registration and attestation Web site but in a separate section following your attestation on the core and menu set measures. The numerators and denominators for the CQMs must be generated by the CEHRT for Stage 1 MU, and the certification of the EHR reflects the CEHRT's ability to generate these reports. The accuracy, however, is not guaranteed by the certification of the EHR. By attesting to this, you are not certifying that the data are accurate.

The quality measures will remain the same for 2013 (as in 2011 and 2012), and EPs are required to report on six of the 44 measures selected by CMS. There are two reporting methods available for Stage 1 measures in 2013 though—either by attestation or through the PQRS EHR Incentive Program Pilot for EPs, if you are participating in the pilot.

Beginning in 2014, all Medicare-eligible providers in their second year and beyond of demonstrating MU must report their CQM data electronically to the CMS. Medicaid providers will electronically report their CQM data to their state.

Although the core measure regarding CQMs has been eliminated in 2014 and the CQMs will no longer be reported during the MU attestation process, all EPs are still required to report CQMs to the CMS in order to demonstrate MU in 2014 and beyond. The reporting will be directly to the CMS, not through the attestation process.

For 2014, the three-month reporting period is fixed to the calendar year quarters in order to align with existing CMS quality measurement programs for all Medicare providers. Therefore, EPs will need to report the quality measures in 2014 for a 90-day period that corresponds to calendar year quarters. In subsequent years, the reporting period for CQMs will be the entire calendar year for EPs.

All EPs, regardless of their stage of MU reporting in 2014, must report on nine of 64 measures and select their CQMs from at least three of six Department of Health and Human Services (HHS) National Quality Strategy domains listed below.

The HHS National Quality Strategy Domains

Patient and Family Engagement

Patient Safety

Care Coordination

Population and Public Health

Efficient Use of Health Care Resources

Clinical Processes/Effectiveness

Please refer to the CMS Stage 1 vs Stage 2 Comparison Table for Eligible Professionals in Appendix A for further specifications.

Provide Clinical Summaries: Eligible Professionals

Table 4-13 identifies objectives and thresholds to meet the MU measure for providing clinical summaries.

TABLE 4-13

MU Measure: Clinical Summaries

Objective	Stage 1 Core Measure	Stage 2 Core Measure
Provide clinical summaries for patients for each office visit.	Clinical summaries to be provided to patients for more than 50% of all office visits within 3 business days.	Clinical summaries to be delivered to patients for more than 50% of all office visits within 1 day of visit.

Why Is This Measure Relevant?

Research has shown that adults only retain approximately 10% of information they learn by listening,[7,8] which is concerning considering the amount of information that is discussed with patients during their office visit. The clinical summary (or after-visit summary) is an important tool to provide patients with a source of information, including things such as their medication list and medication allergies, which they can share with other providers on their care team, as well as diagnostic tests ordered or recommended, referral information, and future appointment date and time. The summary is also important for family members who may be caregivers of children or elderly family members.

Staff

In many practices, clinical summaries are printed near the checkout desk, and the staff delivers the summaries to patients at checkout. In some practices, the provider prints the summary and discusses it with the patient at the end of the visit. Practices with a patient portal and a patient population that is actively using the technology could send the clinical summaries electronically to the patient via the portal.

What to Do

Although this MU measure only requires clinical summaries to include the medication list, medication allergy list, the problem list, and any diagnostic test results, a useful clinical summary would include some additional information such as:

- Date of visit
- Name of provider
- Practice contact information
- Current vital signs
- Medication list
- Medication allergies
- Problem list
- Instructions given during the visit
- Medication changes
- Test results that may be available at the time of the visit
- Tests ordered or suggested
- Referral information
- Follow-up appointment information

Keep these issues in mind regarding clinical summaries:

- Clinical summaries are generally a paper summary of the patient visit handed to patients at checkout on the day of their visit with their provider.
- The ability to customize what information appears on the clinical summary should be a feature every EHR system has available.
- The clinical support staff will most likely document some of the information that will appear on the summary, such as the vital signs taken during the rooming of the patient, and they may verify the patient's medication list and medication allergy list, which is information identified to satisfy the measure.
- One challenge to EPs is completing sufficient electronic documentation during the visit such that it will appear on the clinical summary at the end of the patient visit and satisfy the requirements of the measure.
- Ideally, the EP is using the EHR in the examination room to document the visit, provide patient education, and receive CDS.
- During the visit, the EP may update the problem list based on the findings at the visit and may order new medications, diagnostic tests, or referrals in the EHR. The clinical summary, when printed in the examination room, allows the EP to review the information with the patient and answer any questions the patient may have.
- Having any instructions that were discussed with the patient during the visit and any suggested follow-up with the provider appear on the clinical summary can be very useful to both patients and caregivers.

Please refer to the CMS Stage 1 vs Stage 2 Comparison Table for Eligible Professionals in Appendix A for further specifications.

Some common barriers to meeting the clinical summary measure and possible strategies to address resistance are listed in Table 4-14.

T A B L E 4-14

Common Barriers to Clinical Summaries

Barrier	Strategy
Staff resistance	Educate staff and share rationale for clinical summary
	Train staff how to present clinical summary to patient, explaining the value of the information to patient, family, and other providers
	Locate printer near checkout desk
	Include staff in workflow redesign
	Monitor measure calculation. If <50% of visits are receiving a clinical summary, determine if the staff has stopped handing out summaries to all patients
Provider resistance	Educate provider about rationale for clinical summary
	Provide talking points for discussion with patient
	Support provider's adoption of point-of-care documentation
	Prioritize electronic documentation of new prescriptions or medication changes, orders for laboratory tests, diagnostic tests, referrals, follow-up appointment timeline, and any patient instructions
	Enlist provider input into customization of summary content and appearance
Cost of paper and toner	Customize summary to print on one page
	Order backup supply of toner and paper
	Explore implementing a patient portal
Patient resistance	Ensure staff and provider buy-in
	Provide talking points for staff to discuss clinical summary with patients
	Don't ask patients if they want the clinical summary
	Provide summary to patient with positive reinforcement of value to patient and caregivers
HIPAA concerns	Educate patients of their responsibility to keep health information private
	Consider adding waiver of provider/practice responsibility to protect privacy once health information is given to patient to consent form

Educating the patient about the value of the clinical summary is important, but resolving any existing staff and provider resistance to the summaries is essential for the messaging to the patient to be perceived as sincere and the true benefits of the summary to be realized by both the practice and patients and families.

My [clinical summary] handout put all of this in a patient-friendly format with very little extra physician work during the visit. Now I am focusing more on maximizing this communication, because my patients are delighted with the handout. The clinical summary has become the culmination of the visit—something tangible that patients get for their time and money. I communicate better, the patients are happier, and I qualify for the bonus![8]

—Robert Lamberts, MD

Perform Medication Reconciliation: Eligible Professionals

Table 4-15 identifies objectives and thresholds to meet the MU measure for performing medication reconciliation.

TABLE 4-15

MU Measure: Medication Reconciliation

Objective	Stage 1 Menu Set Measure	Stage 2 Core Measure
The EP who receives a patient from another setting or provider of care, or believes an encounter is relevant, should perform medication reconciliation.	The EP performs medication reconciliation for more than 50% of transitions in care in which the patient is transitioned *into* the care of the EP.	Medication reconciliation is performed at more than 50% of transitions in care.

Why Is This Measure Relevant?

Health care in the United States is known for the silos of information that exist, with information residing with the various providers or facilities where the patient received medical care. It can be challenging for any one provider or facility to have access to, for example, an up-to-date medication list at the time of a medical intervention.

This menu set measure for Stage 1 MU addresses the need for medication reconciliation, especially when a patient transitions from an outside provider or facility back into the care of the EP. Patient safety is at risk when providers of care are prescribing new medications and are unaware of the other medications a patient is also taking. Frequently, providers rely on patients or families to provide an accurate and up-to-date list of medications. (Stage 2 incorporated this measure into the summary-of-care document.)

In many communities, communication between providers or facilities regarding the movement of patients from one facility to another is inconsistent or infrequent. As providers and organizations embrace new models of care that are more patient-centered and coordinated, sharing patient information between providers of care will expand and improve. MU requirements are facilitating some of those changes.

To satisfy the medication reconciliation measure, the provider needs to be aware that a patient is transitioning from another provider or facility. Ideally, the patient is scheduled for an appointment within 3 to 10 days of discharge or transition to reconcile the medications that the patient is currently taking, to address any gaps in understanding, to make changes that may be necessary, and to update the patient's medication list through medication reconciliation.

Staff

Satisfying the medication reconciliation MU measure, in the true spirit of the measure, requires that medication reconciliation take place between the provider and the patient, an interaction that can affect patient safety and outcomes and may prevent some medication-related readmissions. Ideally, medication reconciliation is performed by the provider during a patient visit that has been scheduled in a timely manner after the patient has transitioned back into the care of the EP from another provider or facility.

What to Do

To satisfy the medication reconciliation measure, the provider first needs to be aware that a patient is transitioning from another provider or facility. Consider how you will reliably receive notification of discharge, or discharge summaries, from the facilities most often providing care for your patients.

Although some vendors have added convenient check-off boxes in their EHRs that are designed to feed the medication reconciliation report for MU, this documentation may be occurring while the medical assistant is rooming the patient and verifying the patient's medication list.

There is also a need to document the patient encounter as one that is related to a transition in care, and the documentation needs to be in a structured field for the EHR to calculate the numerator and denominator for this measure. Determine where that documentation should take place in your CEHRT.

Some questions or thoughts to consider when implementing the requirements of this measure are:

- Is medication reconciliation currently done regularly between the provider and patients in your practice?
- Do medical assistants currently verify information with patients during intake, such as medication list and medication allergies, and document preventive screenings that may have been done outside of the practice?
- Is this process considered medication reconciliation in your practice?
- Does your staff know how to indicate in your EHR that a patient encounter is following a transition in care? Is this done consistently and are all staff trained?
- Are EPs aware of how and where to document in the EHR that medication reconciliation has occurred between the patient and the EP during the visit?
- Will the documentation be reportable for the EHR calculation for this measure?

Please refer to the CMS Stage 1 vs Stage 2 Comparison Table for Eligible Professionals in Appendix A for further specifications.

Test Electronic Exchange of Clinical Information: Eligible Professionals

Table 4-16 identifies objectives and thresholds to meet the MU measure for testing the electronic exchange of clinical information.

TABLE 4-16

MU Measure: Electronic Exchange of Clinical Information

Objective	Stage 1 Core Measure	Stage 2
Capability to electronically exchange key clinical information among providers of care and patient-authorized entities (medication list, problem list, medication allergy list, diagnostic test results).	Perform at least one test of certified EHR technology's capacity to electronically exchange key clinical information.	This measure is removed, effective in 2013. The requirement to exchange information is incorporated into the summary of care core measure requirement for transitions in care and referrals.

Why Is This Measure Relevant?

This MU measure is the starting point for being able to share patient information via HIE between multiple providers of care outside of your own organization.

Staff

For the purposes of Stage 1 MU, the EPs in 2011 and 2012 needed to attest that they performed the test of sending electronic information from their certified EHR to another provider with a distinct certified EHR. The *test* of sending electronic information will no longer be required.

What to Do

Consider the following when preparing to share information within the EHR electronically:

■   The CEHRT has the capability to produce a continuity of care document (CCD) or continuity of care record (CCR) to export a limited set of health information to an outside provider or organization (a legally separate entity) that is using a separate, distinct certified EHR.

■   Most vendors have training materials showing the process for creating and exporting the CCD/CCR using their product. Check with your vendor or trainer.

The test to exchange information was required in 2011 and 2012, but the measure to test was eliminated for attestations in 2013. The requirement to exchange information electronically has been incorporated into the Stage 2 summary of care core measure.

Provide Summary of Care Records: Eligible Professionals

Table 4-17 identifies objectives and thresholds to meet the MU measure for providing summary of care records.

TABLE 4-17

MU Measure: Summary of Care Record

Objective	Stage 1 Menu Set Measure	Stage 2 Core Measure
The EP who transitions a patient to another setting or provider of care or refers a patient to another provider of care should provide a summary of care record for each transition of care or referral.	The EP who transitions or refers a patient to another setting or provider of care provides a summary of care record for more than 50% of transitions of care or referrals.	Summary of care document is provided for more than 50% of transitions in care and referrals, with at least 10% sent electronically. One needs to be sent electronically to a recipient with a different EHR vendor or sent to the CMS test EHR.

Why Is This Measure Relevant?

Each provider or facility retains most documentation regarding the care or services they provided to patients. A lack of communication and sharing of information with other providers of care has resulted in repeated diagnostic testing and procedures being performed when patients are seen by a variety of providers in different locations. This lack of coordination of care is challenging for providers, frustrating for patients, and expensive.

The summary of care record will provide a vehicle for sharing information between providers and facilities, including medication and medication allergy lists, problem lists, and diagnostic test results, and should facilitate better coordination of care and safer, less expensive care with better outcomes. Sharing of information, whether by paper, fax, or phone, is better than not sharing information at all. As we move forward in our use of technology, Stage 2 will require sharing some of this information electronically, including with providers outside of your organization using different EHR technology.

Staff

A clear understanding of who will be responsible for completing and sending the summary of care record will facilitate meeting this measure's threshold. Many EHRs have electronic referral templates. EPs usually contribute the specific reason for requesting the referral or transfer and would most easily document the necessary and pertinent information. The clinical staff, with knowledge of both the particular EHR technology and the patient, can also facilitate the sharing of appropriate information in collaboration with the EP. Consistency in the information to be included on an electronic referral form across the health care information systems would facilitate the exchange of pertinent information between providers and facilities.

What to Do

To ensure that the majority of, if not all, referrals or transitions in care from one provider to another or from one provider to a facility are accompanied by a summary of care record, an understanding of your technology, workflow, and staff roles will be necessary.

A few questions to consider when addressing this measure:

- Are most of the referrals generated during a patient visit or outside of a patient visit?
- Who on the staff is currently responsible for documenting the specifics of a referral?
- What information do you currently send with your patient or to a consulting provider or facility? Last visit note? List of medications, allergies, problem list, and some recent diagnostic test results?
- How does your EHR facilitate sending that information? Is it easy to attach electronic documents of your choosing to the referral template in your EHR?
- What role does the staff play in preparing and sending this information?
- How often does your office receive or make calls seeking missing information that is needed to care for your patients?
- Does your office have a referral coordinator whose main responsibility is preparing and sending referral information, obtaining authorizations, and gathering information? If not, who does this work?
- Does your EHR have a "medical summary" feature? Are you able to select which information you'd like sent with a particular referral?
- If you can customize, is the information on the summary the same for all referrals? Are you able to restrict information on a problem list from being included?
- Have you started to create or are you aware of standardized electronic transition of care documents being created in your community or state?
- How is summary of care information shared with outside agencies or providers of care?
- Is any training needed to optimize the use of the existing functionality for referrals and summary of care records in your EHR?

The summary of care core measure in Stage 2 has three requirements.

1. The provider sends a summary of care record for more than 50% of transitions of care and referrals.
2. The provider electronically transmits a summary of care record for more than 10% of transitions of care and referrals.
3. At least one summary of care record is sent electronically to a recipient with a different EHR vendor or to the CMS test EHR.

The summary of care record is an important tool to achieve widespread improvement in the coordination of care and to facilitate higher-quality, less-costly health care. Work with staff and your EHR vendor to design a workflow that is efficient, consistent, and reliable and that optimizes the use of technology to share important information with those who need it. Redesign the workflow if it is not delivering the results you seek. Implement a workflow that is well understood and that will deliver a useful summary of care record the majority of the time.

Please refer to the CMS Stage 1 vs Stage 2 Comparison Table for Eligible Professionals in Appendix A for further specifications.

Provide Patient-Specific Education Resources: Eligible Professionals

Table 4-18 identifies the objective and thresholds to meet the MU measure for providing patient-specific education resources.

TABLE 4-18

MU Measure: Patient-Specific Education Resources

Objective	Stage 1 Menu Set Measure	Stage 2 Core Measure
Use certified EHR technology to identify patient-specific education resources and provide those resources to the patient, if appropriate.	More than 10% of all unique patients seen by the EP are provided patient-specific education resources.	Use EHR to identify and provide patient education. Threshold remains at 10%.

Why Is This Measure Relevant?

In an effort to engage patients and families in their health care, patient education is an important means to inform patients about their medical condition, medications, or diagnostic tests and to encourage them to more actively self-manage their health or condition.

Staff

The EP most likely selects or recommends the educational materials to be provided to the patient, depending on the patient's current educational needs. The EP may print and review the materials with the patient while in the visit, the materials may be printed and provided to the patient at checkout, or the materials may be reviewed by the clinical staff with the patient following the EP visit. Whoever selects the patient-specific educational materials, either suggested by the EHR technology or recommended by the EP, needs to ensure that documentation of the materials provided to the patient is recorded in the appropriate field as structured data. This is necessary to calculate the distribution for meeting this MU measure.

What to Do

An EHR is able to store electronic versions of educational handouts a practice already routinely provides to its patients and can also access health information via the Internet or via EHR vendor products.

- In some EHRs, the system gathers information from a patient's demographics, such as age, and from his or her diagnosis codes and renders suggestions to the EP of available and appropriate patient-specific educational materials.
- The practice may also be able to customize EHR templates and order sets based on diagnosis and/or age so the EHR will prompt the EP with options to select appropriate educational resources during the patient visit.
- In order for the educational materials selected for and provided to a particular patient to be captured in the EHR, the staff must have a clear understanding of how and where to document the materials given to that patient.
- There may be a list of resources and check-off boxes to select, or recording the selection may be linked with printing the materials.
- The patient portal may also be a way to electronically send educational information to patients, and whether that method of delivery is calculated for this measure needs to be clearly understood and verified by your EHR vendor.
- If setup is required before this linkage will occur, or prior to options being available within order sets and templates, your practice should decide which diagnoses or tests are of highest priority for patient education materials to be distributed to patients and designate them as a priority for customization.

As the threshold for this measure is only 10%, this measure is really just laying the groundwork for the availability, use, and electronic documentation of educational materials provided to the patient from within the EHR. As portal adoption and use increase, patient education will be made available to the patients more frequently via the patient portal.

Some questions to consider when operationalizing this measure:

- Does your EHR have educational materials or linkage to materials already available within the EHR system you have?
- If not, do you have the option to purchase a subscription to an educational resource service or is the EHR vendor planning to make educational materials available in a future upgrade?
- Do you have any paper handouts that you currently use that you would like saved as electronic documents within your EHR?
- Are they available in different languages appropriate for your patient population?
- Who usually decides what educational materials the patient is to receive? EP? Nurse?
- Does a staff member currently provide patient education to patients before or after a patient visit?
- If an EP selects the materials, does the EP also print and review them with the patient or are they printed and provided to the patient at checkout?
- Do the staff in your practice need any training to access educational materials and correctly document their distribution?
- If the EHR will change the workflow for your staff and/or EPs, will they be redesigning their workflow to accommodate the changes? Will the new workflow allow them to complete the selection, documentation, and distribution of educational materials efficiently?

■ Has your EHR vendor explained how this needs to be done in order for the EHR to calculate your numerators and denominators for the MU reports?

As mentioned previously, adults only retain 10% of information presented to them by listening.[9] The information being told to or discussed with a patient at a medical appointment may be new information. By providing written educational information specific to an individual patient's circumstances, the EP has a tool to engage patients and families in their health care and to fill the communication gaps when important information is only conveyed verbally.

Please refer to the CMS Stage 1 vs Stage 2 Comparison Table for Eligible Professionals in Appendix A for further specification.

Now let's explore the role the checkout desk staff plays in helping to satisfy the MU measures.

Patient CheckOut: CheckOut-Desk Staff

The staff at the checkout desk may have a supportive role for a few of the MU measures. One key responsibility may be to facilitate an EP meeting MU by handing patients their clinical summaries at the end of each provider visit, if the provider isn't taking that responsibility. Educating staff on the value of the clinical summary to patients, families, and caregivers will provide them with knowledge they need to confidently explain the reason for the clinical summary and answer some of the questions patients may have. Staff's commitment to their role at the checkout desk and their consistency in providing all patients with a copy of the summary can make or break an EP's ability to meet this MU measure.

Prescriptions. The checkout-desk staff may distribute printed copies of prescriptions to patients at checkout, if a patient requests a paper copy or if there was a reason that e-prescribing was not appropriate or available.

Patient Education. The checkout-desk staff may provide patients with copies of patient-specific education resources that the EP may have discussed with the patient and sent to the printer at the checkout desk. They may also have a role assisting the patient with booking tests, appointments, or procedures that the EP has ordered.

Electronic Copy of Health Record. The checkout-desk staff may also receive requests from patients for, and distribute to them, electronic copies of health information, a Stage 1 measure that will be revised beginning in 2014 with the new standards and certification criteria for EHRs. In 2014, Stage 1 will require providing patients with electronic access to their health information, along with the ability to view, download, and transmit their health information.

Meeting MU is a team effort. By adopting a team approach to meeting the MU measures, all staff shares in the responsibility to correctly document patient health information in the EHR and optimize the use of the EHR as a tool to assist them to manage patient populations and provide high-quality care.

SATISFYING MEANINGFUL USE MEASURES OUTSIDE OF THE PATIENT VISIT

Some of the MU measures' required processes are done by practice staff but not in direct connection to a patient visit. Many of these measures are important as you begin to use the data in the EHR for managing populations of patients and for sharing information that is important to public health.

Generate Patient Lists

Table 4-19 identifies the objective and thresholds to meet the MU measure for generating patient lists.

TABLE 4-19

MU Measure: Patient Lists

Objective	Stage 1 Menu Set Measure	Stage 2 Core Measure
Generate lists of patients by specific conditions to use for quality improvement, reduction of disparities, research, or outreach.	Generate at least one report listing patients of the EP with a specific condition.	Generate at least one report listing patients of the EP with a specific condition.

Why Is This Measure Relevant?

Changing the way health care is delivered by managing populations of people who share a common chronic disease or offering services to a population identified in your community will require planned outreach to patients and a more proactive approach. Providers or organizations will identify patients who need a service and offer it to them.

Using an EHR with structured data and reporting capabilities opens the door to identifying patients who, for example, share a common diagnosis, need preventive cancer screening, or require immunizations. Having the capability to generate patient lists is the foundation for beginning to manage populations, practice medicine more proactively, and improve the health of populations.

Staff

As medical practices transform to become PCMHs, team members will work to improve the quality of care they deliver and may identify groups of patients for outreach. Any staff member who is trained in running reports through the practice-management system or registry can generate patient lists if your organization has access to the functionality. Some organizations run reports centrally, and at nonpeak times, so as not to slow the system. The ability to do this with paper charts was limited to billing system data, payer opportunity lists, or recall lists a practice may have instituted.

What to Do

With appropriate training, and to the degree that structured data exist in an EHR, this measure is a meaningful yet simple menu set measure to select and meet for Stage 1 MU. This will be a core measure in Stage 2.

■ Enter a query into your practice-management, scheduling, or EHR system for a patient population pertinent to your practice, such as a list of all patients with diabetes or a list of all patients with diabeties who have an HbA_{1c} level of more than 9%.

■ Save a copy of the patient list that is generated for your supporting documentation for attestation.

■ The patient list that you generate for this measure could be the list of patients that you generate for the patient-reminder measure.

Please refer to the CMS Stage 1 vs Stage 2 Comparison Table for Eligible Professionals in Appendix A for further specifications.

Send Patient Reminders

Table 4-20 identifies the objective and thresholds to meet the MU measure for sending patient reminders.

TABLE 4-20

MU Measure: Patient Reminders

Objective	Stage 1 Menu Set Measure	Stage 2 Core Measure
Send reminders to patients per patient preference for preventive/follow-up care.	More than 20% of all patients 65 years old or older or 5 years old or younger were sent an appropriate reminder during the EHR reporting period.	Use EHR to identify and provide reminders for preventive/follow-up care for more than 10% of patients with two or more office visits in the last 2 years.

Why Is This Measure Relevant?

Patients are accustomed to being reminded about an upcoming appointment, whether via a phone call, a post card, or a reminder call from an automated call system service. The spirit of this MU measure is to remind Medicare-eligible patients and parents of young children that they may be due for some preventive immunizations, tests, or follow-up and to facilitate the use of technology to identify those in need and to generate the reminders. If elderly people receive flu vaccines and the pneumococcal vaccine as recommended[10] or if childhood immunizations are administered according to the recommended schedule,[11] the incidence of preventable diseases or seasonal outbreaks can be significantly reduced. If patients with chronic diseases, such as diabetes or hypertension, are reminded to have the appropriate follow-up, recommended care could be provided to prevent complications or worsening of their condition.

Staff

Depending on the reason for the reminder, administrative staff members are most likely tasked with preparing or doing this outreach if it is by mail. Clinical staff may be more apt to be tasked with calling patients to encourage the recommended actions or to discover existing barriers.

What to Do

The patient-reminder measure is one of the 10 menu set measures for Stage 1 MU, of which attestation to 5 is required. This measure specifies that the reminders be sent using the method of communication *per patient preference*. Prior to ONC certification of EHRs, some EHRs had the ability to designate the phone number at which a patient would prefer to be contacted. Registration in the system could capture home, work, and cell phone numbers by clicking a box next to the preferred contact method.

As patients become more mobile and technology advances, more options for communication and documentation exist. The staff member who registers the patient in the practice-management/EHR system needs to capture the preferred method of contact, such as designating a certain phone number, mailing address, texting number, e-mail address, portal, or other method, if reasonable. If there isn't a check box to indicate the patient's preference, staff and providers should receive training to know where to enter and/or find this information. The providers and staff should discuss and agree on where this information will be captured in the system.

If this is selected as one of your five menu set measures, the following issues should be considered when operationalizing this MU measure.

- Staff should begin to capture the patient's preferred method of receiving communication from the practice as soon as possible, and it should be done consistently.

- There should be agreement on the type of reminders to be sent to patients, particularly patients 65 years and older and 5 years and younger, in order to meet the measure's 20% threshold to send appropriate reminders to those patients during the reporting period.

- The denominator for this measure is a count of all of your patients who are 65 years and older and 5 years and younger and most likely only those with records existing in your EHR.

- The first year Stage 1 reporting period is only 90 days in length. Consider whether you would be able to send enough appropriate patient reminders via the patients' preferred method of communication during those 90 days to exceed 20% of the *total number* of your patients within those age groups.

- The Stage 1 Year 2 reporting period is 365/366 days. This measure may be more achievable during the longer reporting period if you have been capturing the preferred method of communication since Year 1.

- Your EHR should be able to generate lists of patients in need of immunizations, tests, or follow-up and within defined age groups, which should facilitate the staff sending out the patient reminders.

- Understand how your EHR captures the information necessary to calculate your performance on this measure.

This measure changes in Stage 2:

- This is a core measure in Stage 2, so it must be met to achieve MU.
- The EHR is to be used to identify and provide reminders to patients (no age group specified) who need preventive or follow-up care.
- The patient population to receive reminders changes to patients who have had two or more office visits within the past two years.
- The threshold to meet this measure in Stage 2 is more than 10% of patients identified (1) as needing preventive or follow-up care and (2) as having had two or more office visits in 2 years receiving a reminder during the reporting period.
- The reporting period for all EPs in 2014 is 90 days.

As the health care system focus turns more toward preventive care and population health, providing reminders will become a very important part of delivering recommended care to your patient population. To satisfy this measure, your practice will need to understand the specifics of this measure and how your EHR calculates the denominator (patients with two office visits in the past two years) and the numerator (the number of reminders sent). It will be important to develop a plan to implement a reminder system that is a regular part of your practice activities to meet the needs of the changing health care environment and to meet this measure.

Please refer to the CMS Stage 1 vs Stage 2 Comparison Table for Eligible Professionals in Appendix A for further specifications.

Incorporate Laboratory Results as Structured Data

Table 4-21 identifies the objective and thresholds to meet the MU measure for incorporating lab results as structured data.

TABLE 4-21

MU Measure: Clinical Lab Test Results

Objective	Stage 1 Menu Set Measure	Stage 2 Core Measure
Incorporate clinical laboratory test results into EHR as structured data.	More than 40% percent of all clinical laboratory test results ordered by the EP during the EHR reporting period, whose results are either in a positive, negative, or numerical format are incorporated in certified EHR technology as structured data.	Threshold increases to more than 55% of all clinical laboratory test results.

Why Is This Measure Relevant?

Structured data are the information that appears in reports. Although there has been some talk about technology being developed that will search free text for important data points or information, most registries and queries today require data to be entered as structured data to be available to populate reports. Laboratory results are some of the data that are important to monitor and manage for patients with several chronic conditions, such as diabetes, cardiovascular disease, and hyperlipidemia. The structured data are also important to run patient lists, as previously discussed, to outreach to patients in need of certain tests to manage chronic diseases. That outreach may depend on their laboratory results. As the health care system moves from a volume-based reimbursement model to value- or quality-based reimbursement, laboratory results will need to be entered into the EHR as structured data to be able to monitor the quality of care being delivered.

Staff

As previously mentioned, the medical assistant or nurse will most likely have to understand the data needed to monitor quality and how to enter noninterfaced laboratory results into the EHR, such that the data will be reportable. Almost any EHR users in a practice, with appropriate permissions, could receive the training on how to enter certain laboratory results being sent to the practice from noninterfaced laboratories, faxed results, mailed results, and results mentioned in consult reports into structured data fields. Providers, too, should understand the process for entering important laboratory results as structured data into the EHR.

What to Do

Clearly defining the process and the staff who are responsible for entering noninterfaced laboratory results into the EHR is very important for monitoring quality. If your practice does not have one or more laboratory interfaces delivering structured laboratory results into your EHR, selecting this measure as one of your five menu set measures to meet Stage 1 MU should probably be reconsidered. Here are some further considerations:

■ To meet this measure, the only laboratory test orders under consideration are those that have a positive, negative, or numerical result. The certified EHR may have a method of calculating the number of tests ordered and resulted as structured data. If your EHR does, determine how that calculation is done.

■ If you do not have interfaces that you are confident will meet the needed threshold of more than 40% of results entered into the EHR as structured data, then calculating the number of tests ordered by each EP and counting how many of those tests had the results manually entered into the EHR as structured data is cumbersome. And how does one count those results? If a comprehensive metabolic panel is ordered and only 1 or 2 of the 26 individual results are manually entered, does that count as one laboratory order with results entered as structured data or not?

■ It is important for your practice to implement a process and invest the time necessary for manual data entry if individual results that are faxed or mailed to your practice are needed to monitor your quality performance, such as HbA_{1c} or low-density lipoprotein (LDL) results. If manual entry of thousands of individual results for the purpose of meeting this MU measure is the driver, your practice will need to determine if the resources exist to satisfy this measure or whether another menu set would be more easily met.

Reference earlier discussions in this chapter on how to change from a paper workflow to an electronic workflow for detailed information regarding workflow considerations for laboratory orders and results.

Stage 1 and Stage 2 MU requirements involving structured laboratory data will be getting a lot of attention over the next few years.

■ For Stage 1 MU, this measure is an option as one of the five menu set measures needed to meet MU. Consideration needs to be given to the ease of calculating and meeting this measure, particularly if you do not have at least 40% of your tests ordered and results sent via an electronic interface.

■ In Stage 2, this measure is now a core measure and the threshold rises to 55% of the results being entered as structured data. This magnifies the importance of laboratory interfaces sending results into your EHR as structured data, making laboratory data available for sharing electronically with other providers of care, as well as for monitoring quality and improving patient care.

■ By moving this measure to a core measure and increasing the threshold, the message is clear that having laboratory results as structured data is important to the quality and cost of the care we deliver. Interfaces need to be created between the laboratories your patients use and your EHR to facilitate the delivery of structured results. For a variety of reasons, vendors and cost have been the biggest barriers to these interfaces being available, particularly to small practices. We can hope that EHR vendors are working with laboratories to make these interfaces more feasible.

Providers who are feeling the pressure to meet MU to avoid Medicare payment adjustments should contemplate reducing the number of laboratories they use to those laboratories that will provide and deliver results electronically, and as structured data, into their EHRs.

Please refer to the CMS Stage 1 vs Stage 2 Comparison Table for Eligible Professionals in Appendix A for further specifications.

Provide Electronic Health Information to Patients

Table 4-22 identifies the objective and thresholds to meet the MU measure for providing patients with a copy of health information.

TABLE 4-22

MU Measure: Electronic Copy of Health Information

Objective	Stage 1 Core Measure	Stage 2
Provide patients with an electronic copy of their health information upon request (including diagnostic test results, problem list, medication list, medication allergy list).	More than 50% of all patients who request an electronic copy of their health information are provided it within 3 business days. This measure will change in 2014.	Electronic copy of health information is incorporated into the electronic access measure.

Why Is This Measure Relevant?

Providing patients with electronic copies of their health information enables them to transport their information easily, share that information with other providers, or to have it available to them in their personal health record (PHR). As paper medical records were primarily viewed as the providers' records, the electronic record is, in some ways, shifting the ownership of the information in the medical record to the patient. With this information, there is hope for increased patient and caregiver engagement and improved sharing of information by the patients with many of their providers of care. This may facilitate appropriate decision making and a reduction in repeated testing owing to lack of information or results or knowledge of tests and procedures that have already been done.

Staff

The role of check-in and checkout staff in providing electronic information to patients was addressed earlier. Depending on the size of your practice, there may be other staff members who may be appropriate for providing the copies to patients if they request a copy.

What to Do

Although most patients are not aware, they can request a copy of their electronic health information from your office. To meet this Stage 1 core measure, more than 50% of all patients who request a copy must have it provided to them within 3 business days. This requires that your office have an agreed-upon process. Important things to consider to operationalize this measure include:

■ You should develop a process for documenting the name of the patient requesting a copy, the date of the request, and the date it is mailed or provided to the patient. Most likely this will be a manual log of some kind, unless your staff can create a way to capture this information electronically in your EHR, such that the information you need for attestation will be available.

■ It is critical to decide who will be responsible for documenting the requests. If it involves more than one staff member, plan where the log will be kept and who will be responsible for creating and sending or delivering the copy within 3 business days.

■ The EP should accommodate patient requests according to the HIPAA Privacy Rule.

■ Your office should have a small supply of USB fobs or CDs or the ability to post to a patient portal or upload to a PHR, as the patient prefers.

■ The information that must be provided electronically is limited to the information that exists electronically or is accessible from the certified EHR technology and is maintained by or on behalf of the EP, according to the CMS fact sheet for the measure. At a minimum, this would include medication list, medication allergy list, problem list, and any diagnostic test results.

Please refer to the CMS Stage 1 vs Stage 2 Comparison Table for Eligible Professionals in Appendix A for further specifications.

Provide Patients With Electronic Access to Their Records

Table 4-23 identifies the objective and thresholds to meet the MU measure for providing patients with timely electronic access to their health information.

T A B L E   4-23

MU Measure: Patient Electronic Access

Objective	Stage 1 Menu Set Measure	2014 New Stage 1 Changes	Stage 2 Core Measure
Provide patients with timely electronic access to their health information (including laboratory results, problem list, medication lists, and allergies) within four business days of the information being available to the EP.	At least 10% of all unique patients seen by the EP are provided timely electronic access to their health information subject to the EP's discretion to withhold certain information.	In 2014, this will be a Stage 1 core measure. New Objective 50% of patients seen by EP have electronic access to their health information and have the ability to view online, download, and transmit their health information.	Provide online access for more than 50% of patients seen by EP, with more than 5% of the patients accessing their information.

Why Is This Measure Relevant?

The portal is an important tool to involve patients in their care and to give them electronic access to their health information. For those attesting to Stage 1 MU in 2011, 2012, and 2013, the patient electronic access measure was/is an optional measure for providers to select as one of their five menu set measures. For practices with a patient portal, choosing this measure makes sense, especially if their patient adoption or registration to use the portal is going well. As portals mature and adoption spreads, portals integrated with an EHR will offer patients the ability to request prescription refills or an appointment, view laboratory and diagnostic test results, access patient education materials, ask questions of their provider, pay bills, have an actual electronic-visit with their provider, or download and send their information to whomever they choose.

Staff

As the use of portals increases, different staff will access the portal to communicate with patients. The front-desk staff may receive the requests for appointments. Nursing staff or providers may receive requests for prescription refills and referrals and respond to questions from patients. The staff who formerly called patients with their laboratory results will most likely see that activity greatly reduced as more laboratory results and diagnostic test results are posted to the portal. The portal is an important means to greater patient engagement and increased patient satisfaction. Many studies have shown that phone volume decreases when portal use increases.[9,11] Increased portal use by patients will most certainly change the current activity in physician practices today.

What to Do

The decision to implement a portal is often related to whether a provider's EHR vendor offers a portal as part of its system. This MU measure was an optional menu set measure for Stage 1 in 2011 and 2012 and is an optional menu set measure in 2013. You should only select this as one of your five menu set measures if you plan to have a portal available for your entire reporting period. The measure only requires that you have a portal available should a patient want to access the portal. The measure has no requirements to register a certain percentage of your patients or for them to use the portal. The CMS Patient Electronic Access measure specification sheet[13] states:

> The objective and measure focus on the availability of access and the timeliness of data, not utilization. The EP is not responsible for ensuring that 10 percent request access or have the means to access, only that 10 percent of all unique patients seen by the EP could access the information if they so desired.

In 2014, the Stage 1 core measure on providing patients with electronic copies of their health information upon request and this menu set measure on providing patients with electronic access will change to one core measure requiring that more than 50% of patients have the ability to view online, download, and transmit their health information. Stage 2 in 2014 will require all of the patient capability mentioned above and also that more than 5% of patients have actually accessed their information. The message is loud and clear through these changes: Providers will need to have a portal available for their patients in order to successfully attest to MU in 2014.

There are some key considerations to successfully implement and engage patients to use the portal. As more practices implement portals, more lessons will be learned, but here are some things to consider:

- Make sure you have a clear understanding of what the portal will cost to implement and to maintain. It will be necessary to have a Web site for your practice where patients can easily access the portal or a URL that is patient-friendly.

- Patient e-mail addresses are required for patients to register and use the portal effectively. If not already taking place, start having your staff collect patient e-mail addresses on check-in or registration. The staff will need to understand why they are asking patients for their e-mail addresses and they need to be prepared to answer those concerns in a way that will promote the use of the portal in a positive way.

■ Creating a consent form and getting patients to sign the consent and register online for the portal is challenging. Be prepared to have "help desk" or staff available to assist patients with the process and to troubleshoot when they call with registration issues.

■ As part of the consent process, patients will need a username and password to access the portal. Consider what the process will be to provide new passwords when patients forget theirs. You must ensure that it is actually the patient who is requesting and to whom you are sending the password. Some practices or groups require that each patient who wishes to have a portal account have his or her own e-mail address and portal account. Challenging implementation and consent issues involve custody rights, parental access to teenage children's records (which may vary by state), and the ability for a spouse or adult caregiver to request usernames and passwords for accounts other than their own. These and other similar parental, custody, and privacy laws vary from state to state.

■ When you are ready to register patients for the portal, prepare banners or signs for your office that promote the benefits of signing up for the portal. Some providers have tried sending out large mailings to get their patients to sign up for portal accounts and have gotten disappointing results from their efforts.

■ Determine who is going to monitor and receive portal messages and whether you will have portal messages centrally triaged to the appropriate staff or providers. As there are a variety of uses for the portal, many staff may be involved.

■ Decide which features you will start with. Some early adopters allow patients to request prescription refills or request an appointment or a referral via the portal.

■ Suggestions from the EP to patients to sign up so that their laboratory results can be sent to them via the portal, allowing them to view their results sooner, have been found to be effective.

■ Understand the features and options available with your portal and whether or not you can select which features are available to patients. If you are not quite ready to have patients sending electronic messages to you through the portal, other features, such as sending reminders to patients on the portal, may not work without the e-messaging functionality enabled.

■ After you, your staff, and the patients have adjusted to having the portal available, adding features will require preparation but less "selling" than when initially registering patients. Other popular uses of portals are to send patients educational materials, clinical summaries, or reminders (three important MU measures), which saves staff time and printing costs. The portal can facilitate an easier way to satisfy these measures than printing copies for patients. Some practices also allow patients to pay bills and book appointments via the portal.

By giving patients access to their information electronically, MU enables patients and families to become more engaged in their health care by having access to their health information and having the ability to share that information with others.

Please refer to the CMS Stage 1 vs Stage 2 Comparison Table for Eligible Professionals in Appendix A for further specifications.

Protect Electronic Health Information

Table 4-24 identifies the objective and thresholds to meet the MU measure for protecting electronic health information.

TABLE 4-24

MU Measure: Protect Electronic Health Information

Objective	Stage 1 Core Measure	Stage 2 Core Measure
Protect electronic health information created or maintained by the certified EHR technology through the implementation of appropriate technical capabilities.	Conduct or review a security risk analysis in accordance with the requirements under 45 CFR 164.308(a)(1) and implement security updates as necessary; correct identified security deficiencies as part of a risk-management process.	Conduct or review security analysis and incorporate in risk-management process.

Why Is This Measure Relevant?

Security of electronic health information, especially in the current environment of increased implementation and use of EHRs, has been identified as a priority as one of the core measures required to meet MU. The security risk analysis draws attention to the security of electronic personal health information, in particular the confidentiality, integrity, and availability of the information.

Staff

All staff members and EPs have a responsibility to follow existing policies and to keep electronic health information secure. The person responsible for performing the security risk analysis will most likely vary at each practice and organization.

What to Do

Privacy and security of electronic health information are covered in detail in Chapter 1. A brief overview of the tasks that need to be completed to satisfy this core MU measure is below.

- Perform a security risk assessment of your practice or organization to identify any security deficiencies or potential risks to electronic protected health information (PHI).
- Complete a walk-through assessment at each physical location, and identify any security deficiencies at each location.
- If your practice is part of a larger medical group with organizational policies and a central information technology department, some of the security risk analysis may be performed for your practice. A walk-through should still be performed at your practice location to identify potential or existing threats to the security of PHI.
- Document an analysis of the identified security deficiencies and potential threats, taking into consideration the likelihood and severity of these threats.
- Develop and document a plan to address any deficiencies identified during the analysis.
- Implement security updates as necessary, and correct identified security deficiencies prior to or during the EHR reporting period.

- Stage 2 requires that you incorporate the security risk analysis into your risk-management process.
- Hiring an outside consultant or firm to complete this risk analysis is not a requirement of the measure.
- This measure requires EPs to attest that they have conducted or reviewed a security risk analysis prior to or during the reporting period.

Please refer to the CMS Stage 1 vs Stage 2 Comparison Table for Eligible Professionals in Appendix A for further specifications.

Submit Electronic Data to Immunization Registries

Table 4-25 identifies the objective and thresholds to meet the MU measure for submitting data to immunization registries electronically.

TABLE 4-25

MU Measure: Immunization Registry Data Submission

Objective	Stage 1 Menu Set Measure	Stage 2 Core Measure
Capability to submit electronic data to immunization registries or immunization information systems and actual submission according to applicable law and practice. New Stage 1 language added is "except where prohibited."	Perform at least one test of certified EHR technology's capacity to submit electronic data to immunization registries and follow up submission if the test is successful.	Successful ongoing transmission of immunization data.

Why Is This Measure Relevant?

With increased national use of CEHRT, the ability to electronically submit immunization data to immunization registries has increased. Many states have immunization registries or an immunization information system (IIS) to centralize immunization data. According to the CDC, an IIS combines immunization information from different sources into a single record and is able to provide official immunization records for school, day care, and camp entry requirements. An IIS can also help immunization programs to identify populations at high risk for vaccine-preventable diseases and to target interventions and resources efficiently. Because the CMS is encouraging electronic submission of immunization data for this measure, information will begin to flow to area IISs, which opens up new opportunities for better data for population health outreach and research.

Staff

Most likely your practice already has a clinical staff member who has been responsible for submitting immunization data to your local public-health agency or immunization registration program. It would be appropriate for the same staff, with proper training, to assume the responsibility to transmit immunization data electronically. Accuracy of the immunization data that will be exported from your EHR will require all staff and providers to be properly trained to accurately enter immunization data into the EHR.

What to Do

CEHRTs have functionality available to enable submission to public-health immunization registries. Below are some things to consider if you are planning to select this measure as one of your five menu set measures.

- ONC certification is not a guarantee of interoperability with any particular IIS, as local regulations or standards may require additional configuration.

- CEHRT is able to retrieve immunization data from the EHR, utilizing specific standards, and export that information to allow eligible providers to meet this MU measure.

- The validity of the immunization information coming out of the EHR is dependent on accurate information being entered correctly into reportable fields in the EHR when administering immunizations.

- Ongoing monitoring of the accuracy of staff documentation should be implemented to identify any issues, so that training can be offered to correct any inconsistency or inaccuracies.

- EPs should check with their immunization registry to determine if it is capable of receiving data electronically. If not, an exclusion is available for this menu set measure in Stage 1.

- Some public-health agencies require you to contact them to prearrange the test submission.

- You need to retain documentation for 6 years from the public-health agency indicating that you tried, succeeded, or did not succeed in sending immunization data. Any screen shots you can capture of your process would also be recommended as supporting documentation.

- If you are going to select this measure as one of your five menu set measures for Stage 1 and claim an exclusion, obtain documentation from your local public-health agency and/or your EHR vendor if you are unable to submit information, particularly if your local agency is not ready to accept electronic submission of data or if your EHR does not have compatible Health Level 7 (HL7) exchange standards.

Please refer to the CMS Stage 1 vs Stage 2 Comparison Table for Eligible Professionals in Appendix A for further specifications.

Critical Point

This measure does *not* require that you purchase and install, usually at additional expense, any interfaces or bridges that your EHR vendor may tell you are necessary. The EHR has been certified as to its ability to meet Stage 1 MU. New 2014 certification criteria have been developed for EHR products.

Submit Electronic Syndromic Surveillance Data

Table 4-26 identifies the objective and thresholds to meet the MU measure for submitting data to immunization registries.

TABLE 4-26

MU Measure: Syndromic Surveillance Data Submission

Objective	Stage 1 Menu Set Measure	Stage 2 Menu Set Measure
Capability to submit electronic syndromic surveillance data to public-health agencies and actual submission according to applicable law and practice. New Stage 1 language added is "except where prohibited."	Perform at least one test of certified EHR technology's capacity to provide electronic syndromic surveillance data to public-health agencies and follow-up submission if the test is successful.	Successful ongoing transmission of syndromic surveillance data.

Why Is This Measure Relevant?

With increased national use of certified EHR technology, the capability to submit syndromic surveillance data to public-health agencies is improving. The following explanation of syndromic surveillance was published in the CDC's *Morbidity and Mortality Weekly Report* in September 2004[14]:

> Syndromic surveillance has been used for early detection of outbreaks, to follow the size, spread, and tempo of outbreaks, to monitor disease trends, and to provide reassurance that an outbreak has not occurred. Syndromic surveillance systems seek to use existing health data in real time to provide immediate analysis and feedback to those charged with investigation and follow-up of potential outbreaks.... Syndromic surveillance systems might enhance collaboration among public-health agencies, health care providers, information-system professionals, academic investigators, and industry. However, syndromic surveillance does not replace traditional public health surveillance, nor does it substitute for direct physician reporting of unusual or suspect cases of public health importance.

Although syndromic surveillance was developed for early detection of a large-scale release of a biologic agent, current surveillance goals reach beyond terrorism preparedness. Medical-provider reporting remains critical for identifying unusual disease clusters or sentinel cases. Nevertheless, syndromic surveillance might help determine the size, spread, and tempo of an outbreak after it is detected or provide reassurance that a large-scale outbreak is not occurring, particularly in times of enhanced surveillance (eg, during a high-profile event). Finally, syndromic surveillance is beginning to be used to monitor disease trends, which is increasingly possible as longitudinal data are obtained and syndrome definitions are refined.

The fundamental objective of syndromic surveillance is to identify illness clusters early, before diagnoses are confirmed and reported to public-health agencies, and to mobilize a rapid response, thereby reducing morbidity and mortality.[14]

Staff

Physicians, physician assistants, nurse practitioners, and nurses are aware of their reporting responsibilities regarding communicable diseases, cancer, and other public-health issues.

As technology development and use expand, the sources of syndromic surveillance data are sure to also expand. Staff assistance in gathering and submission of the information most likely varies from practice to practice. The primary responsibility to report resides with the physician.

What to Do

CEHRTs have functionality available to enable submission of syndromic surveillance data to public-health agencies. Below are some things to consider if you are planning to select this measure as one of your five menu set measures in Stage 1 or one of your three menu set measures in Stage 2.

- ONC certification is not a guarantee of interoperability with any particular public-health agency, as local regulations or standards may require additional configuration.
- CEHRT is able to retrieve data from the EHR, utilize specific standards, and export that information to allow eligible providers to meet this MU measure.
- The value of the information coming out of the EHR is dependent on accurate information being entered correctly into reportable fields in the EHR.
- Ongoing monitoring of the accuracy of staff documentation should be implemented to identify any issues, so that training can be offered to correct any inconsistency or inaccuracies.
- EPs should check with their local public-health agency to determine if it is capable of receiving data electronically. If not, an exclusion is available for this menu set measure in Stage 1.
- Some public-health agencies require you to contact them to prearrange the test submission.
- You need to retain documentation for 6 years from your local public-health agency indicating that you tried, succeeded, or did not succeed in sending syndromic surveillance data. Any screen shots you can capture of your process would also be recommended as supporting documentation.
- If you are going to select this measure as one of your five menu set measures for Stage 1 and claim an exclusion, obtain documentation from your local public-health agency and/or your EHR vendor if you are unable to submit information, particularly if your local agency is not ready to accept electronic submission of data or if your EHR does not have compatible HL7 exchange standards.
- Stage 2 retains this measure as a menu set measure for ongoing submission of syndromic surveillance data, assuming that you were successful in Stage 1 and can continue that process.

Please refer to the CMS Stage 1 vs Stage 2 Comparison Table for Eligible Professionals in Appendix A for further specifications.

Critical Point

This measure does *not* require that you purchase and install, usually at additional expense, any interfaces or bridges that your EHR vendor may tell you are necessary. The EHR has been certified as to its ability to meet Stage 1 MU. New 2014 certification criteria have been developed for EHR products.

Use Secure Messaging With Patients

Table 4-27 identifies the objective and thresholds to meet the MU measure for using secure messaging with patients.

T A B L E 4-27

MU Measure: Secure Messaging

Objective	New Stage 2 Core Measure
Use secure electronic messaging to communicate with patients on relevant health information.	A secure message was sent using the electronic messaging function of CEHRT by more than 5% of unique patients (or their authorized representatives) seen by the EP during the EHR reporting period

Why Is This Measure Relevant?

Improving quality and efficiency and engaging patients and families in their health care are some of the goals of the EHR Incentive Program. The reality is that patients lead busy lives and manage their own health and chronic conditions the majority of the time. Patients with diabetes self-manage their condition nearly 95% of the time.[15]

Primary-care practices are very busy, and phone volume is high. Secure messaging facilitates asynchronous communication, allowing patients to communicate with their provider when it is convenient for them. As the primary-care shortage grows, messaging improves patients' access to their provider and the practice and, in a variety of studies, has been shown to improve patient and provider/staff satisfaction.[16]

Patients with diabetes can use secure messaging to send their home glucose-monitoring results to their provider. Patients with hypertension can securely send their home blood-pressure measurements. In both cases, medications could be adjusted without a face-to-face visit with the provider. More and more patients want access to their provider via the Internet, and secure messaging use in practices is growing.

Partially in response to the MU incentives, the EHR adoption rate across the country has accelerated over the past few years. Policy makers have made a strong statement by adding secure messaging as a core measure for MU Stage 2. As more providers adopt secure messaging to meet Stage 2 MU, and as patients and families become more engaged, improvement in quality, efficiency, access, and provider and patient satisfaction are anticipated results.

Staff

Secure messaging cannot be implemented in a busy practice without thoughtful planning. Staff and EPs will be affected, adjustment to workflows will be needed, and responsibilities will change. Patients will need to be encouraged to sign up for the portal, and the benefits of secure messaging will need to be explained. Policies will need to be created and consents written and signed by patients. Password distribution and management plans will be implemented, and staff will need to triage the messages coming into the practice via secure messaging.

As with EHR adoption, EPs will have concerns about how secure messaging will affect the care they provide and their productivity—and thus their paycheck. Their fear of endless e-mail threads with patients will not materialize, but until patient adoption of secure messaging catches on, the phones will still ring and the patients will still come into the practice. For a time, secure messaging will be an added challenge to their day, but with support, this too shall pass, and patients and providers will be the beneficiaries.

What to Do

Security, consent, registration, and message management will all need to be addressed prior to implementation of secure messaging. Portal use was introduced as an optional menu set measure in Stage 1, paving the way for the required use of the portal in Stage 2. Secure messaging is done through the portal, although enhanced features may be required. Important considerations when implementing secure messaging are listed below.

- Explore the features and functionality of your portal with your vendor.
- If you have not yet implemented a portal, ask about the secure messaging capability, security, and reporting features of the portal products you are vetting.
- Secure messaging has been in use at some practices for many years.[17] If possible, talk to the staff and providers in a few of these practices. They most likely have learned some valuable lessons.
- Look for features that can provide read receipts and time/date stamps, so that you will know if a message has been read.
- Understand how the messages will be saved into the EHR. Can it be done easily?
- Will any additional language need to be added to your portal consent? Will you include the ability for the practice to withdraw patient access?
- Will you put information on your Web page regarding the proper use of secure messaging or will that information be printed and given to the patient? You should include a statement about secure messaging *not* being an appropriate way to communicate in an emergency.
- Will you require each patient to have his or her own e-mail address? How will you know if it is Mr. Smith or Mrs. Smith who is writing to you?
- How will you handle caregiver consent? Pediatric patients or families with children? Custody issues can pose some challenges.
- At what age do young adults have the right to restrict the sharing of information in your state?
- What will your process be for resetting passwords or providing new passwords to patients? How can you be sure it is the patient who is requesting and receiving it? Ask your vendor or other practices how they have handled the above situations.
- How will you know if a patient has signed the consent for secure messaging or portal use, particularly if you have been capturing e-mail addresses ahead of implementation of your portal? Does your EHR or portal facilitate that?
- Who will help patients register? Who will explain secure messaging to the patients? Will you create a brochure to hand out? Will you have signs/banners in your office to encourage registration?
- Will a staff member triage the messages, respond to some, and route others to the appropriate staff member or EP?
- Will you have a policy that states the timeframe in which the patient will receive a response? Will you monitor adherence to the policy?
- Will there be an expectation that all messages will be reviewed prior to the end of the business day?

- What are the reporting capabilities of your portal? Will you be able to run reports to see the number of patients using secure messaging? By EP?
- Do the reports separate portal activity (prescription refill requests, appointment requests, referral requests) from the messages to EPs?
- Will you be able to monitor the age of patients who are using the portal? What health conditions they have?

When trying to learn anything new, there is a period of adjustment before you'll feel comfortable using the technology and having it fit smoothly into your daily workflow. The learning curve is not as steep as with EHR implementation, but EPs still appreciate one-on-one training to feel comfortable that they are using the technology correctly.

Each EP will figure out how to add responding to messages from patients into his or her workday. Many EPs find that it is easier than playing "phone tag" with patients and find that e-mail conversations are shorter. They also like the fact that the electronic conversations are documented, unlike phone conversations.

Although a fair amount of planning is required, using secure messaging is no more difficult than using regular e-mail. Setting expectations with patients from the start and having the discipline to keep the e-mail exchanges with patients focused on health care issues will serve you well. Payers should realize the benefits of using secure messaging, particularly with patients with chronic diseases, and begin to reimburse for the medical decision making and management that will happen virtually.

NEW STAGE 2 MENU MEASURES

In Stage 2, providers must choose three of six available measures. Five of the measures are new to Stage 2. The syndromic surveillance measure from Stage 1 continues as a menu set measure option in Stage 2.

Accessing Imaging Results Through CEHRT

Table 4-28 identifies the objective and thresholds to meet the MU measure for accessing imaging results through CEHRT.

T A B L E 4-28

MU Measure: Imaging Results

Objective	Stage 2 Menu Measure
Imaging results consisting of the image itself and any explanation or other accompanying information are accessible through certified EHR technology.	More than 10% of all tests whose result is one or more images ordered by the EP during the EHR reporting period are accessible through certified EHR technology.

Why Is This Measure Relevant?

EPs order imaging tests primarily to assist in their diagnostic process. Many patients arrive at appointments where the EP does not have the results of tests that were ordered or is not aware that a test had already been done and then reorders the test to assist the diagnostic process. Not only is this frustrating to EPs, but it is inconvenient, frustrating, and costly to the patient and the health care system. Although the threshold for this new measure is low at 10% of all tests ordered with an image result, it is setting the stage for EHR vendors, hospitals, and imaging facilities to develop products and interfaces to give EPs access to this information. This will be the foundation for increased expectations of access to and sharing of information among providers and facilities of care.

Staff

Staff will be involved in a variety of ways but most likely in checking to make sure the results of the tests are available for the EP. The process for this will depend on whether the results are accessed via a portal or are interfaced into the EHR. The EP most likely will be the one accessing the images and results.

What to Do

When using an EHR, CPOE should be used to enter any medication, laboratory order, or radiology order so that tracking of the status of the order can be done. If the imaging orders are entered and sent to the facility electronically, an expectation would be that the imaging results would be returned to the ordering EP for review and sign off within the EHR. If a specialist is ordering the test, the PCP ideally should be copied on the results so that he or she is aware of tests being done.

The 2014 ONC certification criteria for EHRs define the required functionality within the EHR system. Interfaces exist today in some organizations, and the interpretation of the imaging test is delivered via an interface electronically into some EHRs. A link to access the images and narrative interpretation through the CEHRT and access to scanned images and reports satisfy the measure requirements.

Exclusions are available for providers who order fewer than 100 tests whose result is an image during the EHR reporting period or if a provider has no access to electronic imaging results at the start of the EHR reporting period.

Capture Family History as Structured Data

Table 4-29 identifies the objective and thresholds to meet the MU measure for capturing family history as structured data.

T A B L E   4-29

MU Measure: Family History

Objective	Stage 2 Menu Measure
Record patient family health history as structured data.	More than 20% of all unique patients seen by the EP during the EHR reporting period have a structured data entry for one or more first-degree relatives.

Why Is This Measure Relevant?

As more research is done to expand the knowledge of diseases that have a genetic component, first-degree relative family history will be an important factor in delivering preventive health care, diagnosing disease, and researching treatments to alter the onset or course of the disease. The requirement for the family history to be entered into the EHR as structured data builds on the requirements for structured data in Stage 1 criteria to enable the identification of patients with certain family histories. With the family history entered as reportable data, running a query to identify female patients whose mother had breast cancer or patients with a family history of colon cancer might prompt targeted or more frequent screening.

Staff

Family history is often captured on patient registration forms, and the data entry into the EHR may be done by administrative staff. Medical assistants or nurses may gather the information when rooming the patient, or EPs may discover information during their interview and visit with patients. As portal use increases, patients may be submitting health history and family history information to the practice via the portal. Staff will have the responsibility to enter this information into the EHR if the information is not imported directly into the EHR as structured data.

What to Do

Most EHRs have had the capability to capture family history for some time. EPs are accustomed to writing the family history in their paper medical records or dictating the family history for transcription or entry directly into the EHR. Although this information is being captured, it may not be captured as structured or reportable data. Consider the following suggestions for family history documentation in the EHR.

- It is important for all staff and EPs to receive training in how and where to properly enter family history into the EHR as structured data.
- Identify the staff in your practice whose responsibility it will be for gathering and documenting family history as structured data.
- During chart preparation, have staff check for the presence of family history information in the EHR.
- The measure specifies that more than 20% of all unique patients seen by the EP during the EHR reporting period have structured-data entry for one or more first-degree relatives.
- Design the workflow to efficiently capture the family history on a consistent basis.
- Updating this information is also important to keep the records accurate.
- The only exclusion for this measure is if an EP has no office visits during the EHR reporting period.

Use CEHRT to Submit Cancer Information to Registries

Table 4-30 identifies the objective and thresholds to meet the MU measure for reporting cancer to registries using CEHRT.

TABLE 4-30

MU Measure: Report Cancer Cases

Objective	Stage 2 Menu Measure
Capability to identify and report cancer cases to a public-health central cancer registry, except where prohibited, and in accordance with applicable law and practice.	Successful ongoing submission of cancer case information from CEHRT to a public-health central cancer registry for the entire reporting period.

Why Is This Measure Relevant?

Cancer is one of the leading causes of death in the United States. Increased reporting to cancer registries, in conjunction with increased EHR use, will expand the ability to use the data to identify patterns and trends in occurrence and treatment of this prevalent disease. Large regional registries receive deidentified data and compile data related to geographic and demographic trends. Local registries facilitate tracking of patients diagnosed with cancer, especially to make sure they are not lost to follow-up, and to explore trends in occurrence and treatment patterns and effectiveness.

Staff

Local and state regulations may designate certain EPs as mandated reporters of cancer diagnoses. In many cases, hospitals are required to report new diagnoses. In the ambulatory space, EPs who diagnose and treat cancer will be the most likely to report. Coordination of care among all providers of care and their staff and coordinating the effort to report will be shared by many in the health care system.

What to Do

To operationalize this measure, the responsibility and capability to electronically report to a cancer registry need to be ascertained. There are exclusions to this measure that also should be taken into consideration.

- Clarify your individual or your organization's obligation to identify and report cancer cases to a public-health cancer registry.
- Determine if the public-health agency to which your practice would report is capable at the start of your reporting period of receiving electronic cancer case information in the specific standard required for your EHR.
- Enlist the help of your staff to communicate pertinent information on a regular basis to your local hospital's registry system or to the designated centralized cancer registry.

Report to Specialized Registries Using CEHRT

Table 4-31 identifies the objective and thresholds to meet the MU measure for reporting to specialized registries.

TABLE 4-31

MU Measure: Specialized Registry

Objective	Stage 2 Menu Measure
Capability to identify and report specific cases to a specialized registry (other than a cancer registry), except where prohibited, and in accordance with applicable law and practice.	Successful ongoing submission of specific case information from certified EHR technology to a specialized registry for the entire EHR reporting period.

Why Is This Measure Relevant?

Increased reporting to specialized registries, in conjunction with increased EHR use, will expand the ability to identify patterns and trends in occurrence and treatment of a variety of diseases for which there are registries that can accept the data. Regional registries may receive deidentified data to compile related to geographic and demographic trends. Local registries may facilitate tracking of patients diagnosed with specific diseases to make sure they are not lost to follow-up and to explore trends in occurrence and treatment patterns and effectiveness.

Staff

In an ambulatory setting, EPs who diagnose and treat specified cases will be the most likely to report. Coordination of care among all providers of care and their staff and coordinating the effort to report will be shared by many in the health care system.

What to Do

To operationalize this measure, the responsibility and capability to electronically report to a specialized registry need to be ascertained. There are exclusions to this measure that also should be taken into consideration.

- Clarify your individual or your organization's obligation to identify and report specific disease cases to a specialized registry.

- Determine if the agency to which your practice would report is capable at the start of your reporting period of receiving electronic case information in the specific standard required for your EHR.

- Enlist the help of your staff to communicate pertinent information on a regular basis to your local hospital's registry system or to the designated specialized registry.

Record Electronic Progress Notes

Table 4-32 identifies the objective and thresholds to meet the MU measure for recording electronic progress notes.

T A B L E   4-32

MU Measure: Progress Notes

Objective	Stage 2 Menu Measure
Record electronic notes in patient records.	Enter at least one electronic progress note created, edited, and signed by an eligible professional for more than 30% of unique patients with at least one office visit during the EHR reporting period. Electronic progress notes must be text-searchable. Nonsearchable notes do not qualify, but this does not mean that all of the content has to be character text. Drawings and other content can be included with searchable text notes under this measure.

Why Is This Measure Relevant?

Progress notes capture the provider-patient visit and tell the story about the encounter. The majority of EPs in small practices who adopt EHRs are using the technology to capture demographics, billing information, vital signs, review of systems, as well as the progress notes from the patient visit. Progress notes in the hospital setting have a lower adoption rate, primarily owing to the variety of personnel who document in the medical record of patients cared for in the hospital setting and the complexity of the technology required to do this well.

The searchable parts of the visit report are usually in all the areas of the record mentioned above, but the more EPs use dictation and free-text narrative, the less often reportable data are captured during the visit. The specific language of this measure states that the 2014 ONC certification requires functionality that will allow free-text notes to be searchable, which will expand the capability to search reports of patient encounters for certain symptoms, findings, and impressions. This capability will provide access to more than the current structured data fields of problem list, medication list, allergy list, and vital signs and what has been built into order sets and templates for documenting the visit. Perhaps it will increase the use of technology by EPs who are resistant to using templates and check-off boxes to capture their patient visits in the EHR.

Staff

In ambulatory practices, EPs are most frequently documenting progress notes. In the hospital setting, nurses, hospitalists, respiratory therapists, interns, residents, attending physicians, covering physicians, and many others document the patient's stay in the hospital. Patient visit encounters in the ambulatory space are most often a visit with a physician, nurse practitioner, physician assistant, or nurse, and the progress notes are entered into the patient record during the encounter.

What to Do

If you are an EP using a certified EHR in an ambulatory practice, this measure is most likely one of the three menu set measures you will select to meet Stage 2 MU. Practices that have enlisted the help of regional extension centers to implement an EHR and/or achieve MU are receiving advice on how to do chart abstraction and chart migration as part of their preimplementation and postimplementation plan. Once practices have begun to retire paper charts, the entire patient visit needs to be entered into the EHR as the electronic record becomes the legal record, which includes documenting progress notes in the EHR.

Documenting in the EHR while in the examination room with the patient is the most beneficial way for EPs to receive alerts and patient-specific reminders during the visit, both of which are forms of CDS. Consider some of the following suggestions to meet this measure.

- If progress notes aren't currently being documented in the EHR, provider assistance and training should focus on understanding the EP's current use of the EHR while in the examination room.

- Seek efficiencies, such as creating favorites lists for each EP and order sets and templates for frequently seen diagnoses and chronic diseases.

- History of present illness (HPI), review of systems, and the care plan, including entry of orders into the EHR for medications, laboratory tests, referrals, follow-up, and patient education, are some things EPs can document most easily while in the examination room with the patient.

- EHRs vary greatly in their ease of use, which may affect the amount of documentation done while in the examination room, and many EPs continue to document or dictate the HPI and their impression at the end of the day.

- To meet this measure, there needs to be at least one progress note created, edited, and signed for 30% of the unique patients with at least one office visit during the reporting period. Documenting an entire visit in the EHR for all of your patients will far exceed the 30% threshold for progress notes.

- There are no exclusions for this measure; therefore, it is required for all EPs to meet MU.

SUMMARY

In this chapter, we have attempted to put each MU measure into perspective as to why it is meaningful to those of you who practice medicine and take care of patients every day. The measures emphasize the proper entry of your documentation and your staff's documentation into your EHR, such that the EHR can function as more than a repository. By meeting these measures, you have created a strong foundation on which to build expanded use of the technology to improve care, safety, efficiency, and so much more.

What's in It for Physicians?

- Meeting Stage 1 MU raises EP awareness of the way information needs to be entered into the EHR for it to be available for reporting. Although the thresholds were low and fairly easily achieved in Stage 1, the thresholds increase in Stage 2, which will require monitoring performance, and staff involvement and understanding, to achieve the higher thresholds.

- The requirements of MU are gradually leading EPs and the health system toward effectively using technology as a tool to improve health care in many ways. Ultimately, documenting correctly and using the tools the technology provides to support EP decision making will become common practice, and MU will be seen as general operating procedure, not a separate requirement to meet. Striving to achieve MU also helps provide additional EHR training that EPs wished they had when they had implemented their EHR system. Therefore, achieving MU and leveraging their EHR system simultaneously is hopefully leading EPs back to enjoying the practice of medicine.

What's in It for Staff?

- As with the EPs, MU provides staff with the framework for using the technology to benefit patients and the delivery of care. In many cases, staff acquires new skills, realize greater job satisfaction, and gain experience that could propel their career in different directions. Working to achieve MU fosters a healthier team approach to patient care delivery, generates leaders in the practice, and is the beginning of empowering the staff to take an active role in improving the quality, safety, and outcomes for their patients and their families.

What's in It for Patients?

- Patients are ultimately the beneficiaries of a better coordinated delivery system. EPs and staff using the technology well will access the information to improve care, engage patients and their families, and break down the information silos that frustrate patients as they maneuver the health care system.

ACTION ITEMS

1. Create a priority list of the workflows that your practice plans to redesign to improve efficiency and patient safety and to incorporate the EHR into your everyday workflow in your practice.
2. Review each core measure, and discuss staff responsibilities for each measure.
3. Obtain training, as needed, for all staff to accurately document the information for each measure in your EHR.

4. Decide which menu set measures your practice can most easily meet. Communicate to staff which measures have been selected for Stage 1.
5. Determine your access to your practice's MU reports by discussing with your EHR vendor. Monitor your performance on a regular basis leading up to attestation.
6. Communicate to staff that Stage 1 measures are the building blocks for Stages 2 and 3. Sustaining the Stage 1 measures is essential to meeting further MU stages. Redesign workflows as needed, if the current workflows are not resulting in consistent documentation.

REFERENCES

1. Yin, RK. *Case Study Method: Design and Methods.* 3rd ed. Thousand Oaks, CA: Sage, 2003. Cited by: Ramaiah M, Subrahmanian E, Sriram RD, Lide BB. Workflow and electronic health records in small medical practices. *Perspect Health Inf Manage.* Spring 2012;1-16. 2012;9:1d. Epub2012 Apr 1. Accessed September 17, 2012. .
2. Centers for Disease Control and Prevention, Preventive Care and Screening: Screening Mammography, PQRI 112, NQF 0031. www.cms.hhs.gov/PQRI/20_AlternativeReportingMechanisms. asp#TopOfPage. Accessed August 4, 2012.
3. ———. Features. Tobacco Control Saves Lives and Money. www.cdc.gov/Features/Tobacco ControlData/. Accessed August 4, 2012.
4. Institute of Medicine. *To Err Is Human: Building a Safer Health System.* 1999. www.iom.edu /~/media/Files/Report%20Files/1999/To-Err-is-Human/To%20Err%20is%20Human%201999%20 %20report%20brief.pdf. Accessed February 8, 2013.
5. Baron JM, Dighe AS. Computerized provider order entry in the clinical laboratory. *J Pathol Inform.* 2011;2:35. Published online August 13, 2011. doi:10.4103/2153-3539.83740. Accessed December 30, 2012.
6. The National Academies. Medication errors injure 1.5 million people and costs billion of dollars annually: report offers comprehensive strategies for reducing drug-related mistakes. [news release from the National Academies]. July 20, 2006. www8.nationalacademies.org/onpinews/newsitem .aspx?RecordID=11623. Accessed August 20, 2012.
7. National Training Coordinating Council (NTCC) and AARP/Legal Counsel for the Elderly, Inc. What's so special about teaching adults? *Fast Track Training Series* (Vol 8). Washington, DC: AARP/LCE National Training Project; 1993. www.fastfamilysupport.org/fasttraining/Other /teachingadults-whattrainersneedtoknow.pdf. Accessed July 23, 2012.
8. Lamberts R. Clinical summaries: a valuable part of Meaningful Use requirements. February 22, 2012. Physicians Practice Web site. www.physicianspractice.com. Accessed July 29, 2012.
9. Emont S. Measuring the Impact of Patient Portals: What the Literature Tells Us. May 2011. California Healthcare Foundation Web site. www.chcf.org/~/media/MEDIA%20LIBRARY%20Files/PDF/M /PDF%20MeasuringImpactPatientPortals.pdf. Accessed February 7, 2013.
10. Centers for Disease Control and Prevention. Closing the Gap Report. www.cdc.gov/features /preventiveservices/clinical_preventive_services_closing_the_gap_report.pdf. Accessed November 27, 2012.
11. ———. Immunization Schedules, 2012. www.cdc.gov/vaccines/schedules. Accessed November 27, 2012.
12. McCarthy D, Mueller K, Wrenn J. Issues Research, Inc. Kaiser Permanente: Bridging the Quality Divide With Integrated Practice, Group Accountability, and Health Information Technology. The Commonwealth Fund. June 2009. www.commonwealthfund.org/~/media/Files/ Publications/Case%20Study/2009/Jun/1278_McCarthy_Kaiser_case_study_624_update.pdf. Accessed February 7, 2013.

13. Centers for Medicare & Medicaid Services. Eligible Professional Meaningful Use. Menu Set Measures: Measure 5 of 10, Stage 1. November 7, 2010. www.cms.gov/Regulations-and-Guidance/Legislation/EHRIncentivePrograms/downloads/5_Patient_Electronic_Access.pdf. Accessed November 27, 2012.

14. Henning, KJ. What is syndromic surveillance? *MMWR Morb Mortal Wkly Rep.* September 24, 2004;53(suppl);5-11. www.cdc.gov/mmwr/preview/mmwrhtml/su5301a3.htm. Accessed January 30, 2013.

15. Liederman E, Lee JC, Baquero VH, Seites PG. Physician-patient Web messaging: the impact of message volume and satisfaction. www.ncbi.nlm.nih.gov/pmc/articles/PMC1490042. Accessed December 30, 2012.

16. Leong, SL, Gingrich, D, Lewis, PR, Mauger, DT, and George, JH. Enhancing doctor-patient communication using email: a pilot study. *J Am Board Fam Med.* 2005;18(3):180-188.

17. iHealthBeat. What Percentage of U.S. Doctors Connect With Patients Online via E-Mail, Secure Messaging? www.ihealthbeat.org/data-points/2010/what-percentage-of-us-doctors-connect-with-patients-online-via-email-secure-messaging.aspx#ixzz2JIU4I2u2. Accessed February 7, 2013.

## chapter 5

Surviving Attestation

WHO SHOULD READ THIS CHAPTER?

This chapter is for all eligible professionals (EPs) who want to understand what needs to be done to ensure a successful attestation after months of implementing workflow changes, documentation changes and expanded use of their electronic health records (EHRs) in the care of their patients. This is also for the staff who facilitates the changes and understands data entry and how reports are generated from the EHR and want to see their EPs successfully attest when their 90- or 365-day reporting period is complete.

What you will learn in this chapter:
- How to anticipate the numbers needed for attestation and how they might be generated
- How to appreciate some challenges to combining different sources of data
- The types of documentation to retain to support your attestation of meeting the measures
- How to minimize delays in, or roadblocks to, your ability to attest
- Items to be aware of as you prepare to attest online
- The average time between attestation and delivery of payment and possible reasons for delay
- What's in it for
  - Providers
  - Staff
  - Patients

The culmination of your Meaningful Use (MU) reporting period is the act of electronically attesting to the Centers for Medicare & Medicaid Services (CMS) that you have met the requirements for MU. Attestation is completed electronically through the EHR Incentive Program Registration & Attestation Web site, which can be accessed at www.cms.gov/Regulations-and-Guidance/Legislation/EHRIncentivePrograms/RegistrationandAttestation.html.

In Chapter 4 we discussed in detail each MU measure and the workflows associated with meeting the measures. Assuming that workflows have been successfully implemented and that staff and eligible professionals (EPs) have been documenting consistently in the electronic health record (EHR), the data needed for attestation should be ready to populate reports with the numbers needed to successfully meet MU. This chapter will cover the possible sources of the numbers needed for attestation, the importance of ongoing monitoring of performance, the challenges or delays that may be encountered, and tools and tips to successfully attest.

GENERATING THE NUMBERS

Each MU measure has its own specific measurement criteria and thresholds. While some measures are based on the total number of patients seen and the percentage of those for whom you have documented what the measure requires, other measures look for the total number of unique patients seen during the reporting period who have been the focus of a particular action or documentation. And some measures don't count patients at all but look at actions instead.

If the certified EHR product that you are using is able to produce data based on the measure criteria, then the effort required for you to calculate the numerators and denominators needed for attestation is much less than if you need to manually account for the calculation of the measures. Attesting for MU means that you can answer yes or no or can produce numerical proof in the form of numerators and denominators that you have performed the action required in each measure and meet or exceed the threshold percentage required by the measure.

Table 5-1 displays the stages and reporting periods for attesting to MU.

T A B L E   5-1

Meaningful Use Stages and Reporting Periods

	Stage 1 Year 1	Stage 1 Year 2	Stage 1 Year 3	Stage 2 Year 1	Stage 2 Year 2	Stage 3 Year 1
Eligible years	2011, 2012, 2013, 2014	2012, 2013, 2015	2013 (Only for those whose first year of reporting was 2011)	2014	2015	2016
Reporting period	90 consecutive days in same calendar year	365/366 consecutive days in same calendar year	365 consecutive days in same calendar year	90 consecutive days in same calendar year	365 consecutive days in same calendar year	TBD
		If Stage 1, Year 2 in 2014				
		90 consecutive days in same calendar year				
EHR certification	ONC-ATCB / ONC-CEHRT	ONC-ATCB/ ONC-CEHRT	ONC-CEHRT	ONC-CEHRT 2014 Certification	ONC-CEHRT 2014 Certification	TBD

Abbreviations: EHR, indicates electronic health record; ONC-ATCB, Office of the National Coordinator for Health Information Technology–Accredited Testing and Certification Body; ONC-CEHRT, ONC–certified EHR technology; and TBD, to be determined.

As discussed in Chapter 4, you must meet 15 core measures, 5 menu set measures, and 6 clinical quality measures (CQMs) to achieve Stage 1 MU. Table 5-2 illustrates the distribution of answer types for attestation.

TABLE 5-2

Answer-Type Distribution for Stage 1 MU Measures

	Numerator/ Denominator	Yes/No	Measures with Exclusions
Core measures (15)	10	5	5
Menu set measures (Choose 5 of 10)	6	4	8
Clinical quality measures (Report 6 of 44)	44	0	0

For Stage 2 MU attestation, you must meet 17 core measures, 3 menu set measures, and 9 CQMs. Table 5-3 illustrates the distribution of answer types for attestation to meet Stage 2 MU.

TABLE 5-3

Answer-Type Distribution for Stage 2 MU Measures

	Numerator/ Denominator	Yes/No	Measures with Exclusions
Core measures (17)	13	4	12
Menu set measures (Choose 3 of 6)	3	3	A menu set exclusion will not count as meeting a measure in Stage 2 if there are other measures that the eligible professionals could have selected and met.
Clinical quality measures (Report 9 of 64)	64	0	0

To meet the initial Office of the National Coordinator for Health Information Technology (ONC) Authorized Testing and Certification Body (ATCB) certification criteria, EHR products were required to be able to electronically produce the numerators and denominators for the CQMs, and EPs were required to report those numbers during attestation as generated by the certified EHR. The current EHR certification requirements do not stipulate that numerators and denominators for MU core and menu set measures need to be reported as generated by the certified EHR. This allows EPs to manually generate numerators and denominators for those measures if desired.

Despite the lack of a requirement to do so, many EHR vendors have provided users with electronic calculations for all core and menu set measures. Unlike the CQMs requirement, EPs are allowed to add additional information from other sources to the core and menu set measure calculations if they would prefer to submit different numerators and denominators. For Stage 2, all vendors need to have their EHRs recertified according to

ONC Certified Electronic Health Record Technology (CEHRT) 2014 certification, and electronic calculation and generation of the numerators and denominators for all core and menu set measures is a requirement to meet 2014 certification criteria.

Some EHR vendors provide the capability for you to run reports to show your performance on the measures by inserting a period of time and the corresponding dates of your choosing (eg, 90 days, June 15–September 15). Other EHR vendors only provide access to performance information for periods of 90 days, but only in full-month increments (eg, June 1–August 31) and there may be a waiting period of a few weeks to a month or more after the end of the month to receive this report.

Critical Point

It is important for you to know whether you can run your own reports on your MU measures when you want to, and for a period of time of your choosing, or whether you are dependent on the vendor for such reports.

As shown in Tables 5-2 and 5-3, most of the core and menu set measures will be reported as numerators and denominators when you attest. The denominator for most measures is either the total number of patients seen or the total number of unique patients seen during the reporting period. As Stage 1 is focused on the appropriate capture of data in EHRs to enable reporting and facilitate using the information to manage the care of patients, many of the measures look at the frequency with which information is captured as structured or reportable data on patients seen during the reporting period. Consistent documentation in the appropriate data fields by everyone across your practice will allow you to meet the thresholds necessary for successful attestation.

Because thresholds are met by documenting in the EHR, choosing to include patients who are not in your EHR makes little sense. If some of your patients still have paper records and have not been seen since you implemented the EHR, you most likely would not want to include their records. If you have some patient records in a noncertified EHR and some in a certified EHR, it would most likely be easiest to report only on those in the certified EHR.

Critical Point

To be eligible to participate in the Medicare and Medicaid EHR Incentive Program, you must have 50% of your total patient encounters at locations where CEHRT is available. If the total number of patient encounters is less than 50% at locations with a certified EHR available, you are not eligible to participate in this program.

You will be asked repeatedly as you attest whether the data were extracted from *all* of your patient records or whether the data were extracted *only* from patient records maintained using CEHRT.

The exclusion criteria, when exclusion is available, are based on *all* patient records, so read carefully and make sure you are eligible for any exclusion based on all patient records. The e-prescribing and computerized provider order entry (CPOE) measures are good examples. For them, the exclusion is for EPs who write fewer than 100 prescriptions during the reporting period. The measure would count all prescriptions written by an EP during the reporting period, not just those written for the patients in the certified EHR.

The calculation would include prescriptions written for patients the EP may see in a nursing home that does not have CEHRT. You would need to count those prescriptions written outside of the EHR and add them to the prescriptions ordered in the CEHRT, which will be calculated for you, to decide if you meet the exclusion criteria.

CALCULATING NUMERATORS AND DENOMINATORS

Many of the MU measures stipulate that EPs are permitted but not required to use only the patients whose records are maintained using CEHRT to calculate their performance to meet MU. The CMS does not stipulate that EPs must calculate the measure that way. If you wish to include information about patients whose records are on paper, then your method of calculation must be consistent for all of your measure calculations. Table 5-4 illustrates the measure criteria for the core MU measure regarding smoking status.

TABLE 5-4
Record Smoking Status

Objective	Measure	Exclusion
Record smoking status for patients 13 years old or older.	More than 50% of all unique patients 13 years old or older seen by the EP have smoking status recorded as structured data.	Any EP who sees no patients 13 years or older.

Recording smoking status as structured data can only be accomplished by documenting in the reportable field in the electronic record, but the CMS also states: "The provider is permitted, but not required, to limit the measure of this objective to those patients whose records are maintained using certified EHR technology."

If for some reason you want to calculate all of the unique 13-year-old patients seen during the reporting period, with paper or electronic records, and add them together for your denominator, then you would still need to exceed the 50% threshold of patients who have their smoking status documented in the EHR as structured data. Table 5-5 is an example of what a calculation might look like using both EHR and paper chart information.

TABLE 5-5
Calculation of Smoking Measure

Record Smoking Status Core Measure	Unique 13-Year-Olds Seen During Reporting Period	Number With Smoking Status Recorded as Structured Data	Numerator ÷ Denominator = %	MU Threshold >50%
Electronic documentation only	145	75	75 ÷ 145 = 51.7%	Meets measure
Paper and electronic documentation	165	75	75 ÷ 165 = 45.5%	Does not meet measure

The e-prescribing measure is another example of a measure whose calculations might include data from the EHR as well as outside data. The denominator for that measure is the number of permissible prescriptions written during the reporting period by the EP. If the EP works in more than one office or location, and every location does not have an EHR (eg, a nursing home), then the calculation of the total number of permissible prescriptions written, and those sent via e-prescribing, may be affected. If the EP is trying to claim exclusion from this measure, then the total prescriptions written by the EP, wherever they were written, cannot exceed 100. This measure takes into consideration all permissible prescriptions written by the EP during the reporting period, not just the prescriptions written in the EHR.

The CPOE measure has the same exclusion criteria, and an EP's ability to claim exclusion could also be affected if he or she writes prescriptions while working at various locations. For Stage 2, the language for the exclusion changes to read that the EP can claim exclusion if he or she has written fewer than 100 *medication orders*.

Your EHR vendor's software is going to calculate the measures using the data entered into your EHR, and your results are dependent on the vendor's interpretation of the measures. If a calculation doesn't make sense to you, refer to the vendor's MU documentation, because the vendor's interpretation may not match how you would interpret the measure or how CMS interprets the measure. Your EHR is required to have ONC ATCB certification to meet MU, and the calculations generated by your EHR are your documentation of proof of performance on the measures. Accurate or not, this potential for misinterpretation or inaccuracy of data is one area of weakness discovered during the early reporting periods. Hopefully, 2014 certification criteria will correct these inaccuracies.

There are some calculations for measures done by EHRs that generate a numerator larger than the denominator, such as the menu set measure on clinical laboratory test results, which involves entering laboratory results as structured data. The CMS acknowledges that "imperfection" and asks that the numbers entered by the EP for attestation reflect a numerator that is at least equal to the denominator when the provider is attesting. The attestation system will not allow you to enter a numerator larger than a denominator for any measures. This is explained further in the section on Minimizing Surprises and in the CMS Frequently Asked Questions, which is available at https://questions.cms.gov/faq.php?id =5005&faqId=3823.

DOCUMENTATION OF PROOF

The CMS will be performing audits of EPs. Most of these audits in 2013 will be desk audits. An EP may receive a letter from an attorney's office containing a request for the specific documentation of proof that the CMS would like sent. The timeframe for responding to such a request is 2 weeks. Capturing the necessary information to support your attestation *and* saving it in case of audit are worthwhile efforts prior to attesting.

When you are ready to attest, calculate your performance or obtain the report of your performance from your EHR on the MU measures for the 90-day period or full calendar year, depending on your reporting year. Make sure, for the 90-day period in particular, that all core measure calculations meet or exceed the threshold for MU. The menu set measures you have chosen must also meet the indicated thresholds. If not, you should adjust your 90-day period until such time as the report shows that you have met the measures.

As mentioned previously, some EHRs allow you to run reports for any period of time you enter. Other EHR vendors supply the reports to you. If the report on one 90-day period does not meet all of the measures, a month later the vendor will run a report on the next 90-day period, delaying your possible attestation for at least a month. Unless you can do intermittent checks on your own performance, you may be unaware that your performance has not met the required thresholds.

The report generated from your EHR will be your proof of the numerators and denominators on most of the measures. Retain a copy of this report for each provider, and make sure the reporting period indicated on the report is the period of time that you will be reporting when you attest.

An example of the type questions you will be asked at the time of attestation is shown in Figure 5-1. A "must-have" resource is the EP Attestation User Guide, which takes you step by step through the attestation system materials, and is available in the ancillary material, which is also available at www.cms.gov/Regulations-and-Guidance/Legislation /EHRIncentivePrograms/RegistrationandAttestation.html.

FIGURE 5-1

CPOE Attestation Page in the EP Attestation User Guide

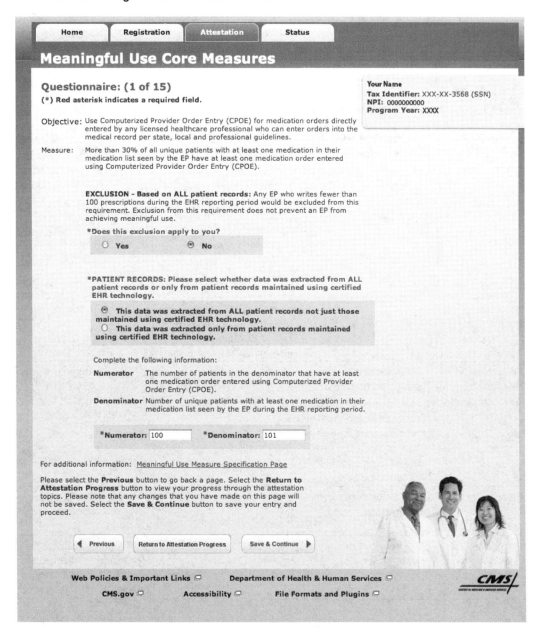

Some of the MU measures do not have numerator and denominator answers. For many of the measures that involve electronically sending information, you must attest that you have satisfied the measure requirements. There is documentation that you should try to create at the time you are sending the information or trying to send the information.

Most EHR vendors have written some type of MU guide for meeting the measures using their EHR. For measures such as the menu set measure in Stage 1 to send immunization information to your public-health agency's immunization registry or immunization information system, there is usually guidance explaining how to create the document that you will send. Capture screen shots of each step of the process as proof that you attempted or completed sending information. Documentation from the receiving entity would also be good information to have in your file.

Table 5-6 suggests the documentation you should consider generating and retaining for 6 years, per the CMS, in case of an audit for Stage 1 and Stage 2 measures. Table 5-7 suggests documentation for the new Stage 2 measures. Most important is the report generated from your EHR of the numerators and denominators necessary for attestation that also indicates the dates of the reporting period for which you are attesting.

TABLE 5-6

Stages 1 and 2 Documentation to Retain

Stage 1 Core Measures	Suggested Stage 1 Documentation	Exclusion Documentation	Changes for Stage 2
CPOE	EHR report of numerator/denominator	EHR report that represents all prescriptions written during the reporting period; if not, retain proof/calculations of prescriptions written outside of the EHR The number of prescriptions written totaling fewer than 100 must be entered when claiming exclusion to this measure	EHR report of numerator/denominator; will include three numerators and denominators for prescriptions, laboratory orders, and radiology orders entered using CPOE
Drug-to-drug/drug-to-allergy interaction check	Screen shot of an alert generated by your EHR Your attestation is your legal certification that you met this measure by stating that this functionality was turned on for the entire reporting period.	None	Incorporated into clinical decision interventions measure
Problem list	EHR report of numerator/denominator	None	Incorporated into the summary of care measure
Permissible prescriptions (e-Rx)	EHR report of numerator/denominator	Same as for CPOE	EHR report of numerator/denominator; will include proof of drug formulary checks

(continued)

T A B L E   5-6 (continued)

Stages 1 and 2 Documentation to Retain

Stage 1 Core Measures	Suggested Stage 1 Documentation	Exclusion Documentation	Changes for Stage 2
Medication list	EHR report of numerator/denominator	None	Incorporated into the summary of care measure
Medication allergy list	EHR report of numerator/denominator	None	Incorporated into the summary of care measure
Demographics	EHR report of numerator/denominator	None	EHR report of numerator/denominator
Vital signs	EHR report of numerator/denominator	Attestation is certifying that you either did not take care of any patients 2 years of age or older or that this is outside the scope for your specialty. Your specialty will be documented in the attestation system. You could run a registry report for the reporting period for patients 2 years or older and keep a copy or screen shot showing the result of the query.	EHR report of numerator/denominator Exclusion criteria changes, separating blood pressure from height and weight and applying to patients 3 years or older. Same type of proof suggested for exclusion.
Smoking status	EHR report of numerator/denominator	Same as vital signs except patients 13 years of age or older	EHR report of numerator/denominator
Report CQMs	You are attesting that you will follow through and submit the CQMs in that section of the attestation. If you don't, you will not meet MU, hence you will not be audited.	None	CQM reporting will be done electronically according to CMS specifications outside of attestation.
Clinical decision support rule	Screen shot of an alert generated by your EHR that is not a medication alert Your attestation is your legal certification that you met this measure by stating that this rule was turned on for the entire reporting period.	None	Screen shots of the required five clinical decision interventions chosen by you plus drug interaction checks

(continued)

T A B L E   5-6 (continued)

Stages 1 and 2 Documentation to Retain

Stage 1 Core Measures	Suggested Stage 1 Documentation	Exclusion Documentation	Changes for Stage 2
Electronic copy of health information	Keep a dated log for each week of reporting period indicating patient name, date of request, date delivered to patient, and type of electronic copy provided (thumb drive, CD, portal, PHR). If no requests, enter "none" each week and sign or initial by staff. Retain with other reports.	None	EHR report of numerator/ denominator for patients having access and for patients accessing information Screen shots of capabilities of portal
Clinical visit summary	EHR report of numerator/ denominator	A report showing that you had no office visits during the reporting period	EHR report of numerator/ denominator
Exchange of clinical information	This measure was deleted after 2012.	None	Incorporated into patient access measure
Protect electronic health information	Documentation of a security risk assessment being done prior to or during the EHR reporting period and annually thereafter Documentation of the analysis of the assessment and a mitigation plan to address any potential threats/risks A documented plan to address the deficiencies found during the assessment and the actions taken to correct them Policies and procedures with identified sanctions, a recorded inventory of technology, and proof of audits should also retained.	None	Same documentation as Stage 1: Document showing the security risk analysis as part of your risk-management process

(continued)

TABLE 5-6 (continued)

Stages 1 and 2 Documentation to Retain

Stage 1 Menu Set Measures	Suggested Stage 1 Documentation	Exclusion Documentation	Changes for Stage 2
Drug formulary check	Screen shot of a drug formulary report generated by your EHR Your attestation is your legal certification that you met this measure by stating that this functionality was turned on for the entire reporting period.	None	Incorporated into the e-Rx measure
Incorporate laboratory results	EHR report of numerator/denominator	Documentation of laboratory tests ordered that do not have positive, negative, or numeric results	EHR report of numerator/denominator
Patient list	Copy of patient list that was generated Your attestation is your legal certification that you generated a list of patients with a specific condition during the reporting period.	None	Copy of patient list report generated
Preventive reminders	EHR report of numerator/denominator	Same as vital signs and smoking status except report showing no patients 65 years or older or 5 years or younger	EHR report of numerator/denominator
Electronic access (portal)	EHR report of numerator/denominator	Report showing that you did not order or create information that would be included in medication list, medication allergy list, problem list, or laboratory results	EHR report of numerator/denominator for patients having access and for patients accessing information Screen shots of capabilities of portal
Patient education	EHR report of numerator/denominator	None	EHR report of numerator/denominator
Medication reconciliation	EHR report of numerator/denominator	Report or log showing you did not receive any patients in transition back to your practice	EHR report of numerator/denominator

(*continued*)

T A B L E   5-6 (continued)

Stages 1 and 2 Documentation to Retain

Stage 1 Menu Set Measures	Suggested Stage 1 Documentation	Exclusion Documentation	Changes for Stage 2
Summary of care record	EHR report of numerator/ denominator	Report or log showing you did not transfer or refer any patients during the reporting period	EHR report of numerator/ denominator for two calculations Documentation of proof that one summary was electronically sent to a recipient with a different EHR vendor or to the CMS test EHR
Immunization data submission	Screen shots of (1) the document electronically generated, (2) the documentation ready for export, (3) the acknowledgment that it was successfully sent or not, and (4) documentation from the public-health agency that received your submission Your attestation is your legal certification that you performed the test.	Letter from EHR vendor stating that the standards to send/receive in its product do not meet the standards in place at the IIS; documentation from your public-health agency of the standard it uses	Proof that ongoing submissions are successfully sent to your public-health agency
Syndromic surveillance data submission	Screen shots of (1) the document electronically generated, (2) the documentation ready for export, (3) the acknowledgment that it was successfully sent or not, and (4) documentation from the public-health agency that received your submission Your attestation is your legal certification that you performed the test.	Documentation that indicates that your public-health agency is not ready to accept the data submission or that standards for submission are not compatible	Proof that ongoing submissions are successfully sent to your public-health agency

Abbreviations: CMS, indicates Centers for Medicare & Medicaid Services; CPOE, computerized provider order entry; CQMs, clinical quality measures; EHR, electronic health record; e-Rx, electronic prescription; IIS, immunization information system; and PHR, personal health record.

TABLE 5-7

New Stage 2 Measures Documentation to Retain

New Stage 2 Core Measure	Suggested Stage 2 Documentation	Exclusion Documentation
Secure messaging	EHR report of numerator/ denominator Screen shot of deidentified secure message	Report showing no office visits during the reporting period or documentation that more than 50% of patients live in an area with limited broadband capability
Imaging results	EHR report of numerator/ denominator	Documentation that fewer than 100 tests that would result in an image were ordered or that there was no access to electronic imaging results at the *beginning* of the reporting period
Family history	EHR report of numerator/ denominator	Documentation of no office visits during the reporting period
Syndromic surveillance	See Stage 1 menu set measure	Documentation that you do not collect any syndromic surveillance data or that the public-health agency cannot receive, receive in a timely manner, or receive in a specific standard required by CEHRT at the *beginning* of the reporting period
Cancer case reporting	Same type of documentation as public-health measures in Stage 1	Documentation that you do not directly diagnose or treat cancer or that the public-health agency cannot receive cancer information as per other registry exclusion criteria
Specialized registry	Same type of documentation as public-health measures in Stage 1	Documentation that you do not diagnose or treat any disease associated with a specialized registry or sponsored by a national specialty society for which the EP is eligible or that the public-health agency cannot receive as per other registry exclusion criteria
Progress notes	EHR report of numerator/ denominator	None

Abbreviations: CEHRT indicates certified electronic health record technology; EHR, electronic health record; and EP, eligible professional.

Critical Point

Exclusions for menu set measures in 2014 will no longer count toward the number of menu set objectives needed to meet MU. If you meet the exclusion criteria for all five menu set measures with exclusions, then the progress note measure must be met to meet MU.

If there are multiple EPs from your practice who will be attesting and they all use a common certified EHR in *one shared practice location*, the testing for the public-health measures would only have to occur *once* for a given CEHRT. All EPs should retain proof of testing the submission of data in their own attestation documentation, as it will be individual EPs who may be selected for audit. The core measure to protect electronic health information could also be addressed at the practice level with documentation of the assessment, analysis, and plan completed once for the practice location and reviewed by all EPs at that location prior to attestation.

MINIMIZING SURPRISES

If you are not working with the regional extension center in your area and haven't secured the services of a consultant who can assist you with your attestation, then many surprises can be avoided by setting aside some time to prepare. Designate time to review your data and the specific requirements for each measure to make sure you have completed everything within the stipulated timeframes. The CMS Stage 1 vs Stage 2 Comparison Table for Eligible Professionals and Stage 2 Overview Tipsheet are great resources to use when checking your data. These are available in Appendix A.

It is important for you to monitor your performance on all of the Stage 1 (15) and 2 (17) core measures and for those menu set measures you have chosen to report on for Stage 1 (5 of 10) or Stage 2 (3 of 6). By periodically checking on how close you are to meeting the thresholds, it will be easier to focus your attention on those particular measures where you are not meeting the thresholds, to adjust workflows, and to educate the staff responsible for the documentation or action in a timely manner to satisfy the measure.

One measure where many EPs find themselves falling short of the required more than 50% threshold at the end of their 90-day reporting period is the clinical summary measure. Often, the checkout-desk staff is responsible for printing and providing patients with a clinical or visit summary at the end of their appointment. Many checkout staff will ask patients if they would like a copy of the summary. As most patients are not aware of the reason for, or usefulness of, a clinical summary, if staff ask a simple yes/no question with no additional explanation, many patients just answer "no" to receiving another piece of paper, and the conversation ends.

When performance on the measure is checked, the EPs, who thought patients were receiving a summary at checkout, are surprised to find that they are not meeting the measure. This can be easily corrected if the measure calculations are being monitored during the period of time leading up to attestation and the staff is following through on handing the summary to all patients. The 90-day average on each measure must meet or exceed the thresholds in order to meet MU. The 90-day period you thought was going to be your reporting period may need to be adjusted based on your findings.

Educating your staff about the purpose and usefulness of the clinical summary and about the MU requirement provides them with the knowledge they need to comfortably offer patients the summary at the end of the visit. As a result, they will be able to more confidently explain the usefulness and features of the summary to the patients at checkout and be more apt to hand out more clinical summaries. When the measure is recalculated, you will most likely see an increase in the percentage of visits at which patients did receive a clinical summary.

The CMS fact sheet for this measure explains other options for providing the clinical summary to patients. If the summary is not delivered at checkout, then a process for delivering a copy within 3 business days of the visit would need to be implemented in order to satisfy this measure for Stage 1. See Appendix A for further information.

Some possible ways to deliver a copy of the summary to patients within 3 business days of their visits are as suggested below.

1. Hand patients a clinical summary at the end of their visit.
2. Upload a summary to the patient's personal health record (PHR), a CD, or a USB fob at checkout.
3. Send a summary to the patient portal, and instruct patients in how to retrieve it.
4. Send a summary to the patient through secure e-mail.

This measure continues as a Stage 2 core measure, but in Stage 2, the summary must be delivered to patients within 1 business day of their visit. This short delivery window will narrow the options.

Hopefully, you registered for the EHR Incentive Program long before you intend to attest. Many EPs encounter some bumps along their way to successful registration because they have forgotten their user names or passwords for the Provider Enrollment, Chain, and Ownership System (PECOS) or need to apply for a National Plan and Provider Enumeration System (NPPES) identifier. If you have kept those in a safe place, have been gathering your data, and have assembled some supporting documentation, then you are getting close to being able to attest.

Double check your numerators and denominators, and compile all of your supporting documentation. Make sure your patient list was run during the reporting period and is time and date stamped (for audit purposes). If you have any concerns or questions about whether you have interpreted the measure correctly, talk with your EHR vendor or your peers, or access the information that is available online on the EHR Incentive Program Web site at www.cms.gov/Regulations-and-Guidance/Legislation/EHRIncentivePrograms/Down loads/EP-MU-TOC.PDF.

Now that everything is in place, you're almost ready to document that you have completed the requirements to be a meaningful user. Figure 5-2 is a flow chart that depicts the order of the steps you will go through to attest.

If you have been monitoring your performance on the measures and have been meeting the thresholds, one surprise you may encounter when attesting is the number of extra questions you will be asked during the data entry portion of your attestation. There are three valuable tools to help you prepare for these questions. The first tool is the Eligible Professional (EP) Attestation Worksheet for Stage 1 of the Medicare Electronic Health Record (EHR) Incentive Program in which you manually enter your numerators and denominators for the core and menu set measures. It is available in Appendix B and at www.cms.gov/Regulations-and-Guidance/Legislation/EHRIncentivePrograms/downloads /EP-Attestation-Worksheet.pdf.

FIGURE 5-2

EP Medicare Attestation Flow Chart

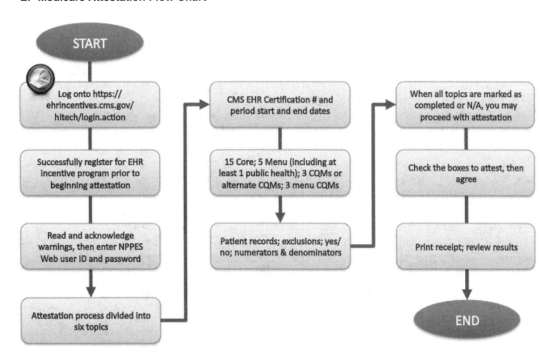

The second tool is the MU Attestation Calculator. This is an electronic tool that simulates what you will encounter when you enter the CMS site to attest. Numerators and denominators are entered into the tool and a summary of which measures you passed or failed, based on the data entered, will be provided at the end. The CQMs are not included. This tool is available at www.cms.gov/apps/ehr.

The third tool is the CMS Attestation User Guide for Eligible Professionals. This is an excellent tool that provides a screen shot of each screen you will encounter when you log in to attest. The guide walks you through the process of getting to where you will enter the data to attest, including all 15 core measures, 10 menu set measures, and 9 CQMs—3 core, 3 alternate core, and 3 other randomly chosen measures. This tool is available as part of the ancillary material of this book and at www.cms.gov/Regulations-andGuidance/Legisla tion/EHRIncentivePrograms/downloads/EP_Attestation_User_Guide.pdf.

When reviewing the guide, pay attention to the questions asked during attestation, particularly on the measure to provide an electronic copy of health information to patients within 3 business days, if they have requested a copy. If you have not received any such requests, you will be claiming exclusion from this measure. Once you answer that the exclusion *does* apply to you, you will not need to enter zeros for the numerator and denominator. Also, proceed carefully when answering the questions on the public-health measures to accurately reflect your ability to meet the exclusion criteria for these measures.

When you have completed entering your information for the core measures, you will begin the menu set measure section of attestation. First, you will have to designate which measure you have chosen for the required public-health measure, and then you will designate the four other menu set measures you have chosen to submit by checking the box next to each measure you have chosen. There are two exclusions to consider on each public-health measure and a third question to answer on two measures with yes/no answers—drug formulary and patient list. Read carefully before selecting your answers.

If you have selected clinical laboratory test results as one of your menu set measures, some EHRs produce reports that indicate that there were more laboratory results entered as structured data (numerator) than there were tests ordered (denominator). The attestation site will not allow you to enter a numerator larger than a denominator. For example, some EHRs count a CBC order as one order but then count the individual values returned via interface into the EHR in the calculation of the numerator. The CMS has asked that if you encounter this situation, you should enter the numerator as the same number that is the denominator. For potential audit purposes, make sure you indicate on your EHR-generated report what number you reported as your numerator, especially if the number is different from that is on your EHR-generated report.

Once you have completed the menu set measures, another area of caution is the order in which you enter your numerator and denominators. For the core and menu set measures, the numerator is entered first and then the denominator for each measure. For CQMs, the data-entry order reverses and the denominator is entered first, and then the numerator for each measure is entered. The clinical quality measures also have a requirement to enter the number of patients excluded from the measures, so look for those numbers on the report you have generated from your EHR—for example, patients with bilateral mastectomy excluded from the denominator of the mammogram quality measure.

Review the Attestation User Guide before attestation day, so you can prepare yourself for the questions you will be asked and the information that you will need to enter.

Thus far, you've been provided with some areas of caution, your numbers suggest that you have met the required thresholds, you've completed the tests to print or send electronic health information, and your security risk analysis has been written and deficiencies have been addressed. Congratulations! You are ready to attest.

HITTING THE SUBMIT BUTTON

MU attestation is an individual attestation by providers that reflects their use of the EHR for the patients they have seen during the reporting period in relation to the measures. You've worked hard to reach this point, and resubmitting your attestation because you have entered something incorrectly is not an easy process. Attest at a time and in a place where you can concentrate and complete the attestation without interruption. If all goes smoothly, the attestation will take less than the hour of time set aside.

The following list includes suggestions to simplify your attestation process.

- Print a copy of your 90- or 365-day report from your EHR for the measures.
- Gather your user name, password, and EHR certification number, and assemble these near the computer.
- It may be helpful to have someone with you who can read the numbers to you for each measure and to double check that the numerators and denominators have been entered correctly. Some of the questions you will need to answer may seem confusing at the time, and it can be helpful to have an extra pair of eyes in the room. Print an extra copy of your 90- or 365-day report for the person assisting you.
- Log in to the registration and attestation system, and click on the attestation tab.
- You should see your name, tax identification number, and National Provider Identifier, all of which were entered when you registered for the EHR Incentive Program.
- Click "Start Attestation," and you will then be prompted to enter your EHR certification number and the dates of your reporting period.
- If you are reporting Year 1, Stage 1, make sure the dates include at least 90 days in the same calendar year for the reporting period.
- Make sure that the dates of your reporting period on your EHR reports are the same dates you are entering into the attestation system.
- Complete the entry of your numerators and denominators for all core, menu set, and CQMs and carefully answer all of the questions asked.
- After you save your last CQM report, you will be sent to a screen that will indicate if all of the topics for attestation have been completed.
- This is your last opportunity to review or edit the information you have entered before you attest. Select any of the measure list tables to review your entered information.
- Select the "Edit" button if you find any errors in data entry.
- Select "Continue to Attest" if you are ready to attest.
- Review the attestation statements, and if you agree with the statements and are ready to attest, check the box next to each statement and click "Agree."
- If you are not ready to submit your attestation, click "Disagree," and you will be sent to the home page. The information you entered will be saved in the system.
- If you are ready to attest, you will click "Yes" after reviewing the information on the confirmation page.
- Read and agree to the attestation disclaimer.
- If your attestation was accepted and successful, you will receive a submission receipt. Print the receipt, and file it with your supporting documentation for this attestation.
- If you receive a rejected submission receipt, you did not demonstrate MU with the information submitted. You can review a summary of the measures and see which measure(s) were rejected.

- If you understand where the error occurred, you can resubmit your attestation, but it cannot be for the same 90-day period. Therefore, the reports from your EHR need to be rerun to reflect the new dates of attestation and any changes in numerator and denominator data.

- When ready to attest, you will go through the entire process again, hopefully resulting in an accepted submission.

WAITING FOR THE CHECK

Congratulations! Your hard work and your staff's hard work have allowed you to meet the MU requirements. The CMS has indicated that you can expect to receive your check within 4 to 8 weeks of successful attestation. The CMS does, however, have a requirement for each EP to reach $24,000 of Medicare-allowable charges before it will pay the incentive. The first-year incentive was 75% of the $24,000, or $18,000, in the Medicare program for meeting MU through 2012. If your first year of attesting is in 2013, the maximum incentive payment for Year 1 will be $15,000, or 62.5% of the $24,000 threshold.

If you attest early in the year, perhaps in April after completing a 90-day reporting period from January to March, and you have not reached the $24,000 of Medicare-allowable charges, you can still attest, but the CMS will hold issuance of the check until such time as you meet the $24,000 threshold. If you are an EP who sees few Medicare patients, it may take the majority of the calendar year to reach the threshold. Again, you can attest at any point that you have met the measures, but you may have a delay in receiving the payment from the CMS. Likewise, if you reach year end and have not met the $24,000, the CMS will issue a check for a percentage of the amount of allowable charges you reached, depending on the reporting year.

If you are registered for the Medicaid EHR Incentive Program, states are required to issue a check within 45 days of verifying that an EP has successfully attested. Medicaid payments are based on the year of reporting and the percentage of Medicaid patients according to regulation. The first-year payment is the largest. Payment amounts are lower through the rest of the payment years and are not dependent on consecutive years of meeting MU, as in the Medicare program. Also unlike the Medicare program, there are no payment reductions in the Medicaid program.

Your Medicare attestation submission receipt includes your attestation tracking information. If you believe you have met the $24,000 threshold and you do not receive your check within 4 to 8 weeks, have this tracking information handy for your phone call with the EHR information center help desk, which is available Monday to Friday from 8:30 AM to 4:30 PM in all time zones by calling 888-734-6433.

The check will arrive eventually, but remember that, in order to avoid a Medicare payment reduction, you must continue to meet MU in consecutive years. So enjoy your success, and then clarify when your next reporting period will begin and whether there are new measure requirements to learn about.

If 2013 is your first reporting year for Stage 1, then your reporting period is 90 days. If 2013 is your second reporting year for Stage 1, then you need to meet the measures for the full 2013 calendar year. No matter which stage or year of reporting, in 2014 all EPs will have a 90-day reporting period to account for the expected learning curve for vendors and EPs alike, who will face using a certified EHR that has been reconfigured to meet the new 2014 certification criteria. Please refer to Table 1-3 for the payment schedule for participants in the Medicare EHR Incentive Program.

SUMMARY

The documentation process to achieve Stage 1 MU is the foundation for EPs and their staff to document in the EHR and for them to be meaningful users of EHR technology. Successful attestation is facilitated by looking ahead to understand what needs to be completed or documented long before the end of a 90-day reporting period is reached, monitoring your performance regularly, and making changes as needed to meet the measure thresholds. This chapter has provided hints, lessons learned, and caution signs learned through the EP attestations of 2011 and 2012 and suggested many tools to assist you in your attestation. The knowledge shared has hopefully provided a map and smoothed the sometimes bumpy road to meeting MU to successfully attest and prepared you for the changes ahead.

What's in It for Physicians?

■ Attestation is the culmination of learning the requirements of participation in the EHR Incentive Program and working hard to meet the thresholds for the measures. If you have successfully attested, your EHR now has structured data that will allow you to run reports and give you access to information about your patients that you have not had previously, particularly if you are an EP in a small medical practice.

■ If you have successfully attested, the CMS will be sending you a check for your efforts to defray some of the costs associated with adopting the technology. Stage 2 builds on what you learned in Stage 1, and Stage 3 will build on Stage 2 and further advance the use of technology to assist you in the management of your patient populations.

What's in It for Staff?

■ The staff has been integral to any providers who have implemented the workflows necessary to meet all of the MU measures in their practice. It is hoped that the staff and EPs have worked together as a team to meet the measures, have learned the importance of consistency in their documentation in the EHR, and are enjoying their role in the practice using the EHR to document the care of their patients. MU is a journey toward providing better health care, and staff plays an important role in EPs' success in meeting MU.

What's in It for Patients?

■ If a patient's EP has successfully attested to MU of a certified EHR, the EP is alerted at the time of the visit if there are tests the patient is due for, the patient's medication list can be searched in the event of a medication recall, and his or her health information will be available in a format that will allow electronic exchange of information with other EPs on the patient's care team.

■ As MU stages progress, patients will have access to their health information electronically and be able to contact their provider using secure messaging. Their EPs will have access to the information they need to make good decisions, especially if patients have transitioned from one provider to another or from one facility to another.

ACTION ITEMS

1. Learn how to access your MU reports in your EHR. Determine whether or not you can run the reports when you want to monitor your progress on meeting the MU measures.

2. Run reports or obtain access to the information on how you are currently doing on meeting the measure thresholds, and then work as a team to improve where needed.
3. Print the tools mentioned in this chapter, and use them to prepare for attestation.
4. Save the documentation suggested in this chapter to support your attestation in case you are audited.
5. Check with your biller or run a report to know whether you have reached the $24,000 Medicare-allowable charges to date or in the previous year, so you will know if your check from the CMS will be arriving within 4 to 8 weeks after attestation.
6. Continue to monitor your practice's performance on meeting the measures, as the thresholds will increase and the measures will change as you progress through the MU stages.
7. Celebrate your accomplishment as a team.

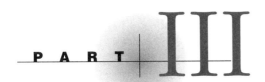

Clinical Aspects of Meaningful Use What Physicians Need to Consider: Patient Engagement and Leveraging Tools to Manage Outcomes

Physicians and their practices will undergo significant changes in both workflow and processes as they implement electronic health records (EHRs) and successfully attest to the Meaningful Use (MU) measures. With change comes opportunity. Physicians often do not have the luxury of stepping back to reflect how best to optimize their practice; MU provides them this opportunity.

In a health care environment that includes medical homes, accountable care organizations, pay for performance, and increasing reporting requirements, how can physicians leverage the EHR to help their practice succeed? Chapters 6 and 7 provide physicians a way to address these broader themes while meeting the MU requirements. They focus on a broader view of the MU themes around patient engagement, outcomes, and population health. These three themes encompass:

- The heart of a practice—the physician-patient relationship
- The nature of the practice—the population seen by the practice
- The practice's effectiveness—clinical outcomes

By combining the three, a physician can leverage the positive impact of the relationship (eg, better health outcomes, less litigation), the more effective management of a business (eg, population-level interventions that provide the largest return to the practice and the patient), and the quality of care delivered.

## chapter 6

Managing the Meaningful Patient Relationship

WHO SHOULD READ THIS CHAPTER?

This chapter should be read by physicians who are interested in thinking more broadly about how to effectively build meaningful relationships with their patients as they move from paper to electronic health records (EHRs). Physicians in all stages of EHR implementation will benefit from reading this chapter as it will inform the selection, implementation, workflow redesign, and use of an EHR and help them meet the "meaningful patient relationship" Meaningful Use (MU) objectives.

What you will learn in this chapter:

- How to build on patient engagement and reinforce a meaningful patient relationship
- How to leverage the meaningful patient relationship to meet MU objectives
- How to assess and redesign relevant workflows to include patient engagement
- What's in it for
  - Physicians
  - Staff
  - Patients
- Action items important for managing the patient relationship.

The physician-patient relationship is the foundation upon which quality care is delivered. The nature of this relationship has a significant effect on patient and family engagement, one of the four major themes driving Meaningful Use (MU).[1] This chapter will provide an overview of the characteristics important to developing a good physician-patient relationship, approaches to incorporating patients and family engagement within the practice, and the related MU measures. The other themes—improving quality, safety, and efficiency and reducing health disparities; improving care coordination; and improving population and public health—are discussed in more detail in Chapter 7.

Studies indicate that successfully engaging patients and families is a key component to providing high-quality health care.[2] Patient engagement is predicated on the establishment of a physician-patient relationship, which, in its ideal form, is based on choice, competence, communication, compassion, continuity, and no conflict of interest—referred to as the six Cs.[3] There are many articles that discuss the nature of this relationship and attributes in more detail. Another list of attributes includes empathy, trust, respect, availability, benevolence, compassion, competence, honesty, integrity, knowledge, reliability, respectfulness, sincerity, and understanding.[4] Moreover, the depth of the patient-physician relationship has been proposed to be a function of knowledge (about each other), trust, loyalty, and regard in the context of continuity of care and consultation.[5] For physicians, these attributes are a given, as all are aligned with the principles of medical ethics.[6] However, the physician-patient relationship has a more profound effect that goes beyond the principles of medical ethics and good bedside manners. A good relationship is positively associated with improved outcomes, increased patient satisfaction, compliance with the medical regimen, and adherence to healthy lifestyles.[2,4,7]

The three core elements of an effective physician-patient relationship include the ability of a physician to:

■   Elicit the patient's perspective.
■   Listen.
■   Facilitate shared decision making.

To obtain a true understanding of a patient's perspective about his or her illness and/or concerns, the physician needs to ask the right questions.

What to Do: Obtain a Patient's Perspective

One approach, the BATHE technique,[8] focuses on obtaining a more comprehensive assessment of a patient's situation by asking the following four questions and closing the exchange with empathy:

■   Background: What is going on in your life?
■   Affect: How do you feel about it?
■   Trouble: What troubles you the most?
■   Handling: How are you handling that?
■   Empathy: That must be very difficult.

Asking these questions will provide the physician with significant insights into the patient's state of mind but also enable the physician to effectively focus on the patient's priority issue (what troubles you most). However, this exchange is not effective without listening to what the patient and/or caregiver is saying. Listening is not only an essential component of clinical data gathering and diagnosis, but is also a healing and therapeutic agent and a means of fostering and strengthening the patient-physician relationship.[9] Last, patients need to be a partner in the decision-making process. To facilitate the patient's active participation in his or her own care, physicians should be able to apply underpinnings of behavioral change, which is especially important for chronic and preventable diseases. For example, the physician can apply the five "As" of patient counseling: assess, advise, agree, assist, and arrange. Making patients a partner in care (that is, enabling participatory care) is highly positively correlated with patient satisfaction, regardless of race or gender.[10]

As noted above, shared decision making is a core element of patient engagement and the physician-patient relationship.[11,12] For patients to make health care decisions and act on information provided by the physician, they need to understand and consider the courses of action available, the chances of both positive and negative outcomes, and their importance and desirability. Shared decision making supports not only patient-centered care as discussed by the Institute of Medicine,[13] but also informed consent. The physician should work with the patient (and caregiver) to reinforce joint priority setting and care planning throughout the patient-physician relationship. This should be documented within the electronic health record (EHR) and become part of the clinical summary shared with the patient as part of meeting the MU objectives discussed later.

What to Do: Implement a Process That Facilitates Shared Decision Making
Make sure to develop a process that incorporates the essential elements necessary to shared decision making[14] and implement appropriate tags into the visit documentation template.

- Define/explain the problem
- Present options
- Discuss pros/cons
- Clarify patient values/preferences
- Discuss patient ability
- Discuss recommendations
- Check patient's understanding
- Make or explicitly defer decision
- Arrange follow-up

Based on the nature of the practice and the disease/problem profile of the practice's patients, reflect on how best to reinforce and streamline this process.

HOW MU OBJECTIVES RELATE TO PATIENT ENGAGEMENT

There are a total of six measures (Stages 1–3) that align with the patient engagement MU theme. Table 6-1 provides a high-level overview of the six measures associated with patient engagement, expected results to the practice, and potentially relevant practice processes. Three of these objectives revolve around sharing information, captured within an EHR, with the patient and/or family. The other three cover the following different themes:

- Providing relevant educational resources to patients about their condition
- Reinforcing communications between the physician and the patient
- Enabling patients to participate in the electronic documentation process

T A B L E 6-1

Summary of MU Measures Aligned With Patient Engagement, Expected Results, and Clinical Practice Process

Measure	Description	Expected Results	Practice Touch Points
Stage 1			
Stage 1 core measure #12: electronic copy of health information	Provide patients with an electronic copy of their health information (including diagnostics test results, problem list, medication lists, medication allergies) upon request.	Increases practice efficiency: Time to make an electronic "copy" is likely a more cost-effective and efficient approach to providing clinical records than photocopying medical records. Improves shared decision making through increasing transparency	Office staff process: office staff to make an electronic copy or provide online access Physician process/review of history: physicians to support scenarios within their workflow where patients bring electronic copies of their health information to a visit

(continued)

T A B L E   6-1 (continued)

Summary of MU Measures Aligned With Patient Engagement, Expected Results, and Clinical Practice Process

Measure	Description	Expected Results	Practice Touch Points
Stage 1 core measure #12 (continued)		Increases access to patient clinical information. Patients can share the information with their other health care providers, which is important if no other clinical data exchange option is available or practical.	
Stage 1 core measure #13: clinical summaries	Provide clinical summaries for patients for each office visit.	Supports shared decision making

Reinforces discussions and treatment | Physician's process/documentation: Physicians will enter data for the clinical summary with components relevant to the patient; physicians will need to ensure that they finish their documentation as soon as possible (ideally, before the patient leaves).

Office staff process: (ideally, at end of visit) office staff to provide a copy of the clinical summary to the patient |
| Stage 1 menu set measure #5: patient electronic access | Provide patients with timely electronic access to their health information (including laboratory results, problem list, medication lists, and allergies). | Supports shared decision making

Reinforces discussions and treatment

Increases access to patient clinical information. Patients can share the information with their other health care providers, which is important if no other clinical data exchange option is available or practical. | Office staff process: office staff to ensure patients are provided access to their health information

Physician process/review of history: physicians to support scenarios within their workflow where patients bring electronic copies of their health information to a visit |
| Stage 1 menu set measure #6: patient-specific education resources | Use certified EHR technology to identify patient-specific education resources and provide those resources to the patient if appropriate. | Supports shared decision making

Reinforces discussions and treatment | Clinical process/patient education: clinical staff to provide educational resources to patients |

(continued)

T A B L E 6-1 (continued)

Summary of MU Measures Aligned With Patient Engagement, Expected Results, and Clinical Practice Process

Measure	Description	Expected Results	Practice Touch Points
Stage 2			
Stage 2 core measure: secure electronic messaging to patients	Use secure electronic messaging to communicate with patients on relevant health information.	Supports patient-physician communication Improves efficiency of practice as compared with phone calls	Practice process/between clinical appointments: office staff to implement process to support message routing; physician will need to respond to patient messaging that becomes part of the EHR.
Proposed Stage 3			
Patient-submitted data	Provide patients with ability to submit information.	Improves efficiency of practice as patients can update their information themselves Supports shared decision making	Office staff process: providing patients with access Physician process: review with patients and confirm

INCORPORATING MU SHARED DECISION MAKING INTO THE CLINICAL PRACTICE

If you are committed to improving the patient-physician relationship at the practice level, it is important to: (1) embed patient workflow into the clinical workflow practice; (2) consider patient (and caregiver) tools when looking at EHR and other health information technology (IT) solutions for the clinical practice; and (3) proactively obtain feedback on process and leverage that information to improve practice processes. We touch on each of these separately below. There are many ways to reinforce patient engagement, from before the visit to after the patient leaves the office.

The starting point is to consider a patient's workflow as part of the clinical workflow assessment and redesign for EHR selection, EHR use, and MU attestation.

Previsit: Scheduling Patient Visits

The process of a patient scheduling a visit has important ramifications to the patient-provider relationship. When you provide patients the ability to schedule an appointment online, you enable direct patient engagement and may support additional capabilities such as data self-entry (eg, presenting complaint/purpose of visit, updating of insurance information) and reminder support (automated appointment reminders via e-mail, voice mail, notice on portal, integration to patient's calendar). Although providing online scheduling is not an MU measure, Stage 3 measures propose allowing patients to enter information electronically, such as caregiver data. Moreover, supporting online scheduling will not only benefit the patient, but it can also improve the efficiency of the physician practice.

What to Do: Provide Patients the Ability to Schedule Appointments Online

First you need to capture workflow and requirements:

■ Identify optimal workflow, functionality, and processes to support online scheduling.

- ■ Determine scope of patient control: For example, if a practice would like patients to make a request for an appointment time, the system will need to generate a confirmation request to the front-office staff. Once confirmed, the system will need to notify the patient that the appointment was successfully booked. This is different from a workflow that enables a patient to directly schedule an appointment for an open time slot. In that instance, the front office does not need a product that enables a support-and-approval process. Practices will need to determine different scenarios relating to scheduling, and assess which aligns best with their practice.

- ■ Set policies: Should patients be allowed to see any physician in the practice? Who can schedule for a patient? Can patients cancel appointments online? If so, how close to the appointment? Is the patient automatically billed in advance for a scheduled appointment and does the patient lose that money if he or she does not show up?

Next you need to assess your technical options. Based on the workflows and requirements you have identified, you should prioritize the functionality you need in a system. Use that information as the basis to either compare different systems or assess whether a particular system can support your needs. Some functionality that may prove relevant and should be considered includes:

■ Does the office practice-management system (PMS) provide an online patient portal? If so, can EHR functionality be integrated into it?

■ Can the PMS enable online patient scheduling? If not, are there electronic patient scheduling software applications that integrate into the PMS?

■ Does the system automatically associate the patient with his or her "primary" physician? Does it support a broad range of actions such as requesting a time slot, scheduling, bill paying, and/or canceling (within a set timeframe)?

■ Does the system support the ability of the front office to block slots as needed for each clinician in the practice?

■ Are appointment reminders supported? This includes electronic notification to a patient (text or automated voice) or reminder for the front-office staff to call the patient.

■ It may be difficult to find unintegrated PMS and EHR systems that can provide an integrated patient portal. Are there clinical office Web-hosting sites that can integrate different application portals onto one site?

Capturing Patient Data

One of this first things a patient is asked to do at the physician's office is to fill out a paper form asking for clinical information such as family and personal history, risk factors, medications, and allergies. Providing the patient with a capability to enter this information either through a patient portal *before* a visit or electronically during the visit will not only facilitate patient-physician engagement but can improve the efficiency of the practice. The ability of patients to submit information electronically (eg, family history, functional status, medical devices) is being proposed as a Stage 3 measure. This is consistent with the increasing focus on having patients directly interact through electronic means, such as secure messaging, online portals, and personal health records (PHRs).

What to Do: Enable Patients to Electronically Enter Information Into the EHR/PMS

You need to set workflow, define functionality, and develop processes to manage the patient data.

- Determine what information should be entered by the patient. (Consider starting with the current intake forms and expand from there.)
- Determine who first reviews the information for accuracy with the patient. If it will be the physician, no other review is needed. How are data entry and interpretation errors addressed?

Patient Check-in

When a patient arrives at the office, consider what information is needed from the patient.

What to Do: Leverage Electronic Devices for Patient Use to Support Practice Workflows

You need to assess the need for and mode of patient data entry.

- If the practice provides patients with forms to fill out (eg, updating information such as allergies, medications, family history), consider replacing the paper version with an electronic one.
- If the data already exist, can these forms be prepopulated? Like most physicians, patients often complain when they need to fill out the same information over and over again.
- In thinking through hardware and software (EHR applications, portals, PMS), consider having an electronic device in the waiting room (eg, kiosk, secured tablet) for patients to use to fill out the forms. These tools can also be used to deliver educational information and decision aids to patients and their families as they wait.
- Determine how the data are denoted as entered by the patient and how they relate to the information entered by the physician.
- Determine whether or not the data entered can be confirmed as being reviewed by the physician or other clinician. Does the system copy the data into the clinical component of the record? How are changes dealt with?

Physician Documentation

The information discussed with the patient should be captured as part of the clinical note when appropriate. Although patients have had the right to get copies of their medical records since the enactment of the Health Insurance Portability and Accountability Act (HIPAA), including notes (with some exceptions), as a result of MU, patients will receive a clinical summary for each visit. This is an important shift in practice and requires that the physician take this fact into consideration when documenting the encounter. As a result, the clinical summary should support not only the needs of the clinician, but also those of the patient.

What to Do: Write the Clinical Summary With the Patient in Mind

There are several important considerations related to writing clinical summaries.

- Understand how the EHR builds the clinical summary to be shared with the patient (vs other physicians) and what is or is not customizable.

- Consider information necessary to support patient engagement and shared decision making (as discussed earlier).

- Ensure that documentation of the visit is completed as soon as possible. The benefit of completing it before the patient leaves is that the patient can be given the summary before he or she leaves, saving a potential step needed for office staff to send it to the patient.

- Assess if the EHR system is able to automatically provide the clinical summary via patient portal, secure e-mail, notification of office staff, or some other tools once the physician has completed his or her documentation.

- Be familiar with the scope for the clinical summary stipulated by the Centers for Medicare & Medicaid Services (summarized in Table 6-2), and assess an EHR's capability around it.

- Understand the potential benefits of clinical summaries, such as:

    - For the physician: to ensure the capture of robust data that are needed for other MU objectives and to support the delivery of quality care.

    - For the patient: to remind or inform about details of the clinical visit, including follow-up instructions.

    - For other physicians: to provide up-to-date information that might be relevant in the care of the patient after the visit—for example, in the emergency room.

    - For public health: to provide information about immunizations and other information that might be relevant during a public-health emergency.

TABLE 6-2

Components of a Clinical Summary as Defined by the CMS

Information Type	Description and Benefit	How Generated
Patient name	When printing or providing an electronic copy of a clinical summary, the patient's name should be included as a field. This ensures that the information is linked with the correct patient.	Office staff inputs during patient registration (entered once)
Provider's name[a] and office contact information	Providing contact information makes it easy for patients and other physicians to contact the office.	Office staff inputs during EHR setup (entered once)
Date of visit	It is important to document the date when the office visit occurred. This field is usually generated by the system.	EHR/PMS generated
Location of visit	If there are multiple offices, providing a location is important for the patient and office.	Office staff inputs during EHR setup (entered once) or selected by office staff
Reason for visit	This is also referred to as *chief complaint* and provides documentation as to why the patient came to visit the physician.	Office staff or patient inputs during scheduling; physician confirms

(*continued*)

TABLE 6-2 (continued)

Components of a Clinical Summary as Defined by the CMS

Information Type	Description and Benefit	How Generated
Current medication list[b] (Stage 1 core measure #5)	Providing an updated medication list is critical to helping patients keep track of their medications. Ideally, the medication list provides information not only of the name, dose, and frequency, but also the date first prescribed, which condition (problem) it is for, and any notes on how to take (eg, with food). To support medication reconciliation, there should also be a notation as to when last reconciled.	Physician enters, updates, and maintains (can be supported by other clinical staff).
Current medication allergy list** (Stage 1 core measure #6)	Providing patients with their updated medication allergy list is important. Other allergies are also important to include, such as food allergies. If there are no active medication allergies, an entry still must be made (eg, no known medication allergies). If drug-allergy alerts are enabled, this list should be based on a standard nomenclature. In addition to allergies, there should be a note as to the type of reaction.	Clinical staff enters, updates, and maintains; physician reviews
Vitals signs (Stage 1 core measure #8)	Vitals to be included are height, weight, calculated BMI, and blood pressure (for patients 2–20 years old, provide a growth chart). This provides patients with documentation they can use to track their vital signs.	Clinical staff updates; physician reviews
Procedures	If any procedures were carried out during the visit, they should be noted.	Physician/clinical staff inputs; physician confirms
Clinical instructions	Include written instructions to support verbal directions given. This is important for the patients/caregivers as they can refer to it once they leave the office.	Physician/clinical staff inputs
Problem list[b] (Stage 1 core measure #3)	Providing patients with a list of current and active diagnoses as well as past diagnoses relevant to their current care is important so that the patients can understand their medical problems.	Physician enters, updates, and maintains
Immunizations administered (Stage 1 core measure #9)	Include a list of any immunizations provided to the patient.	Physician/clinical staff inputs
Medications administered	Include a list of any treatment (medication, dose, route, and indication) provided to the patient.	Physician/clinical staff inputs.
Summary of topics covered/considered during visit (Stage 1 only)	It is helpful to summarize what was discussed with the patient from symptoms to treatment choices. This reinforces the patient-physician relationship and serves as a reminder after the visit.	Physician/clinical staff inputs (new)

(continued)

TABLE 6-2 (continued)

Components of a Clinical Summary as Defined by the CMS

Information Type	Description and Benefit	How Generated
Future appointments (time and location of next appointment)	If scheduled, provide time and location of next appointment or recommended timeframe to schedule with supporting information (for example, testing facility, consulting doctor); include scheduling of testing, referrals, next visit.	Office staff (locations can be prepopulated)
Recommended decision aids	Patient decision aids range in scope and complexity. At a basic level they provide information on the disease/condition, options, benefits, harms, scientific uncertainties. More advanced aids can provide probabilities of outcomes tailored to the patient's health risk factors and values clarifications such as describing outcomes in functional terms so that patients can consider which benefits and risks matter most to them.[15]	Physician/clinical staff inputs and provides materials (new)[c]
Future scheduled tests and pending tests (laboratory and other diagnostic test orders)	Summarizing any tests that have been ordered helps avoid duplication of orders and also provides a record of what results are still pending.	Physician inputs orders; office staff facilitates
Diagnostic test results[b] (if received within 24 hours after visit)	It is important for patients to get a copy of all of their test results.	EHR obtained; physician reviewed
Symptoms (Stage 1 only)	Capturing and sharing the symptoms that the patient experienced will reinforce to the patient that the physician listened and can prompt patients to remember if other symptoms were not shared.	Physician/clinical staff inputs
Referrals to other providers[a]	Listing information for patients relevant to referrals will provide them with needed information to schedule them.	Physician orders; office staff facilitates
Demographic information[a]	Providing demographic information (eg, sex, race, ethnicity, date of birth, and preferred language) will enable other health care providers to quickly capture this information and help mitigate errors in patient identification and reduce fraud.	Office staff enters during patient registration (entered once)
Smoking status[a]	Providing smoking status will aid other health care providers in documentation and also allow for multiple intervention points for patients who smoke.	Physician/clinical staff inputs
Care plan fields[a]	Care plan fields, such as goals and instructions, allow for exchange of information related to continuity of care, especially for patients who need additional support such as home health care.	Physician/clinical staff inputs (new)[c]

Abbreviations: BMI indicates body mass index; EHR, electronic health record; and PMS, practice-management system.
[a]Additions made for Stage 2;
[b]Minimum required for Stage 1 (for Stage 2 all information recorded in the EHR for the fields is required).
[c]New denotes documentation that may be a variation from current practice.

Table 6-2 points to an increased documentation burden for physicians in creating the clinical summary. How physicians set up and implement their documentation within the EHR system will significantly affect their business (eg, time needed for documentation). Physicians will need to balance the documentation burden with the business benefit. This includes what can be documented by the patient, nurse, or other office staff. Another critical decision revolves around what is free text vs controlled text (eg, drop-down, checkbox); the latter is critical for reporting. Refer to Chapter 7 for details relating to reporting requirements (eg, clinical quality measure reporting, public-health reporting).

Patient Education

As discussed earlier in relation to patient engagement, providing patients (and caregivers) access to health education resources relevant to them is important to helping them understand their medical problems and which treatment might be best for them. Stage 1 MU menu measure #6 requires that an EHR provide a physician access to patient education aids that are "tailored" to patients based on their problem list, medication list, or laboratory results.

Critical Point

Stage 1 MU menu set measure #6 ensures that the EHR can provide physicians with patient-specific education resources.

- The EHR should support the presentation of identified patient-specific education resources to the physician based on the patient's problem list, medication list, or laboratory results.
- Practices can deliver this to the patient in a range of formats, including hard copy, online via a patient portal, or in a PHR.

The physician office should assess different options for supporting the informational and resource needs of their patients. Physicians should not limit themselves to the resources presented within an EHR. Resources may be important to provide to patients to improve health outcomes and can be made available through patient portals. Some EHRs will allow physicians to upload resources into the system in a way that supports the MU objective. (For MU attestation, the numerator for Stage 2 specifies that only patient-specific education resources identified by the certified EHR technology can be counted, whereas in Stage 1 it does not.)

What to Do: Identify and Provide Relevant Educational Resources to the Patient
Consider the following in preparation for providing patient-specific educational resources.

- Explore what types of resources would be most appropriate for your patient population. For example, in a practice with a significant number of obese or overweight patients, identifying resources for weight-loss programs and/or support groups could be very helpful. Links to these resources can be added to a patient portal. Carefully select these resources, and make sure they are credible.
- Find relevant information for patients that engage them in decision making. For patients and their families who need to make treatment decisions, decision aids have additional benefits that go beyond the other types of information listed. Several randomized controlled trials of patient decision aids show they are better than standard care in terms of[7]:

- Increasing participation in decision making without increasing anxiety
- Improving decision quality
- Improved knowledge of options, benefits, harms
- More realistic expectations of the probabilities of benefits and harms
- Better match between personal values and choice
- Lowering decisional conflict
- Helping undecided people to decide

- Gather or build a set of patient decision aids. Patient decision aids may also play a role in addressing underuse and overuse of options. They have been shown to reduce the uptake of expensive surgical options. They also increase the uptake of colon cancer screening options, which are underused, and lower the rates of prostate cancer screening tests, which are overused.[7] Some resources that you can leverage include:
  - For patients: the Effective Health Care Program (Agency for Healthcare Research and Quality) at http://www.effectivehealthcare.ahrq.gov.
  - For clinicians: the Effective Health Care Program (Agency for Healthcare Research and Quality) at www.effectivehealthcare.ahrq.gov/index.cfm.
  - The Informed Medical Decisions Foundation at http://informedmedicaldecisions.org.
  - The Patient Decision Aids from the Ottawa Hospital Research Institute at http://decisionaid.ohri.ca/index.html.
- Understand the capabilities of the EHR to provide, manage, and present resources.
- When assessing an EHR and/or a patient portal, consider the resources available through it for patient education.
- Find out whether or not materials can be added within the EHR that can leverage the EHR's ability to match resources to the appropriate problem, medication, or laboratory result.
- Determine if there are patient-specific educational resources available in different languages and tailored for different ethnic groups, if relevant to the practice.

Physician-Patient Communication

As discussed earlier, an important aspect of the physician-patient relationship is communication. Communicating with patients in an electronic format, with agreed-to parameters, has been found to improve the efficiency of clinical practices.[16] For example, electronic messaging resulted in decreased phone call volume.[17] Moreover, patients were overwhelmingly satisfied and physicians and staff generally satisfied with the use of Web messaging between patients and the provider practice.[17] Secure messaging is a Stage 2 core measure that supports the asynchronous ability to communicate between the physician and the patient. This secure messaging currently focuses on point-to-point communication (eg, EHR to PHR message or EHR to patient portal message).

What to Do: Engage in Secure Electronic Messaging With Patients
Incorporate guidelines for communications, such as those listed below[18]:

- Establish turnaround times.
- Inform patients about privacy issues.
- Define the types of transactions and sensitivity of subject matter permitted—eg, prescription refill, appointment scheduling.
- Provide subject-line guidance to patients—eg, prescription, appointment, billing.

- Have patients include their name and identification number within the body of the message.
- Configure automatic reply to acknowledge receipt.
- Place all copies of messages, replies, and confirmations of receipt within the EHR.
- Send a message when patient-request is completed—eg, message to the patient that the refill request has been completed.
- Request patients use auto reply to acknowledge that they've read the provider's message.
- Maintain patient mailing lists, but use blind copy feature to maintain privacy.
- Be professional, and make sure content is appropriate.
- Have a signed patient-physician agreement for informed consent for the use of electronic messaging.
- Share communication guidelines and terms.
- Provide instructions for when and how to convert to phone calls or office visits.

Critical Point

A Stage 2 MU core measure requires secure messaging from patients.

- To support increasing physician-patient interaction, Stage 2 focuses on demonstrating patient engagement—specifically, patients sending secure messages to their physician (5% threshold).
- There is an exception available in areas without broadband availability.

WHAT TO CONSIDER WHEN SUPPORTING PATIENT-PHYSICIAN ELECTRONIC COMMUNICATION

Since the communication between the patient and the physician is part of the medical record (documentation) the physician will need to assess how the EHR supports this functionality. For example, if the EHR does not provide the infrastructure for communication, what is the approach to link the communication to the patient record?

Access to Clinical Information

Once a patient leaves the physician office, 40% to 80% of the medical information provided by the physician is immediately forgotten.[19] This is one reason why it is important to provide patients access to their medical record.

What to Do: Provide Patients Access to Their Medical Record
Consider the following in relation to patient access:

- Provide electronic access to the medical record. Providing patients and their caregivers access to their medical information ensures that they will be able to review it when they are home. This includes making an electronic copy of their medical record available to patients for Stage 1 (core measure #12).
- Provide electronic access to test results. Physician offices need to develop appropriate policies and procedures to notify patients of test and diagnostic results so that they will be made electronically available within 4 days (Stage 1 menu set measure #5). This may not be a problem for normal or negative findings. However, some findings may be

more appropriate for the physician to discuss with the patient in person or by phone—for example, a positive HIV test or cancer biopsy.

- Make the clinical summary available to patients. MU requires that patients receive their clinical summary shortly after their visit. Physicians should prepare to make clinical summaries available to their patients within 1 day in Stage 2.

Critical Point

Stage 1 MU core measure #12 focuses on providing patients with an electronic copy of their medical record.

- There is a move to increased electronic interaction with patients. This is true for providing patients access to their medical records. From Stage 1 to Stage 2, the timeline to provide access increases from 3 days to 4 days. However, the scope of the information shared increases.
- There is a difference regarding the electronic format. Stage 1 requires an electronic copy of the patient's information be made available. This could be achieved via, for example, patient portal, PHR, or CD. Stage 2 mandates online access with the ability to download and transmit health information.
- Stage 2 requires that 5% of patients should be accessing their record online.
- This requirement is limited to information that exists electronically in or is accessible from the certified EHR technology. At a minimum, diagnostic test results, problem list, medication list, and medication allergies list must be provided.
- Eligible professionals (EPs) can charge a reasonable, cost-based fee.
- EPs may choose to withhold certain information if substantial harm may arise from disclosure.

Copying Data and Providing the Data to a Patient

Providing patients with an electronic copy of their health information can be accomplished in a variety of ways. The first step in the process is to ascertain how a specific EHR supports patient data downloads and what formats are available. For example, does the information get presented in a document (such as a PDF) format or is an "EHR-viewer" application provided so that the information is seen in a specific format? Can this be saved to a thumb drive or CD/DVD? Can an EHR export data in a specific format (HL7) that can be uploaded into another EHR or a PHR? Can it be sent from one device or application to another? One example is the Blue Button. The Blue Button is an application developed for the Veterans Administration (VA) to support veterans in their ability to download data from their VA PHR. Although started with the VA (My HealtheVet and TRICARE Online), the private sector (eg, UnitedHealth Group, Aetna, and Kaiser) is also adopting it (go to www.va.gov/bluebutton for more information).

What to Do: Determine the Format for Sending Information to Patients
When deciding how to provide electronic information to patients, consider the following issues:

- If you are interested in sending this information via e-mail, there are several additional issues to consider (see guidance on secure messaging earlier in this chapter).[18] Consider getting a patient's informed consent to use e-mail. Encrypt the message; if a patient wants to waive the encryption requirement, make sure that this waiver is captured in the record. Advise the patient to use a personal rather than a work e-mail address.

Work e-mails are *not* private. Make sure to save the e-mails as part of the patient's medical record.

■ Each EHR may have a different process for downloading information about a specific patient. If functionality is limited or the type of data that can be downloaded for a patient is limited, there may be other options. Some EHRs have the ability to embed physician-selected clinical data into a "consult request" letter. This may be a work-around if another mechanism for getting a copy of patient-requested data is not supported.

■ When considering approaches to providing electronic access to clinical information, explore EHR capabilities. For example, does the EHR provide a patient portal functionality? Does it provide a mechanism for electronically downloading patient clinical data onto an electronic medium?

■ Can you select what information is accessible to the patient? If you can select the information to be shared, make sure that the minimum information requirements are met (eg, diagnostic test results, problem list, medication list, and medication allergies list for Stage 1).

■ Determine what ability the EHR has for providing patients with appropriate resources.

Critical Point

Stage 1 MU menu set measure #5 focuses on providing patients with electronic access to their medical information .

■ Patients must have access to their medical information within 4 days after that information is available to the physician unless the physician determines that sharing the results should best be done in person or on the phone.

■ At a minimum, diagnostic test results, problem list, medication list, and medication allergies list must be provided.

■ Physicians may choose to withhold certain information if substantial harm may arise from disclosure.

■ This is no longer a measure for Stage 1 in 2014 as it will be subsumed by Stage 2 MU core measure #12.

■ The measure specifies online access to a patient portal or PHR, but the information can be communicated in other ways if the physician deems it more appropriate.

What to Do: Support Electronic Access to Clinical and Other Related Data

Review the two rights that HIPAA Privacy Rule grants individuals as those rights apply to this measure. They include the ability to:

■ View and obtain a copy of much of their health information, such as:
  ■ Medical records,
  ■ Billing records,
  ■ Enrollment and claims records, and
  ■ Other information used by the covered entity to make decisions about them
■ Have corrections made to such information.

In the context of EHRs and patient portals owned by covered entities, the HIPAA requirements apply. Think about how you will support these requests in an EHR-enabled environment. Consider functionality needed to support a PHR or patient portal.

Critical Point

Stage 1 MU core measure #13 requires the provision of a clinical summary for each patient visit.

- There is a significant reduction in the timeframe for providing the clinical summary from 3 days in Stage 1 to 1 day in Stage 2.
- The information provided to patients must include all the items listed as part of a clinical summary (see Table 6-2). At a minimum, for Stage 1, the information must include diagnostic test results, problem list, medication list, and medication allergies list (similar to Stage 1 core measure #12).
- Physicians may choose to withhold certain information if substantial harm may arise from disclosure.
- For complex patients or where patient visits last several days and the patient is seen by multiple eligible providers, a single summary at the end of the visit can be used.
- Physicians cannot charge a fee for this information.
- The information can be provided in a variety of ways, including patient portal, PHR, CD, thumb drive, secure e-mail, paper copy.

PATIENT/CAREGIVER TOOLS

Providing patients and caregivers tools can provide significant benefits to the physician practice. These tools can range from interactive decision aids that can help improve health outcomes to scheduling applications that can reduce administrative costs. For patients and caregivers to access these tools, physicians will need to provide access through a physician-practice Web site, patient portal, or PHR.

Patient Portal

As MU requirements for patient communications increase, consider patient portals. The term *portal* is often used to describe an access point within the Internet. The portal is a secure Web site that can be the entry point for the patient into an application tied to a physician's EHR, the patient's PHR, or another service. In this chapter, we will refer to the patient portal as a secure Web site where patients can access services and patient health information provided by a physician. It can support interaction and communication between patients and their health care providers. Some of the basic functionality of a patient portal allows patients to:

- Check appointment schedules.
- Request (with preferred dates and times) appointments and receive reminders.
- Review clinical (EHR) data.
- Access clinical information such as laboratory results and clinical summaries.*
- Request prescription refills.
- Fill in documentation/forms.
- Access health-related education materials.*
- Exchange messages with physicians and members of their practice.*
- Access statements, insurance information.

When looking at EHR functionality, keep in mind that the patient portal services listed above will help your office's workflow, improve patient satisfaction, and facilitate attestation of many of the consumer-focused MU measures. (The items marked with an asterisk are related to MU.)

What to Do: Consider Patient/Caregiver Tools When Looking at EHRs and Other Health IT Solutions

When considering a patient portal, keep in mind the following:

- When assessing the different EHR and other health IT solutions, there are many functionalities to consider, including electronic scheduling, communications, patient data entry, resources, and access to clinical information. The core functionality that a physician will need to support any of these functionalities is a patient portal. A patient portal is an access point for a patient to sign into and interact electronically with the physician office. Physicians should identify what functionality is needed to support their patient-engagement workflow and assess the current functionality of an EHR to support these capabilities.

- Ask your EHR vendor for details related to future proposed functionalities and what relevant applications they interface with.

Personal Health Records

A PHR is an electronic record of an individual's health information by which the individual controls access to the information and may have the ability to manage, track, and participate in his or her own care. It also provides the potential to create the individual's longitudinal health history. PHRs also allow patients to capture information created by themselves, such as glucose level, health notes, blood pressure, or over-the-counter-medication use.

There are many different vendors of PHRs being offered to consumers that vary in functionality, cost, data-exchange capabilities with EHRs, educational materials, and health-related applications. If the PHR is offered and/or maintained by a covered health care provider or health plan, it falls under the HIPAA Privacy Rule; otherwise, it does not.[20]

If your patient is using a PHR hosted by a third party, have the patient understand that you have no knowledge or control over the privacy policies of the PHR company, how the information is safeguarded, how the information will be used and disclosed, and how access to the data within the PHR is controlled. If you are asked to send information to the site, it may be wise to have the patient sign a waiver of liability/responsibility.

There may be challenges related to the ability to exchange clinical data between a physician's EHR and the consumer's PHR. It is useful to find out what, if any, PHRs have been interfaced with a specific EHR and if there are any additional costs for supporting data exchange. The data exchange could be as simple as downloading clinical information requested by a patient in a specific format to a thumb drive or CD or it could be as complex as a real-time data exchange between applications through a health information exchange.

OBTAIN FEEDBACK FROM PATIENTS

For physicians and their practices that are committed to developing strong physician-patient relationships and empowering their patients, it is necessary to implement a feedback process.

What to Do: Proactively Obtain Feedback on Processes and Leverage That Information to Improve Them

Continually improve patient-engagement processes by gathering patient experiences, suggestions, and feedback through a variety of methods such as:

- Questions as part of the consultation
- Patient and caregiver interviews
- Postappointment calls to patients
- Complaint review
- Group feedback
- Patient satisfaction surveys
- Patient stories

Physicians and their practice staff should review their findings and address any deficiencies. This can be done by an annual practice assessment.

SUMMARY OF MEANINGFUL USE REQUIREMENTS

It is important for the physician to understand that the MU requirements for patient engagement will continue to grow from Stage 1 to Stage 2 and beyond. Consider the changing requirements as you select, implement, and optimize your workflow. Table 6-3 summarizes the high-level changes that you can expect. Moreover, it also summarizes the technical and format options needed to support them (eg, patient portal). To effectively meet Stage 1 criteria, physicians need either a patient portal or a tethered PHR (tied to the physician's EHR) as part of their office's technical infrastructure.

TABLE 6-3

Summary of High-Level Changes in MU Measures Related to Patient Engagement and Their Implications for Technology Needs

Measure	Stage 1	Stage 2	Directions for Stage 3
Electronic copy of health information	Core measure #12: provide patients with an electronic copy of their health information (including diagnostic test results, problem list, medication lists, medication allergies) upon request. More than 50% of those requesting this information provided it within 3 days	Replaced by Stage 2 core measure 7: patient electronic access (see below under patient electronic access measure)	N/A
Technology:	*Patient portal, PHR, electronic media (eg, CD, thumb drive)*		

(continued)

T A B L E 6-3 (continued)

Summary of High-Level Changes in MU Measures Related to Patient Engagement and Their Implications for Technology Needs

Measure	Stage 1	Stage 2	Directions for Stage 3
Clinical summaries	Stage 1 core measure #13: provide clinical summaries for patients for each office visit. Clinical summaries provided for more than 50% of all office visits within 3 business days	Stage 2 core measure #8: time reduced from 3 to 1 business day; expansion of data fields (eg, demographic, smoking) and removal of others (eg, symptoms)	Make clinical summary pertinent to the office visit.
Technology:	*Patient portal, PHR, secure e-mail, electronic media (eg, CD, thumb drive), or paper copy*	*Patient portal, PHR, secure e-mail, electronic media (eg, CD, thumb drive), or paper copy*	
Patient electronic access	Stage 1 menu set measure #5: provide patients with timely electronic access to their health information (including laboratory results, problem list, medication lists, and medication allergies) within 4 business days of the information being available to the physician. At least 10% of patients provided electronic access	Stage 2 core measure #7: provide patients the ability to view online, download, and transmit their health information within 4 business days of the information being available to the EP. More than 50% of patients provided access and more than 5% of patients view, download, or transmit the information within 4 business days. Expanded information requirements: patient name, provider's name, and office contact information; current and past problem list; procedures; laboratory test results; current medication list and medication history; current medication allergy list and medication allergy history; vital signs (height, weight, blood pressure, BMI, growth charts); smoking status; demographic information (preferred language, sex, race, ethnicity, date of birth); care plan field(s), including goals and instructions and any known care-team members, including the primary-care provider of record	Expectation that if data are generated during the course of the visit that the information should be available within 24 hours. There may be a move to include an automated transmit capability (eg, Automated Blue Button Initiative[21])
Technology	*Electronic access through either patient portal or PHR*	*Electronic access through either patient portal or PHR with additional capability to download and transmit data*	

(continued)

T A B L E   6-3 (continued)

Summary of High-Level Changes in MU Measures Related to Patient Engagement and Their Implications for Technology Needs

Measure	Stage 1	Stage 2	Directions for Stage 3
Patient-specific education resources	Stage 1 menu set measure #6: use certified EHR technology to identify patient-specific education resources and provide those resources to the patient if appropriate. More than 10% of patients provided resources	Stage 2 core measure #13: same as in Stage 1 with a change in how measured: requires that only those patient-specific education resources identified through the certified EHR be counted in the numerator	Provide educational materials in the patient's language.
Technology	*Format not specified*	*Useful format for the patient (such as, electronic copy, printed copy, electronic link to source materials, through patient portal or PHR)*	
Secure electronic messaging to patients	N/A	Stage 2 core measure #17: use secure electronic messaging to communicate with patients on relevant health information. More than 5% of patients sent secure message by a certified EHR. Exception: limited access to broadband	Increase messaging to 10%.
Technology		*E-mail or the electronic-messaging function of a PHR, an online patient portal, or any other electronic means*	
Patient-submitted data	N/A	N/A	Provide patients the ability to submit patient-generated health information to improve performance on high-priority health conditions and/or to improve patient engagement
Technology			*Patient portal or PHR*
Patient able to request amendment	N/A	N/A	Provide patients the ability to request an amendment to their record online
Technology			*Patient portal or PHR, secure messaging*

Abbreviations: BMI indicates body mass index; EHR, electronic health record; N/A, not applicable; and PHR, personal health record.

SUMMARY

Leverage the process of attesting for MU to build infrastructure and workflows to support a meaningful patient relationship. The benefits of doing so translate into improved patient relationships, improved patient outcomes, improved quality measures, reduced medical malpractice rates, and other financial and nonfinancial benefits (eg, pay for performance).

What's in It for Physicians?

- Physicians have an opportunity to benefit greatly from patient engagement and meaningful use of their EHR. As EHR vendors improve functionality to support patient engagement, physicians will benefit. When choosing wisely, optimizing use, and integrating their EHRs with appropriate tools, physicians will be able to achieve:
  - Efficiencies in patient scheduling, insurance updates, and patient intake.
  - Improved patient outcomes as a result of increased patient engagement.
  - Improved patient satisfaction and physician-patient relationships.
  - Streamlined and cost-effective online delivery of patient education and resources.

What's in It for Staff?

- The office staff are critical team members for an effective, positive physician-patient relationship. They work with the patient throughout the process, from setting up an appointment to providing patients copies of their record or health information to scheduling tests and consults to sending them reminders. Moving to leverage EHRs and the enhanced ability to electronically interact with patients will help streamline their work. Patients can electronically make appointments (saving phone calls), fill in insurance and clinical data directly (saving typing it into the system), and access their clinical information. This enables the staff to focus on the content and not on data entry.

What's in It for Patients?

- Patients and their caregivers benefit greatly from the tools and resources being provided by their physician through meaningful use of their EHR. They are able to access their clinical information, download it, and potentially manage it in their own PHR. Their physicians may also provide patients vetted resources and decision aids so that they can be more informed when having to make difficult health decisions and will be able to better manage their own health. All of these activities will enhance patients' relationships with their physicians and ultimately result in better, more satisfying care and better health.

ACTION ITEMS

1. Assess EHR/PMS functionality to support patient engagement—for example, patient portal, educational resources, documentation templates, secure messaging, and data-sharing control (being able to select what information can be shared with the patient and when).
2. Evaluate how well you address the following components necessary to support a strong physician-patient relationship:
   - How effective are you in gaining a patient's perspective?
   - How well do you listen to a patient?
   - How well do you engage a patient as an active partner in his or her care?

3. Assess your interaction and documentation around patient engagement (check **Step** if you perform the step; check **EHR** if you are documenting what you've done in an EHR).

   a. Define/explain the problem   Step ____   EHR ____
   b. Present options   Step ____   EHR ____
   c. Discuss pros/cons   Step ____   EHR ____
   d. Clarify patient values/preferences   Step ____   EHR ____
   e. Discuss patient ability   Step ____   EHR ____
   f. Discuss recommendations   Step ____   EHR ____
   g. Check patient's understanding   Step ____   EHR ____
   h. Make or explicitly defer decision   Step ____   EHR ____
   i. Arrange follow-up   Step ____   EHR ____

   Based on the assessment, determine which steps are missing and how they may be better incorporated into patient interactions and your documentation process.

4. Build processes and workflows to enhance the physician-patient relationship. Include patient workflow in clinical workflow.
5. Enable shared decision making, such as joint priority setting and care planning, and document these activities in the EHR.
6. Create a visit documentation template that captures the essential elements necessary to shared decision making that aligns with the nature of the practice and disease/problem profile of the patient.
7. Develop workflow and processes to enable the patient to get access to the clinical summary in a timely manner.
8. Develop office process for making electronic copies of patient health information.
9. Think about what information that needs to be entered into the EHR can potentially be entered by a patient. This includes any forms the patient or the office staff complete based on what the patient tells them. This could include new patient forms, insurance data, current conditions, family history, and so on. Assess workflow implications and value. If positive, assess technical approaches to support patient data entry. This includes assessing EHR or patient portal capabilities in data capture and integration into the record.
10. Develop office processes to provide patients and caregivers access to their online health information (eg, passwords, rules regarding access by other family members/care-givers).
11. Make sure that online patient access is supported. This includes support for password retrieval, appropriate use guidelines, patient education on how to use, and technical support.
12. Develop process for dealing with electronic health data brought into the practice for the physician to review (eg, have a nonnetworked computer available to view information to minimize risk of virus or a mechanism to upload the relevant information) that meets the needs and style of the office.
13. If your system supports online patient scheduling, determine those hours you want to make available and those that you would like to reserve for consults, calling patients, and so on.
14. Explore resources relevant to your patient population available on the EHR or through other online sources.
15. Assess the ability of the EHR to link to or add external resources in a manner consistent with the MU requirements.

16. Leverage EHRs and other technologies to support patients and gain practice efficiencies (eg, online patient scheduling, patient portals, online patient data-entry forms).
17. Assess clinical summary functionality and how best to ensure that it supports MU attestation requirements.
18. Consider different approaches to support electronic exchange of information with your patients.
19. Develop processes to support secure electronic messaging between the office and patients. Make sure to educate patients about how to use electronic communications.

REFERENCES

1. Health IT Policy Committee. Policy: Meaningful Use Subgroup #3 Improve Care Coordination. August 2012. www.healthit.gov/policy-researchers-implementers/policy-meaningful-use-sub group-3-improve-care-coordination. Accessed August 28, 2012.
2. Berry LL, Parish JT, Janakiraman, R, et al. Patients' commitment to their primary physician and why it matters. *Ann Fam Med*. 2008;6(1):6-13.
3. Emanuel EJ, Dubler NN. Preserving the physician-patient relationship in the era of managed care. *JAMA*. 1995;273(4):323-329.
4. Grant SB. Are there blueprints for building a strong patient-physician relationship? *Virtual Mentor*. 2009;11(3):232-236.
5. Ridd M, Shaw A, Lewis G, Salisbury C. The patient-doctor relationship: a synthesis of the qualitative literature on patients' perspectives. *Br J Gen Pract*. 2009;59(561):e116-e133.
6. American Medical Association. *Principles of Medical Ethics*. Revised June 2001. www.ama-assn.org/ama/pub/physician-resources/medical-ethics/code-medical-ethics/principles-medical-ethics.page?_Accessed January 23, 2013.
7. O'Connor AM, Bennett CL, Stacey D et al. Decision aids for people facing health treatment or screening decisions. *Cochrane Database Syst Rev*. 2009.
8. Stuart MR, Lieberman JA. *The Fifteen Minute Hour: Therapeutic Talk in Primary Care*. Oxford, England: Radcliffe Publishing; 2008.
9. Jagosh J, Boudreau JD, Steinert Y, Macdonald ME, Ingram L. The importance of physician listening from the patients' perspective: enhancing diagnosis, healing, and the doctor-patient relationship. *Patient Educ Couns*. 2011;85(3):369-374.
10. Cooper-Patrick L, Gallo JJ, Gonzales JJ, et al. Race, gender, and partnership in the patient-physician relationship. *JAMA*. 1999;282(6):583-589.
11. Prochaska JO, Velicer WF. The transtheoretical model of health behavior change. *Am J Health Promot*. 1997;12(1):38-48.
12. Ruggiero L, Redding A, Rossi JS, Prochaska JO. A stage-matched smoking cessation program for pregnant smokers. *Am J Health Promot*. 1997;12(1):31-33.
13. The National Academy of Sciences, Board on Health Care Services. *Crossing the Quality Chasm: A New Health System for the 21st Century*. Washington, DC: The National Academies Press; 2001. Available at: www.nap.edu/catalog.php?record_id=10027. Accessed January 23, 2013
14. Makoul G, Clayman ML. An integrative model of shared decision making in medical encounters. *Patient Educ Couns*. 2006;60(3):301-312.
15. Elwyn G, O'Connor AM, Bennett C, et al. Assessing the quality of decision support technologies using the International Patient Decision Aid Standards instrument (IPDASi). *PLoS One*. 2009;4(3):e4705.
16. Wallwiener M, Wallwiener CW, Kansy JK, Seeger H, Rajab TK. Impact of electronic messaging on the patient-physician interaction. *J Telemed Telecare*. 2009;15(5):243-250.
17. Liederman EM, Lee JC, Baquero VH, Seites PG. Patient-physician Web messaging: the impact on message volume and satisfaction. *J Gen Intern Med*. 2005;20(1):52-57.

18. Kane B, Sands DZ; for the AMIA Internet Working Group, Task Force on Guidelines for the Use of Clinic-Patient Electronic Mail. Guidelines for the clinical use of electronic mail with patients. *J Am Med Inform Assoc.* 1998;5(1):104-111.

19. Kessels RP. Patients' memory for medical information. *J R Soc Med.* 2003;96(5):219-222.

20. US Department of Health & Human Services Office for Civil Rights. Personal Health Records and the HIPAA Privacy Rules. www.hhs.gov/ocr/privacy/hipaa/understanding/special/healthit/phrs .pdf. Accessed August 26, 2012.

21. Ricciardi L, Fridsma D. Call for Participation in the Automate Blue Button Initiative: Enhancing Consumer Access to Health Information. *Health IT Buzz Blog.* www.healthit.gov/buzz-blog /electronic-health-and-medical-records/blue-button-initiative-enhancing-consumer-access-health -information. Accessed January 23, 2013.

## chapter 7

Ensuring Long-Term Success: Improving Outcomes Through Meaningful Use

WHO SHOULD READ THIS CHAPTER?

This chapter should be reviewed by physicians who are interested in learning how best to leverage population-level techniques, electronic health record (EHR)–related tools, and change management to improve outcomes and meet the Meaningful Use (MU) objectives. The information covered is relevant to physicians at any stage in the implementation of an EHR. Physicians interested in targeting specific quality measures for improvement will also benefit from reading this chapter.

What you will learn in this chapter:

■ How to leverage MU to meet the needs of the practice
■ How to leverage relevant preventive services to improve outcomes
■ The four critical EHR capabilities for improving outcomes
■ How to align clinical quality measures (CQMs) to most benefit your practice
■ How to apply change management to improve outcomes
■ Why improving outcomes is beneficial for:
  ■ Physicians
  ■ Staff
  ■ Patients
■ Action items important to improving outcomes

Physician offices are operating in a changing health care environment. As part of health care reform (eg, the Patient Protection and Affordable Care Act),[1,2] physicians now face pay for performance, medical homes, accountable care organizations (ACOs), medical error reporting, focus on prevention, patient engagement, quality reporting (eg, clinical quality measures [CQMs]), and Meaningful Use (MU). These changes are driven, in part, by growing cost pressures and the public's realization that they have not been receiving the quality of care they have expected.[3-5] There is an increased expectation that the health care market will reduce health care costs while improving the quality of care being delivered. Electronic health records (EHRs) and their ability to exchange health information are seen as critical tools that support the delivery of safe, high-quality, efficient, and effective care. It is in this context that the Department of Health and Human Services is driving the use of

EHRs through MU objectives implemented over several stages. As you will recall, the MU stages focus on different themes:

- Stage 1 (2011–2012): enable data capture and sharing
- Stage 2 (2014): advance clinical processes
- Stage 3 (2016): achieve improved outcomes[6]

The themes build to support the long-term goal of improving outcomes. As a result, it is becoming more important for physicians and their practices to wisely select, implement, and use an EHR in a manner that can most effectively improve outcomes.

There are many factors relevant to improving outcomes, such as patient and physician behavior, treatment decisions, and supporting tools. Successfully engaging patients and families is a critical starting point in improving outcomes and was covered in Chapter 6. This chapter will focus on how to make decisions throughout the MU process to ensure long-term success by focusing on what is needed to improve outcomes. With this goal in mind, we will discuss the following topics:

1. Assessing the physician and his or her practice
2. Implementing appropriate preventive services
3. Aligning CQMs to the practice
4. Leveraging key EHR capabilities
5. Employing change management

Also discussed will be how to support outcomes at the public-health level (through reporting).

Physicians should ensure that the goals of the physician practice, the practice type, and the population of patients seen are the central point around which EHR selection, work-flow and process changes, EHR implementation, and MU decision making (eg, CQM) are framed. In the light of the physician-practice perspective, implementation of relevant preventive services should position the practice for improved outcomes. In fact, many are aligned with the MU CQMs.

A fully functional EHR is critical to support the delivery of safe, effective, efficient, and quality care to patients. To optimize outcomes, the physician will need to understand and leverage four EHR capabilities most relevant to improving outcomes both within the practice and beyond it. These capabilities are:

1. Data collection
2. Practice-based population health management
3. Clinical decision support (CDS)
4. Communication/data exchange

Each will be described in more detail and presented as part of a recommended process for not only optimizing a practice's approach to implementing these capabilities, but also ensuring that they align, as appropriate, to the priorities and needs of the physician practice.

Physicians need to acknowledge that the EHR is a critical tool for the long-term success of the practice. This success requires that the physician practice learn how to best leverage and use the EHR. Not all physicians will experience the same successes or challenges. Moreover, EHRs can vary dramatically in how well they may be able to support the needs of a physician practice. It is up to physicians and their practice to effectively select, implement, and, ultimately, leverage the appropriate tools to improve outcomes. If the physician practice is not committed to making changes in workflows and other business processes, the EHR cannot be expected to help the practice achieve its goals. This is illustrated by the outcome variations found in the literature. It will take clear goals, commitment, and effort to fully change the status quo and optimize an EHR to gain its maximal potential for the practice. Leveraging change management together with the power of data will help a practice make and maintain these changes. This will be critical to enabling the physician practice to most effectively improve clinical outcomes, the focus of this chapter.

ASSESSING THE NEEDS OF THE PHYSICIAN PRACTICE

The decisions made during the implementation and meaningful use of an EHR will dramatically effect both the financial and practice workflow of the physician practice. It is critical not only that these decisions be guided by the needs and nature of the practice, but also that data be captured as part of the assessment process covered below.

What to Do: Assess the Goals of the Practice and the Population of Patients Served

To effectively position the practice for successful outcomes, both clinical and financial, four aspects of a practice need to be assessed: practice goals, practice characteristics, patient population, and business characteristics. It is the evaluation of each of these, as a practice, that will serve to guide EHR selection and implementation decisions (eg, CDS focus), MU-related decisions (eg, CQM selection), and business decisions (eg, new services).

Practice Goals and Characteristics. It is important for your practice to clearly articulate goals for the short and longer term (eg, provide the best care in the city, join an ACO, sell the practice, or increase revenue). It is also beneficial to understand individual goals from other physicians, clinical staff, and nonclinical staff in the context of the physician practice. Also important is the nature (eg, specialty) of the practice. By confirming and collecting this information, you can gain insights into your practice that will inform decisions relevant to the business, EHR selection and implementation, and change management.

Patient Population. In order to more strategically make decisions relevant to EHR selection, EHR tool deployment (eg, CDS), and CQM selection, it is critical that you understand the nature of your patient population. Gather as much information about your patients as is readily accessible. Information can be obtained through a variety of sources, such as billing, practice-management systems, insurer reports, and EHRs (if implemented). What is the age distribution? What are the most common chief complaints? Chronic conditions? Procedures? Orders? While collecting and evaluating the data about the patients seen by the practice, you should document information about the data:

- Data source (eg, billing)
- How difficult or easy to obtain
- Currency of the data
- Quality of the data
- Format (electronic, *International Classification of Diseases* [*ICD*]–9 code)
- Ability to support analysis (eg, can it be exported to reporting tools such as Microsoft® Excel)
- Gaps

Business Characteristics. Your practice should also assess business aspects, such as payer-negotiated rates, payer mix, services offered, impact of pay for performance, and staffing. This assessment is important because it can help inform the financial effect of changes such as adding services, increasing efficiencies, or improving outcomes.

Informing Direction

It is critical that the physician practice goals, specialty, patient population, and business characteristics are clearly understood, as they will guide the direction the practice will take in terms of setting priorities, which will affect patient outcomes and future success. You should use this information to make decisions as to which CQMs are most appropriate for your practice. Moreover, your practice should have other goals that go beyond MU attestation. These goals and decisions will inform direction relevant to effectively leveraging the EHR capabilities. Only by making these assessments and addressing the points in this chapter can you make a well-informed decision that best meets the needs of the practice and ensure that the tools and processes are in place to optimize success.

PREVENTIVE SERVICES AS A BASE TO IMPROVE OUTCOMES

Significant improvements in health outcomes are tied to the practice's ability to deliver effective preventive services (primary through tertiary, described in Table 7-1). This is highlighted by the fact that many of the CQMs are related to these services.

TABLE 7-1

Preventive Services to Support Practice-Based Population Health (PBPH)

Focus	Aim	PBPH Functionality Needed	Examples
Primary prevention	Prevent a disease from occurring (eg, provide a vaccine to prevent a disease, counsel a patient to stop smoking to prevent emphysema and lung cancer). **This intervention is focused primarily on immunizations and counseling for risk reduction.**	Clinical decision support to target alerts and reminders that support the workflow of the practice around specific activities. This could be targeted at the physician, practice staff, and/or the patient. Subpopulation reports to assess opportunities for delivering services to the group in the most effective manner. Reports to assess effectiveness of the practice in delivering preventive services	When scheduling a follow-up visit for patients, the scheduler gets an alert to inform the patient that he or she will be scheduled for a tetanus booster at the next visit. A practice sends a notice to the patient either electronically or by mail with a list of primary preventive services that are due. A physician seeing a patient gets an alert reminding him or her to ask the patient about smoking cessation. The practice runs a monthly report to assess the number of patients who are smoking, the number who have received counseling to stop, and those who have received treatments (eg, nicotine patches).

(continued)

T A B L E   7-1 **(continued)**

Preventive Services to Support Practice-Based Population Health (PBPH)

Focus	Aim	PBPH Functionality Needed	Examples
Secondary prevention	Find and treat disease early, when the patient is asymptomatic (eg, order mammography to identify early stages of breast cancer so that it can be removed, measure a patient's blood pressure to identify patients who may be hypertensive). **This intervention is focused primarily on screening.**	As above	When scheduling a follow-up visit for a patient, the scheduler gets an alert to inform the patient to schedule a Pap smear. A practice sends a notice to a patient either electronically or by mail with a list of secondary preventive services that are due. A physician seeing a patient gets an alert reminding him or her to order a lipid profile for this high-risk patient. The practice runs a monthly report to assess how well it is delivering its preventive services, eg, percentage of women who receive a mammogram who are eligible to receive one.
Tertiary prevention	Treat and manage patients with clinical illness to minimize complications and maximize health (eg, providing a thiazide diuretic to a patient who is hypertensive to reduce the risk of heart failure and to avoid ischemic stroke). **This intervention is focused primarily on disease management and controlling the progression of a disease.**	Clinical decision support with recommended treatment options, recommendations for monitoring a patient's disease, reporting templates to capture physical findings, ordering templates to support best-practice treatment guidelines, graphs that capture disease measures over time relevant to treatment	The scheduler is prompted to schedule a monthly follow-up appointment for a patient with hypertension to assess the effectiveness of the new medication on the patient's blood pressure. The practice sends a notice to a patient to get a hemoglobin (Hb)A$_{1c}$ test. A physician seeing a patient with diabetes opens up a physical exam template tailored to patients with diabetes. The practice runs a monthly report to assess how well the care of patients with diabetes is being managed as evidenced by their HbA$_{1c}$ levels.

What to Do: Identify the Appropriate Preventive Services to Implement Within Your Practice

Using the knowledge obtained earlier through the practice assessment, identify which preventive services will be a priority for the practice. Develop goals and measures that are relevant to performing these services, the workflow necessary to support them, the role(s) of practice staff, and relevant patient-engagement approaches (described in Chapter 6). Also consider the effect on the business (eg, expected increased time to see patients, staffing costs/savings, payment implications both positive and negative). We will discuss how to leverage an EHR to implement these services later in the chapter. Successfully delivering preventive services to a practice population will result in improved outcome measures, benefits to the practice if it is part of an ACO, reduced liability, and healthier patients.

ALIGNING CLINICAL QUALITY MEASURES TO THE PRACTICE

The Centers for Medicare & Medicaid Services (CMS) describes CQMs as measures of processes, experiences, and/or outcomes of patient care, observations or treatment that relate to one or more quality aims for health care such as effective, safe, efficient, patient-centered, equitable, and timely care. The CMS requires the reporting of a set of CQMs as a way to demonstrate that eligible professionals (EPs) are using EHRs in a meaningful way. Physicians can take advantage of using CQMs to assess their processes in managing the care of their patients and the effectiveness of their interventions in those areas most relevant to them. Currently, physicians are required to choose three core and three alternate CQMs. In 2014, physicians will need to choose nine CQMs. The CMS has a recommended list of nine measures that align with national quality priorities (pediatric and adult) but they are not required. (Stage 1 and 2 CQMs are provided in Table 7-2.) However, the CQMs must cover at least three of the National Quality Strategy domains noted below:

- Patient and family engagement
- Patient safety
- Care coordination
- Population and public health
- Efficient use of health care resources
- Clinical processes and effectiveness

As discussed in earlier chapters, currently there are two options for CQM reporting: attestation or the Physician Quality Reporting System (PQRS). For more information on the PQRS, go to www.cms.gov/Medicare/Quality-Initiatives-Patient-Assessment-Instruments /PQRS/index.html. By 2014, CQM reporting will need to be done through the CMS (with the exception of Medicaid, where it is reported to the state).

There may be additional benefits of reporting CQMs. Check for additional programs focused on quality reporting at the following Web sites: www.cms.gov/Medicare/Quality -Initiatives-Patient-Assessment-Instruments/PQRS/Maintenance_of_Certification_Program _Incentive.html and https://mocmatters.abms.org/default.aspx.

It is important for physicians to find out how an EHR will support CQMs by knowing the answers to the following questions:

- Which CQMs are supported?
- How is attestation for Stage 1 and beyond supported? What about attestation in 2014? Can the reports already support submission to the CMS directly (eg, through the PQRS reporting mechanism)?
- Are there any additional costs associated with CQM collection and reporting?
- If not all of the CQMs are currently supported, when will all those listed for 2014 be supported? Are there additional costs associated with this or is it a standard update?

What to Do: Assess the CQMs That Best Match the Priorities Identified Earlier and Modify if Necessary to Meet the MU Criteria

Compare the priority preventive services you identified earlier in the chapter with the CQM list in Table 7-2. In the event that there are no matches or an insufficient number (either in total or by number of domains), select those CQMs that most align with your business needs and may be the easiest to implement. Once the CQMs have been identified, assess the required measures of the CQMs against the outcome goals and associated measures that you identified as important to meet your business goals (eg, preventive services). If other measures were identified, be sure to include them with the CQMs as part of the practice's broader list of measures. It is critical for the practice not only to make sure to capture CQMs for MU attestation, but also those measures important to the practice's business goals. Make sure to document all measures. Decisions regarding collection of measures, reports, and so on should be deferred until the EHR capabilities have been explored and you have a better sense of what can or cannot be supported.

TABLE 7-2

CQMs Highlighting 2014 Recommended Core Measures (Boldface)[a]

NQF No.	CQM	Description	Domain
NQF 0001* (no longer a measure in 2014)	Asthma Assessment	Percentage of patients 5–40 years of age with a diagnosis of asthma who have been seen for at least two office visits and who were evaluated during at least one office visit within 12 months for the frequency (numeric) of daytime and nocturnal asthma symptoms	
0002 PC*	**Appropriate Testing for Children With Pharyngitis**	**Percentage of children 2–18 years of age who were diagnosed with pharyngitis, received an order for an antibiotic, and received a group A streptococcus (strep) test for the episode**	Efficient Use of Health Care Resources
0004*	Initiation and Engagement of Alcohol and Other Drug-Dependence Treatment	Percentage of patients 13 years of age and older with a new episode of alcohol and other drug (AOD) dependence who received the following. Two rates are reported. a. Percentage of patients who initiated treatment within 14 days of the diagnosis b. Percentage of patients who initiated treatment and who had two or more additional services with an AOD diagnosis within 30 days of the initiation visit	Clinical Process/ Effectiveness
0012* (no longer a listed measure in 2014)	Prenatal Care: Screening for Human Immunodeficiency Virus (HIV)	Percentage of patients, regardless of age, who gave birth during a 12-month period who were screened for HIV infection during the first or second prenatal care visit	
0013* (no longer a listed measure in 2014)	Hypertension: Blood Pressure Measurement	Percentage of patient visits for patients 18 years of age and older with a diagnosis of hypertension who have been seen for at least two office visits with blood pressure (BP) recorded	

(continued)

TABLE 7-2 (continued)

CQMs Highlighting 2014 Recommended Core Measures (Boldface)[a]

NQF No.	CQM	Description	Domain
0014* (no longer a listed measure in 2014)	*Prenatal Care: Anti-D Immune Globulin*	*Percentage of D(Rh) negative, unsensitized patients, regardless of age, who gave birth during a 12-month period, who received anti-D immune globulin at 26–30 weeks' gestation*	
0018 AC*	**Controlling High Blood Pressure**	**Percentage of patients 18–85 years of age who had a diagnosis of hypertension and whose blood pressure was adequately controlled (<140/90 mm Hg) during the measurement period**	Clinical Process/ Effective-ness
0022 AC	**Use of High-Risk Medications in the Elderly**	**Percentage of patients 66 years of age and older who were ordered high-risk medications. Two rates are reported.** **a. Percentage of patients who were ordered at least one high-risk medication** **b. Percentage of patients who were ordered at least two different high-risk medications**	Patient Safety
0024 PC*	**Weight Assessment and Counseling for Nutrition and Physical Activity for Children and Adolescents**	**Percentage of patients 3–17 years of age who had an outpatient visit with a primary-care physician (PCP) or obstetrician/gynecologist (OB/GYN) and who had evidence of the following during the measurement period. Three rates are reported.** **a. Percentage of patients with height, weight, and body mass index (BMI) percentile documentation** **b. Percentage of patients with counseling for nutrition** **c. Percentage of patients with counseling for physical activity**	Popula-tion/Public Health
0027* (no longer a measure in 2014)	*Smoking and Tobacco Use Cessation, Medical Assistance: (a) Advising Smokers and Tobacco Users to Quit, (b) Discussing Smoking and Tobacco Use Cessation Medications, (c) Discussing Smoking and Tobacco Use Cessation Strategies*	*Percentage of patients 18 years of age and older who were current smokers or tobacco users, who were seen by a practitioner during the measurement year, and who received advice to quit smoking or tobacco use or whose practitioner recommended or discussed smoking or tobacco use cessation medications, methods, or strategies*	
0028 AC*	**Preventive Care and Screening: Tobacco Use: Screening and Cessation Intervention**	**Percentage of patients 18 years of age and older who were screened for tobacco use one or more times within 24 months and who received cessation-counseling intervention if identified as a tobacco user**	Popula-tion/Public Health

(continued)

T A B L E 7-2 (continued)

CQMs Highlighting 2014 Recommended Core Measures (Boldface)[a]

NQF No.	CQM	Description	Domain
0031*	Breast Cancer Screening	Percentage of women 40–69 years of age who had a mammogram to screen for breast cancer	Clinical Process/ Effectiveness
0032*	Cervical Cancer Screening	Percentage of women 21–64 years of age who received one or more Pap tests to screen for cervical cancer	Clinical Process/ Effectiveness
0033 PC*	**Chlamydia Screening for Women**	**Percentage of women 16–24 years of age who were identified as sexually active and who had at least one test for *Chlamydia* during the measurement period**	Population/Public Health
0034*	Colorectal Cancer Screening	Percentage of adults 50–75 years of age who had appropriate screening for colorectal cancer.	Clinical Process/ Effectiveness
0036 PC*	**Use of Appropriate Medications for Asthma**	**Percentage of patients 5–64 years of age who were identified as having persistent asthma and were appropriately prescribed medication during the measurement period.**	Clinical Process/ Effectiveness
0038 PC*	**Childhood Immunization Status**	**Percentage of children 2 years of age who had four diphtheria, tetanus, and pertussis (DTaP); three polio (IPV); one measles, mumps and rubella (MMR); three *H influenzae* type B (HiB); three hepatitis B (Hep B); one chicken pox (VZV); four pneumococcal conjugate (PCV); one hepatitis A (Hep A); two or three rotavirus (RV); and two influenza (flu) vaccines by their second birthday**	Population/Public Health
0041*	Preventive Care and Screening: Influenza Immunization	Percentage of patients 6 months of age and older seen for a visit between October 1 and March 31 who received an influenza immunization or who reported previous receipt of an influenza immunization	Population/Public Health
0043*	Pneumonia Vaccination Status for Older Adults	Percentage of patients 65 years of age and older who have ever received a pneumococcal vaccine	Clinical Process/ Effectiveness
0047* (no longer a measure in 2014)	*Asthma Pharmacologic Therapy*	*Percentage of patients 5–40 years of age with a diagnosis of mild, moderate, or severe persistent asthma who were prescribed either the preferred long-term control medication (inhaled corticosteroid) or an acceptable alternative treatment*	
0052 AC*	**Use of Imaging Studies for Low Back Pain**	**Percentage of patients 18–50 years of age with a diagnosis of low back pain who did not have an imaging study (plain X-ray, MRI, CT scan) within 28 days of the diagnosis**	Efficient Use of Health Care Resources

(continued)

T A B L E   7-2 (continued)

CQMs Highlighting 2014 Recommended Core Measures (Boldface)[a]

NQF No.	CQM	Description	Domain
0055*	Diabetes: Eye Exam	Percentage of patients 18–75 years of age with diabetes who had a retinal or dilated eye exam by an eye care professional during the measurement period or a negative retinal exam (no evidence of retinopathy) in the 12 months prior to the measurement period	Clinical Process/ Effectiveness
0056*	Diabetes: Foot Exam	Percentage of patients 18–75 years of age with diabetes who had a foot exam during the measurement period	Clinical Process/ Effectiveness
0059*	Diabetes: Hemoglobin A$_{1c}$ (HbA$_{1c}$) Poor Control	Percentage of patients 18–75 years of age with diabetes who had HbA$_{1c}$ >9% during the measurement period	Clinical Process/ Effectiveness
0060	Hemoglobin A$_{1c}$ Test for Pediatric Patients	Percentage of patients 5–17 years of age with diabetes who had an HbA$_{1c}$ test during the measurement period	Clinical Process/ Effectiveness
0061 (no longer a measure in 2014)*	*Diabetes: Blood Pressure Management*	*Percentage of patients 18–75 years of age with diabetes (type 1 or type 2) who had blood pressure <140/90 mm Hg*	
0062*	Diabetes: Urine Protein Screening	Percentage of patients 18–75 years of age with diabetes who had a nephropathy screening test or evidence of nephropathy during the measurement period	Clinical Process/ Effectiveness
0064*	Diabetes: Low Density Lipoprotein (LDL) Management	Percentage of patients 18–75 years of age with diabetes whose LDL-C was adequately controlled (<100 mg/dL) during the measurement period	Clinical Process/ Effectiveness
0067 (no longer a measure in 2014)*	*Coronary Artery Disease (CAD): Oral Antiplatelet Therapy Prescribed for Patients With CAD*	*Percentage of patients 18 years of age and older with a diagnosis of CAD who were prescribed oral antiplatelet therapy*	
0068*	Ischemic Vascular Disease (IVD): Use of Aspirin or Another Antithrombotic	Percentage of patients 18 years of age and older who were discharged alive for acute myocardial infarction (AMI), coronary artery bypass graft (CABG), or percutaneous coronary interventions (PCI) in the 12 months prior to the measurement period or who had an active diagnosis of ischemic vascular disease (IVD) during the measurement period and had documentation of use of aspirin or another antithrombotic during the measurement period	Clinical Process/ Effectiveness

(continued)

T A B L E 7-2 (continued)

CQMs Highlighting 2014 Recommended Core Measures (Boldface)[a]

NQF No.	CQM	Description	Domain
0069 PC	**Appropriate Treatment for Children With Upper Respiratory Infection (URI)**	**Percentage of children 3 months–18 years of age who were diagnosed with upper respiratory infection (URI) and were not dispensed an antibiotic prescription on or 3 days after the episode**	Efficient Use of Health care Resources
0070*	Coronary Artery Disease (CAD): Beta-Blocker Therapy—Prior Myocardial Infarction (MI) or Left Ventricular Systolic Dysfunction (LVEF <40%)	Percentage of patients aged 18 years of age and older with a diagnosis of coronary artery disease seen within a 12-month period who also have a prior MI or a current or prior LVEF <40% who were prescribed beta-blocker therapy	Clinical Process/ Effectiveness
0073* (no longer a measure in 2014)	Ischemic Vascular Disease (IVD): Blood Pressure Management	Percentage of patients 18 years of age and older who were discharged alive for acute myocardial infarction (AMI), coronary artery bypass graft (CABG), or percutaneous transluminal coronary angioplasty (PTCA) from January 1 to November 1 of the year prior to the measurement year or who had a diagnosis of ischemic vascular disease (IVD) during the measurement year and the year prior to the measurement year and whose recent blood pressure is under control (<140/90 mm Hg)	
0074* (no longer a measure in 2014)	Coronary Artery Disease (CAD): Drug Therapy for Lowering LDL-Cholesterol	Percentage of patients aged 18 years of age and older with a diagnosis of CAD who were prescribed a lipid-lowering therapy (based on current ACC/AHA guidelines).	
0075*	Ischemic Vascular Disease (IVD): Complete Lipid Panel and LDL Control	Percentage of patients 18 years of age and older who were discharged alive for acute myocardial infarction (AMI), coronary artery bypass graft (CABG), or percutaneous coronary interventions (PCI) in the 12 months prior to the measurement period or who had an active diagnosis of ischemic vascular disease (IVD) during the measurement period and had a complete lipid profile performed during the measurement period and whose LDL-C was adequately controlled (<100 mg/dL)	Clinical Process/ Effectiveness
0081*	Heart Failure (HF): Angiotensin-Converting Enzyme (ACE) Inhibitor or Angiotensin Receptor Blocker (ARB) Therapy for Left Ventricular Systolic Dysfunction (LVSD)	Percentage of patients aged 18 years of age and older with a diagnosis of heart failure (HF) with a current or prior left ventricular ejection fraction (LVEF) <40% who were prescribed ACE inhibitor or ARB therapy either within a 12-month period when seen in the outpatient setting or at each hospital discharge	Clinical Process/ Effectiveness

(continued)

TABLE 7-2 (continued)

CQMs Highlighting 2014 Recommended Core Measures (Boldface)[a]

NQF No.	CQM	Description	Domain
0083*	Heart Failure (HF): Beta-Blocker Therapy for Left Ventricular Systolic Dysfunction (LVSD)	Percentage of patients aged 18 years of age and older with a diagnosis of heart failure (HF) with a current or prior left ventricular ejection fraction (LVEF) <40% who were prescribed beta-blocker therapy either within a 12-month period when seen in the outpatient setting or at each hospital discharge	Clinical Process/ Effectiveness
0084* (no longer a measure in 2014)	Heart Failure (HF): Warfarin Therapy Patients With Atrial Fibrillation	Percentage of all patients aged 18 years of age and older with a diagnosis of heart failure and paroxysmal or chronic atrial fibrillation who were prescribed warfarin therapy	
0086*	Primary Open Angle Glaucoma (POAG): Optic Nerve Evaluation	Percentage of patients aged 18 years of age and older with a diagnosis of POAG who had an optic nerve evaluation during one or more office visits within 12 months	Clinical Process/ Effectiveness
0088*	Diabetic Retinopathy: Documentation of Presence or Absence of Macular Edema and Level of Severity of Retinopathy	Percentage of patients aged 18 years of age and older with a diagnosis of diabetic retinopathy who had a dilated macular or fundus exam performed that included documentation of the level of severity of retinopathy and the presence or absence of macular edema during one or more office visits within 12 months.	Clinical Process/ Effectiveness
0089*	Diabetic Retinopathy: Communication with the Physician Managing Ongoing Diabetes Care	Percentage of patients aged 18 years of age and older with a diagnosis of diabetic retinopathy who had a dilated macular or fundus exam performed with documented communication to the physician who manages the ongoing care of the patient with diabetes mellitus regarding the findings of the macular or fundus exam at least once within 12 months	Clinical Process/ Effectiveness
0101	Falls: Screening for Future Fall Risk	Percentage of patients 65 years of age and older who were screened for future fall risk during the measurement period	Patient Safety
0104	Major Depressive Disorder (MDD): Suicide Risk Assessment	Percentage of patients aged 18 years of age and older with a new diagnosis or recurrent episode of MDD who had a suicide risk assessment completed at each visit during the measurement period	Clinical Process/ Effectiveness
0105*	Antidepressant Medication Management	Percentage of patients 18 years of age and older who were diagnosed with major depression and treated with antidepressant medication and who remained on antidepressant medication treatment. Two rates are reported. a. Percentage of patients who remained on an antidepressant medication for at least 84 days (12 weeks) b. Percentage of patients who remained on an antidepressant medication for at least 180 days (6 months)	Clinical Process/ Effectiveness

(continued)

T A B L E   7-2 (continued)

CQMs Highlighting 2014 Recommended Core Measures (Boldface)[a]

NQF No.	CQM	Description	Domain
0108 PC	**ADHD: Follow-up Care for Children Prescribed Atten-tion-Deficit/Hyper-activity Disorder (ADHD) Medication**	**Percentage of children 6–12 years of age and newly dispensed a medication for attention-deficit/ hyperactivity disorder (ADHD) who had appropriate follow-up care. Two rates are reported.** **a. Percentage of children who had one follow-up visit with a practitioner with prescribing authority during the 30-day initiation phase** **b. Percentage of children who remained on ADHD medication for at least 210 days and who, in addi-tion to the visit in the initiation phase, had at least two additional follow-up visits with a practitioner within 270 days (9 months) after the initiation phase ended**	Clinical Process/ Effective-ness
0110	Bipolar Disorder and Major Depres-sion: Appraisal for Alcohol or Chemi-cal Substance Use	Percentage of patients with depression or bipolar dis-order with evidence of an initial assessment that in-cludes an appraisal for alcohol or chemical substance use	Clinical Process/ Effective-ness
0384	Oncology: Medical and Radiation— Pain Intensity Quantified	Percentage of patient visits, regardless of patient age, with a diagnosis of cancer currently receiving chemo-therapy or radiation therapy in which pain intensity is quantified	Patient and Family Engage-ment
0385*	Colon Cancer: Chemotherapy for AJCC Stage III Colon Cancer Patients	Percentage of patients 18–80 years of age with AJCC Stage III colon cancer who are referred for adjuvant chemotherapy, prescribed adjuvant chemotherapy, or have previously received adjuvant chemotherapy within the 12-month reporting period	Clinical Process/ Effective-ness
0387*	Breast Cancer: Hormonal Therapy for Stage IC–IIIC Estrogen Receptor/ Progesterone Re-ceptor (ER/PR)– Positive Breast Cancer	Percentage of female patients 18 years of age and older with Stage IC–IIIC ER/PR–positive breast cancer who were prescribed tamoxifen or aromatase inhibitor (AI) during the 12-month reporting period	Clinical Process/ Effective-ness
0389*	Prostate Cancer: Avoidance of Over-use of Bone Scan for Staging Low-Risk Prostate Can-cer Patients	Percentage of patients, regardless of age, with a diag-nosis of prostate cancer at low risk of recurrence re-ceiving interstitial prostate brachytherapy, external beam radiotherapy to the prostate, radical prostatec-tomy, or cryotherapy who did not have a bone scan performed at any time since diagnosis of prostate cancer	Effective Use of Health Care Resources
0403	HIV/AIDS: Medical Visit	Percentage of patients, regardless of age, with a diag-nosis of HIV/AIDS with at least two medical visits dur-ing the measurement year with a minimum of 90 days between each visit	Clinical Process/ Effective-ness

(continued)

T A B L E 7-2 (continued)

CQMs Highlighting 2014 Recommended Core Measures (Boldface)[a]

NQF No.	CQM	Description	Domain
0405	HIV/AIDS: *Pneumocystis Jiroveci* Pneumonia (PCP) Prophylaxis	Percentage of patients 6 weeks of age and older with a diagnosis of HIV/AIDS who were prescribed *Pneumocystis jiroveci* pneumonia (PCP) prophylaxis.	Clinical Process/ Effectiveness
TBD (proposed as NQF 0407)	HIV/AIDS: RNA Control for Patients With HIV	Percentage of patients 13 years of age and older with a diagnosis of HIV/AIDS with at least two visits during the measurement year, with at least 90 days between each visit, whose most recent HIV RNA level is <200 copies/mL	Clinical Process/ Effectiveness
0418 AC; PC	**Preventive Care and Screening: Screening for Clinical Depression and Follow-up Plan**	**Percentage of patients 12 years of age and older screened for clinical depression on the date of the encounter using an age-appropriate standardized depression screening tool and, if positive, a follow-up plan is documented on the date of the positive screen.**	Population/Public Health
0419 AC	**Documentation of Current Medications in the Medical Record**	**Percentage of specified visits for patients 18 years of age and older for which the eligible professional attests to documenting a list of current medications to the best of his or her knowledge and ability. This list must include all prescriptions, over-the-counters, herbals, and vitamin/mineral/ dietary (nutritional) supplements and must contain the medications' name, dosage, frequency, and route of administration.**	Patient Safety
0421 AC*	**Preventive Care and Screening: Body Mass Index (BMI) Screening and Follow-up**	**Percentage of patients 18 years of age and older with an encounter during the reporting period with a documented calculated BMI during the encounter or during the previous 6 months and, when the BMI is outside of normal parameters, follow-up plan is documented during the encounter or during the previous 6 months of the encounter with the BMI outside of normal parameters** **Normal Parameters: Age 65 years and older BMI ≥23 and <30. Age 18–64 years BMI ≥18.5 and <25.**	Population/Public Health
0564	Cataracts: Complications Within 30 Days Following Cataract Surgery Requiring Additional Surgical Procedures	Percentage of patients 18 years of age and older with a diagnosis of uncomplicated cataract who had cataract surgery and had any of a specified list of surgical procedures in the 30 days following cataract surgery that would indicate the occurrence of any of the following major complications: retained nuclear fragments, endophthalmitis, dislocated or wrong-power intraocular lens (IOL), retinal detachment, or wound dehiscence	Patient Safety

(continued)

T A B L E 7-2 (continued)

CQMs Highlighting 2014 Recommended Core Measures (Boldface)[a]

NQF No.	CQM	Description	Domain
0565	Cataracts: 20/40 or Better Visual Acuity Within 90 Days Following Cataract Surgery	Percentage of patients 18 years of age and older with a diagnosis of uncomplicated cataract who had cataract surgery and no significant ocular conditions impacting the visual outcome of surgery and had best-corrected visual acuity of 20/40 or better (distance or near) achieved within 90 days following the cataract surgery.	Clinical Process/Effectiveness
0575 (no longer a measure 2014)	*Diabetes: HbA$_{1c}$ Control (<8%)*	*The percentage of patients 18–75 years of age with diabetes (type 1 or type 2) who had HbA$_{1c}$ <8.0%*	
0608	Pregnant Women Having Had HBsAg Testing	Percentage of female patients 12 years of age or older who had a full-term delivery during the measurement period who were tested for HBsAg during pregnancy	Clinical Process/Effectiveness
0710	Depression Remission at Twelve Months	Percentage of adult patients 18 years of age and older with a diagnosis of major depression or dysthymia and an initial Patient Health Questionnaire (PHQ-9) score >9 who demonstrate remission at 12 months (defined as PHQ-9 score <5)	Clinical Process/Effectiveness
0712	Depression Utilization of the PHQ-9 Tool	Adult patients 18 years of age and older with the diagnosis of major depression or dysthymia who have a PHQ-9 tool administered at least once during a 4-month period in which there was a qualifying visit	Clinical Process/Effectiveness
TBD PC	**Children With Dental Decay or Cavities**	**Percentage of children ages 0–20 years who have had tooth decay or cavities during the measurement period**	Clinical Process/Effectiveness
1365	Child and Adolescent Major Depressive Disorder: Suicide Risk Assessment	Percentage of patient visits for those patients 6–17 years of age with a diagnosis of major depressive disorder with an assessment for suicide risk	Patient Safety
1401	Maternal Depression Screening	Percentage of children who turned 6 months of age during the measurement year who had a face-to-face visit between the clinician and the child during the child's first 6 months and whose mother had a maternal depression screening at least once when the child was 0–6 months of age	Population/Public Health
TBD	Primary Caries Prevention Intervention as Offered by Primary Care Providers, Including Dentists	Percentage of children 0–20 years of age who received a fluoride-varnish application during the measurement period	Clinical Process/Effectiveness

(*continued*)

TABLE 7-2 (continued)

CQMs Highlighting 2014 Recommended Core Measures (Boldface)[a]

NQF No.	CQM	Description	Domain
TBD	Preventive Care and Screening: Cholesterol—Fasting Low Density Lipoprotein (LDL-C) Test Performed	Percentage of patients 20–79 years of age whose risk factors have been assessed and for whom a fasting LDL-C test has been performed	Clinical Process/ Effectiveness
TBD	Preventive Care and Screening: Risk-Stratified Cholesterol—Fasting Low Density Lipoprotein (LDL-C)	Percentage of patients 20–79 years of age who had a fasting LDL-C test performed and whose risk-stratified fasting LDL-C is at or below the recommended LDL-C goal	Clinical Process/ Effectiveness
TBD	Dementia: Cognitive Assessment	Percentage of patients, regardless of age, with a diagnosis of dementia for whom an assessment of cognition is performed and the results reviewed at least once within a 12-month period	Clinical Process/ Effectiveness
TBD	Hypertension: Improvement in Blood Pressure	Percentage of patients 18–85 years of age with a diagnosis of hypertension whose blood pressure improved during the measurement period	Clinical Process/ Effectiveness
TBD AC	**Closing the Referral Loop: Receipt of Specialist Report**	**Percentage of patients with referrals, regardless of age, for which the referring provider receives a report from the provider to whom the patient was referred**	Care Coordination
TBD	Functional Status Assessment for Knee Replacement	Percentage of patients 18 years of age and older with primary total knee arthroplasty (TKA) who completed baseline and follow-up (patient-reported) functional status assessments	Patient and Family Engagement
TBD	Functional Status Assessment for Hip Replacement	Percentage of patients 18 years of age and older with primary total hip arthroplasty (THA) who completed baseline and follow-up (patient-reported) functional status assessments	Patient and Family Engagement
TBD	Functional Status Assessment for Complex Chronic Conditions	Percentage of patients 65 years of age and older with heart failure who completed initial and follow-up patient-reported functional status assessments	Patient and Family Engagement
TBD	ADE Prevention and Monitoring: Warfarin Time in Therapeutic Range	Average percentage of time in which patients 18 years of age and older with atrial fibrillation who are on chronic warfarin therapy have international normalized ratio (INR) test results within the therapeutic range (ie, time in therapeutic range) during the measurement period	Patient Safety

(continued)

NQF No.	CQM	Description	Domain
TBD	Preventive Care and Screening: Screening for High Blood Pressure and Follow-up Documented	Percentage of patients 18 years of age and older seen during the reporting period who were screened for high blood pressure and for whom a recommended follow-up plan is documented based on the current blood pressure reading as indicated	Population/Public Health

Abbreviations: AC indicates adult set; ACC/AHA, American College of Cardiology/American Heart Association; ADE, adverse drug effect; AJCC, American Joint Committee on Cancer; CQM, clinical quality measure; *H influenzae, Haemophilus influenzae*; HBsAg, hepatis B surface antigen; IPV, inactivated poliovirus; mL, milliliter; MRI, magnetic resonance imaging; NQF, National Quality Forum; PC, pediatric set; TBD, to be determined; and VZV, varicella zoster virus.
[a]Measures with an asterisk denote prior CQMs; those italicized will phase out in 2014. Those without an NQF number are not currently endorsed.

This approach of leveraging CQMs to improve your clinical practice allows you to drive changes to your clinical practice based on your goals and patient population. Details around each of the measures can be obtained from the following Web site: www.cms.gov/apps/ama/license.asp?file=/QualityMeasures/Downloads/EP_MeasureSpecifications.zip. To track the development of CQMs, go to www.cms.gov/Medicare/Quality-Initiatives-Patient-Assessment-Instruments/QualityMeasures/index.html?redirect=/QualityMeasures.

As noted earlier, you should select the CQMs to align with the clinical focus areas that provide you the most value. Once the CQMs have been selected, you should have detailed information collected relevant to the measures, workflow, and so on, as discussed earlier. This information will guide the development of the documentation templates, use of population-level tools (including order sets), decisions on CDS implementation, and how these EHR capabilities will be leveraged.

LEVERAGING EHR CAPABILITIES TO IMPROVE OUTCOMES

As mentioned earlier, EHRs can help support the physician practice in improving outcomes if they are implemented appropriately. The four primary capabilities (data collection, practice-based population health management, CDS, and communication and data exchange) that are important to managing and improving outcomes are discussed below.

Data-Collection Capabilities

Capturing the right data in the correct format is critical to leveraging an EHR to improve outcomes and meet MU quality reporting requirements. Throughout the entire EHR process (from selection to implementation), the physician should pay significant attention to how information is collected and its format to support both the MU measures and the tools critical to supporting outcome improvements. Not paying sufficient attention to the data aspects of an EHR will significantly reduce the long-term value to the physician and the practice. In order to assess and improve outcomes, it is important to understand not only the measures that describe them, but also how to most effectively collect and leverage them. This chapter will not list all of the detailed measures relevant to all outcomes; many are covered elsewhere.

As noted before, a significant benefit of requiring physicians to use Office of the National Coordinator (ONC)–certified EHRs for the MU Incentive Program is that it provides strong market incentives for EHR vendors to provide the technical capabilities needed to support MU. Many of the MU objectives require the capture of specific data. This sets the stage for improving outcomes by supporting relevant data collection, enabling CDS and the capability to explore practice-level outcomes. Table 7-3 summarizes some of the data-collection requirements for MU at a high level.

TABLE 7-3

Data-Collection Requirements^a Related to MU

MU Measure	Types of Data
Demographics	Preferred language, sex, race, ethnicity, date of birth, *gender identity, sexual orientation*
History	Smoking status, family history, *occupational and industry codes, disability status*
Physical exam	Height, weight, blood pressure, body mass index (calculated)
Clinical assessment and intervention	Problem list, counseling (eg, smoking), clinical quality measures, clinical decision support, immunizations, treatment: procedures and medications given (eg, dose, route), clinical summary, care plans (goals, instructions), educational materials
Orders	Structured medication information (eg, medication name, dose, frequency, administration route, duration), allergy nomenclature (eg, allergen, reaction type), medication status (eg, active, discontinued), laboratory/diagnostic test
Results	Laboratory, imaging, diagnostic (eg, impressions)
Patient engagement	Access to clinical information, clinical summaries, laboratory and diagnostic test results, and clinical education materials/decision aids

^aItems in italics are for Stages 2 and 3.

EHRs are required to support the collection of demographics such as preferred language, gender, race, ethnicity, and date of birth. These attributes are often very important to identify target patient populations for preventive services (eg, women 40–69 years of age for breast cancer screening). The proposed Stage 3 recommendations would add occupation and industry codes, sexual orientation, gender identity, and disability status. The measure would require that 80% of all unique patients seen by physicians have demographics recorded as structured data.

Despite the fact that the collection of these data is required for MU, not all measures are associated with a defined data standard. For example, blood pressure measurements may have been coded as a number or an integer. As a result, data collected by one EHR may not be collected in the same format as implemented in another EHR. This may not be much of an issue within a practice but could add challenges if data are exchanged. It is always better to coordinate "standards" with exchange partners before implementation. The EHR certification requirements posted by the ONC provide insight into which of these standards already exist.[7] For more details, go to www.healthit.gov/policy-researchers-implementers/reference-grids-standards-and-certification-criteria.

What to Do: Assess What Type of Measures (Data) Are Critical to the Physician Practice

Based on the assessment of the practice described earlier in this chapter, you should have clear ideas about what measures (data elements) will be important to capture for reporting, running reports (eg, against goals), and/or to enable CDS. You should compare these measures against those that an ONC-certified EHR is required to support. For those measures that are *not* integrated into the EHR, it will be important to consider developing a documentation template that enables the collection of the measure in a standardized way (ie, drop-down or pick list). The more work you do, the more informed the EHR selection process, efficient the implementation, and effective the outcome-improvement strategy.

Ensure that you have a clear understanding of the EHR's ability to capture and store the clinical data. For each data element important for CDS, assess and document relevant information such as:

- Where the data are captured
- Who can enter the data
- Any workflow requirements related to the EHR and the practice around the data capture
- How the data are captured (drop-down, free text, check-box)
- Whether or not the data can be used for CDS and how
- Whether the data can be extracted into a report or exported

Data drive the tools needed to improve outcomes, effectively run the physician practice, and succeed financially in the long term.

Practice-Based Population Health Capabilities

Most physicians deliver care to their patients at the individual patient-physician level. To more effectively manage the care of patients seen by a physician at the practice level, referred to as practice-based population health (PBPH), an appropriate approach and specific tools are needed.

EHR Capabilities Needed to Support Practice-Based Population Health

For physicians and their practices to be successful in the future, they will need to have access to PBPH functionality and know how to effectively leverage it.

PBPH is defined as "an approach to care that uses information on a group ('population') of patients within a clinical practice ('practice-based') to improve the care and clinical outcomes of patients within that practice."[8]

There are many benefits in using a PBPH approach, such as the ability to follow patient disease profiles, perform care-gap analyses,[9] target interventions to improve quality measures, efficiently identify patients for education or outreach, inform negotiations with insurers and other payers, match patients with clinical trial opportunities, send batch messages to specific patients (eg, drug recalls), provide data to guide resource decisions, and expand business opportunities for the practice. A major benefit of MU is that it requires that EHRs have population-level functionality for physicians.

There are at least five major functionalities that are necessary to implement PBPH within a practice according to a 2010 Agency for Healthcare Research and Quality report on PBPH.[8] These major functionalities are summarized in Table 7-4. One additional functionality that is not listed in the table that is critical to the sustainability of a physician practice is the ability to integrate financial information with the clinical data. This will enable physicians to better negotiate value to payers and ACOs.

Critical Point

When selecting an EHR, find out what population-level tools are available. You should reflect on your practice assessment (as discussed earlier) to guide the decision-making process. Key areas to consider are:

- What data are available for evaluation? What are the limitations?
- What data analysis, graphing/visual exploration, and reporting tools are available?

- What data can be readily exported? Can the data be downloaded to Excel or other spreadsheet applications?
- Can queries be easily created? How complex can the queries be? What are the limitations?
- Can the system support a population action for a group of patients—eg, printing (or e-mailing) individual letters for a group of patients?

TABLE 7-4

Major Functionalities Needed to Support Practice-Based Population Health[8]

1. Identify Subpopulations of Patients
Generate lists/reports of subpopulations of patients based on vendor-provided queries of diagnostic codes, laboratory results, medications, and other codified data fields.
Update or revise vendor-provided queries.
Develop new queries to identify subpopulations of patients based on diagnostic codes, laboratory results, medications, and other codified data fields.
2. Examine Detailed Characteristics of Identified Subpopulations
Customize reports to include desired patient information.
Access additional clinical/demographic data about patients within a subpopulation.
Conduct sequential queries to narrow down the initial list of identified patients.
Sort or stratify the list according to severity of condition or degree of risk.
3. Create Reminders for Patients and Physicians
Generate and be able to customize notifications to contact a subpopulation of patients.
Generate and be able to customize reminders for physicians about groups of patients who meet criteria for preventive care or disease management.
Create self-generated reminders to be delivered to the physician's "in-boxes" on specified future dates.
4. Track Performance Measures
Identify clinical patterns within the practice.
Produce reports on how well one physician, one care team, or one practice is meeting quality measures and/or guidelines.
Provide peer comparison reports for one physician, one care team, or one practice.
Customize reports to apply different quality measures to different subgroups of patients.
Designate exclusions using reason codes.
5. Make Data Available in Multiple Forms
Save reports generated by queries.
Export data from queries to other applications.
Print reports.
Provide graphic displays on quality measures and/or guidelines by physician, care team, or practice.
Display trends over time on quality measures and/or guidelines by physician, care team, or practice.

Practice-Based Population Health–Related MU Objectives

Two MU objectives—the patient list and patient reminders—fit under PBPH functionality. One objective requires basic EHR functionality (the ability to generate patient lists), while the other (patient reminders) is more sophisticated and its implementation will depend on the capability of the EHR. You should think about how to leverage these two "capabilities" more broadly to support your prioritized goals.

What to Do: Identify What Lists Are Needed to Implement the Priorities Set by Your Practice

In order to support processes to improve outcomes and manage population health, a core requirement is the ability to generate lists from the EHR. Stage 1 menu set measure #3 requires the ability to generate lists of patients by specific conditions to use for quality improvement, reduction of disparities, research, or outreach. Stage 2 requires the generation of at least one report listing patients with a specific condition. Discussions around Stage 3 include the generation of lists of patients for multiple specific conditions and near real-time dashboards (eg, graphic indicators of outcomes such as percentage of patients with diabetes who have had their yearly comprehensive foot exam) for physicians to use for quality improvement, reduction of disparities, research, or outreach.

As mentioned earlier, the ability to generate patient lists, such as by specific conditions, will help you in assessing the conditions that your practice is addressing. For certification, EHRs have to be able to electronically select, sort, retrieve, and generate lists of patients according to, at a minimum, the data elements included in: problem list, medication list, demographics (preferred language, gender, race, ethnicity, and date of birth), and laboratory test results. When assessing an EHR, it is important to explore the type of report-generating capability provided. This should be guided by your assessment of your overall priorities, not only those that support the MU requirements. Some questions to ask include:

- Can the EHR list all patients who have been seen a certain number of times within a specified timeframe? (This is important for getting the numerators and denominates for MU attestation.)
- What information can be selected and retrieved from the EHR—eg, smoking status, risk factors, family history, surgical history, interventions (eg, smoking counseling)?
- Can a physician create measures that can also be retrieved? (This capability is critical for physicians interested in leveraging outcomes relevant to their business that ONC certification may not require the vendors to support.)
- What format and/or application can this information be exported to?
- Can lists be created with multiple selects and exceptions (eg, women between the ages of 21 and 65 years who have not had a total hysterectomy and have not had a Pap smear in the last 3 years)?
- How does this functionality support patient reminders and other batch patient activities (eg, patient notification, integration with another system)?
- Can the report be done at a practice level? Physician level?
- Do the lists include address, e-mail, and phone number?
- Can report queries be saved? Automatically run (eg, monthly)?

The more robust the tool for exploring the patient population, the more benefit to the practice. However, a system that can download almost any field that is in the EHR into a spreadsheet may be more valuable than one that can show you predesigned graphs on a very narrow set of fields. As noted before, make sure that the system can export to spreadsheet formats or import into other analytic applications (eg, statistical software packages, such as SAS [SAS, Cary, NC], SPSS [SPSS, Chicago, IL]).

Consider how a data-analytic tool can aid your practice in making decisions about how to streamline care around specific interventions, negotiate with insurance companies, prepare for recertification, and assess the relevance of core measures. This capability is also critical to achieve the patient-reminder MU objective. If the data are accessible for exporting for analytics, you will have the option to acquire more sophisticated analytical tools. One important word of caution: When downloading clinical data out of the EHR, it is important to make sure that the data are not identifiable (preferable) or that the system to which it is downloaded has sufficient security measures in place to prevent inappropriate disclosures.

What to Do: Assess and Leverage EHR Capabilities to Support Patient Reminders

The EHR certification requirement to support patient reminders allows users to electronically generate a patient-reminder list for preventive care and/or follow-up care according to patient preferences based on, at a minimum, the data elements included in problem list, medication list, medication allergy list, demographics, and laboratory test results. However, this does not specify how an EHR will support the ability to send patients reminders around preventive and follow-up care. EHR functionality that can be leveraged to meet this MU requirement needs to include patient lists, secure messaging, and data portability. You should carefully assess the capabilities of an EHR to support this measure, which was also discussed in Chapter 6.

Ask the EHR vendor to demonstrate how the system does the following:

- Identifies a patient needing preventive and follow-up care
- Supports the notification of a patient (e-mail, phone call, letter)
- Facilitates scheduling the patient
- Flags if the patient ever received the service or not
- Alerts the physician if the patient being seen requires preventive and follow-up care so that it can be delivered during the current visit or ordered for the next visit, as appropriate (This is a CDS capability discussed in more detail later in the chapter.)

Are clinical rules embedded within the reminder system to identify patients? If so, other questions to ask include:

- What are the rules that support the reminder system to identify patients for follow-up based on? For example, a yearly reminder for patients 6 months or older sent between October and March. The system will need to be able to identify patients within that age range and facilitate sending reminders from October through March to the appropriate contact person using his or her preferred contact preference.
- How are these rules maintained?
- Can additional rules be created?
- Can the reminder and rule history be maintained?
- Can the rules be managed at the physician level or are they at the practice level?
- How can these rules be modified to meet the physician's needs and workflow?

If the EHR available does not have sophisticated CDS rules embedded within it to support a measure, you will have to develop your own processes. Three different approaches, based on EHR capabilities, are discussed below.

- **Population approach:** In this approach, you would identify a preventive service (eg, breast-cancer screening) and use the EHR to generate a list of patients who would be the appropriate recipients of that preventive service (eg, women 50–74 years of age who have not received a mammogram in the last 2 years) and contact them via their preferred method of contact. If such capabilities are not supported by the EHR or the practice-management system, you may be able to leverage other applications to generate letters, e-mails, or a call list to remind patients to schedule their preventive service.

Achieving the preventive service measure while meeting the patient-reminder MU objective is complex and requires the practice to develop a special workflow to support it. The positive attributes of this approach are that it does not require a patient visit to begin the process, can be a bulk process, and can allow for practice workflow optimization (eg, certain services are provided at certain times of the year).

■ **Patient-specific approach:** In this approach you would create order sets for preventive services and/or follow-up care. For EHRs that embed CDS, when the patient is due for a preventive service, you could be alerted during the visit or the order set could be automatically included at the end of the visit. The patient is reminded during the visit and, if the service was not provided, the front desk could make the appointment before the patient leaves. The benefits of this process are that it occurs in the context of delivering care and fits with the workflow. However, patients who do not regularly see you will not get reminders.

■ **Fully automated:** Such a system has CDS embedded within it to match patients with the appropriate preventive services. Once the rule has been "fired," the EHR automatically generates a reminder to the patient based on his or her contact preferences—eg, the system can send an e-mail to the patient, print a letter for mailing by the front office, or send a task to the front office to call the patient to schedule the appropriate preventive services and/or follow-up care. In this scenario, a patient portal would facilitate online scheduling. If the patient does not schedule an appointment, the practice can automate an escalation protocol. The benefits of this process are automation, minimal staff time and effort, and tailored patient reminders.

Clinical Decision Support Capabilities

CDS tools are applications that analyze data to help health care providers make a clinical decision.[10] As the definition implies, CDS requires data that are in a computable format. The only way that this is possible is if data are entered in a specific way, as highlighted earlier. This is why many of the other MU requirements such as demographics, problem list, allergies, and medication list are so important.

There are several types of CDS that support physicians in many different types of activities,[10] as highlighted in Table 7-5. However, implementing CDS needs to be done with great care, and it is very important for physicians to sufficiently understand the capabilities and limitations of CDS functionality within a potential or acquired EHR. The buy-in of the end-users of the functionality is also critical. Implementation of CDS does not guarantee success. For example, CDS for chronic disease management resulted in significant improvements in process of care but less in patient health outcomes.[11] Studies have shown that incentivizing physicians, along with other care-management tools, leads to improved quality of care of patients with chronic diseases (process and outcome measures).[12,13] One interpretation of those studies is that physicians who are incentivized—that is, are motivated to make changes—yield better outcomes. Another example is the inconsistent results found in studies investigating the effectiveness of computerized CDS for improving the delivery of preventive services.[14] How the clinician responds to and uses the tools directly contribute to their effectiveness. In some of the studies, some clinicians turned off alerts for preventive service reminders (eg, mammography), while others ignored them entirely (referred to by some as "alert fatigue"); hence, no improvements in the preventive service rates could be expected. It is also important to understand that EHR CDS functionality may be poorly designed and not conducive to the clinical workflow or the practice type. For example, a nephrologist seeing patients with complex renal conditions will likely not benefit from CDS alerts based on normal renal functioning for medications given to patients with renal insufficiencies.

TABLE 7-5

Three Major Tasks Enabled Through Clinical Decision Support Tools

Task	Type	Description	Benefits/Challenges	Example
Support of data entry	Smart forms	Tailor information collection based on specific patient data or condition	*Benefits:* Streamlines documentation process Improves documentation of services Provides reminders to perform specific activities *Challenges:* "Form/check-box" may be too restrictive for some physicians who prefer narration Time-intensive to develop forms if not already available Potentially "false" documentation Time-intensive to mix and match data elements of form and may not be flexible	Physical exam documentation that is tailored for a specific type of chief complaint or problem—eg, template for a neurological exam
Support of data entry	Order sets, care plans, and protocols	Facilitate the delivery of evidence-based best practices	*Benefits:* Ability to leverage common order sets, care plans, and protocols to gain efficiency Supports evidence-based care guidelines *Challenge:* Time-intensive to create and maintain if not already available	Yearly physical examination laboratory order sets based on patient characteristics (eg, age, risk factors)
Support of data entry	Warnings and alerts	Provide feedback on something entered into the system flagging a potential hazard or recommending action	*Benefits:* Ability to check medication orders for drug-to-drug, drug-to-allergy, and drug-to-medical condition hazards Provides checks for documentation errors Highlights abnormal findings in laboratory results *Challenges:* Alert fatigue Workflow interruptions	Contraindication alert when a physician orders penicillin for penicillin-allergic patient
Assessment	Reference/ knowledge resources	Provide tailored access to relevant information and resources (eg, information button)	*Benefits:* Access to references/resources when most helpful Supports patient-engagement MU measures *Challenge:* EHR vendors may not maintain the currency of the resources.	Reminder to order mammography for female patient along with a link to the US Preventive Service Task Force recommendations

(*continued*)

T A B L E 7-5 (continued)

Three Major Tasks Enabled Through Clinical Decision Support Tools

Task	Type	Description	Benefits/Challenges	Example
Assessment	Expert workup and management advisors	Provide guidance for diagnoses and treatment options	*Benefits:* Supports a physician in the diagnostic process *Challenges:* May result in multiple testing Dependent on strength of algorithm	Recommended workup is provided to assess the etiology of a complex set of symptoms.
Event-based	Data- and time-triggered events	Alert the physician of a new event that occurs asynchronously	*Benefits:* Enables the physician to learn about an abnormal laboratory result or other finding without having the patient in the office Provides reminders of time-driven events such as preventive screenings or monitoring *Challenges:* Too many alerts of a noncritical nature may cause alert fatigue Critical findings may get lost in the informational findings if not appropriately flagged May require additional work if access to the patient record is not seamless	Physician is alerted by the system for a critical laboratory test result.

Abbreviation: MU indicates Meaningful Use.

As highlighted in Table 7-5, CDS can provide the physician many benefits, but there are challenges as well. Physicians should understand the capabilities of an EHR as it relates to these different types of CDS capabilities. Explore how the CDS settings can be modified. For example, can a physician change when an alert is fired based on the severity of potential contraindications? Can alerts be controlled at a specific physician-user level or only for the whole practice? What makes sense for the patient population being seen in the areas of practice that need improvement? How can unhelpful alerts be managed?

Ultimately, CDS systems can help the physician and improve outcomes by ensuring that the physical exam and findings are tailored to the patient's health conditions and that patients receive evidence-based care in a consistent manner, are not exposed to adverse events such as drug-to-drug or drug-to-allergy interactions, and are provided care in a timely manner. Moreover, CDS improves the efficiency of the physician practice by streamlining complex order sets and protocols, facilitating documentation of physical examinations, and providing references when needed in context.

What to Do: Leverage the EHR's Clinical Decision Support Capabilities to Best Support Your Outcome Goals

Stage 1 MU measures touch upon drug-interaction checks and a general CDS rule. However, requirements around CDS will continue to grow through Stages 2, 3, and potentially 4 (see Table 7-6).

TABLE 7-6

CDS-Related MU Objectives

Stage 1	Stage 2	*Direction for Stage 3*
Implement drug-to-drug and drug-to-allergy interaction checks.	Is no longer a separate objective for Stage 2 (part of CDS)	
Implement one CDS rule relevant to specialty-wide clinical priority along with the ability to track compliance with the rule (one CDS rule).	Use CDS to improve performance on high-priority health conditions (five interventions).	*Use CDS to improve performance on high priority health conditions (15 interventions).*

Abbreviation: CDS indicates clinical decision support.

For MU, the CMS defined CDS as "Health IT [health information technology] functionality that builds upon the foundation of an EHR to provide persons involved in care decisions with general and person-specific information, intelligently filtered and organized, at point of care, to enhance health and health care."[15]

This definition is vague and allows for different types of rules to be implemented (eg, renal dosing calculations, recommended testing/treatment). Certified EHRs are required to implement these automated, electronic CDS rules (in addition to drug-to-drug and drug-to-allergy contraindication checking) based on the data elements included in the problem list, medication list, demographics, and laboratory test results. Notifications and care suggestions based upon CDS rules are required to be indicated in real-time. CDS, even when aligned with physician practice priorities, will not guarantee success in improving outcomes. The effectiveness of these tools relies on commitment, workflow optimization, evidence of improvement, and feedback, which will be discussed in more detail later.

Critical Point

MU requires the implementation of CDS interventions.

- Stage 1 requires implementation of one CDS intervention.
- Stage 2 requires the implementation of five CDS interventions, including drug-to-drug and drug-to-allergy checking; this increases to 15 for Stage 3.
- It is up to the physician to determine which CDS interventions to implement.

The CDS MU objective provides a win-win opportunity for your practice. The high-priority health conditions are aligned with CDS supporting the achievement of CQMs, and vendors are required to support them. You need to assess the EHR's CDS capabilities and limitations against the priorities of your practice. Based on this assessment, you will be better able to determine which of the priorities can be supported by the EHR's CDS capability. You will also need to take into account the workflow implications and effectiveness of the CDS rule as it is implemented within the system. The benefits and challenges provided in Table 7-5 should be taken into account during this assessment.

What to Do: Assess CDS Tools Related to Medications and How They May Be Leveraged to Support Practice Priorities

Stage 1 core measure #2 requires physicians to turn on their drug-to-drug and drug-to-allergy interactions checks. This capability is usually a part of an EHR's computerized provider order entry (CPOE) system. Certified EHR systems are to automatically and electronically generate, and indicate in real-time, notifications at the point of care for drug-to-drug and drug-to-allergy contraindications based on medication list, medication allergy list, and CPOE. The system should also provide certain users the ability to adjust notifications provided for drug-to-drug and drug-to-allergy interaction checks. Other related core measures that tie into the CPOE system include drug formulary checks, medication reconciliation, active medication list, and medication allergy list, which are described elsewhere.

CDS integrated into EHRs is not the same across different EHRs. This is also true for the CPOE related drug-to-drug and drug-to-allergy interaction checks that the EHR performs. For example, would you be able to enable alerts for severe reactions (eg, renal failure) and disable alerts for minor reactions (eg, diarrhea)? Before you implement drug-to-drug and drug-to-allergy interaction alerts, it is important to understand the details of the CDS capability of the specific EHR of interest. Below are some issues to explore:

- Ask the vendor to provide details about the nature of the CDS that enables this capability.
- Is it possible to set different levels of sensitivity around drug-to-drug or drug-to-allergy interactions?
- Ask other practices that have implemented this EHR to discuss their experiences with and approach to drug-to-drug and drug-to-allergy alerting.
- For the drug-to-allergy interaction checks, understand the format necessary for the allergies. Allergies not entered in a structured format are unlikely to support drug-to-allergy checking.
- The allergen is important but so is capturing the allergic reaction in a standardized format. Being able to distinguish between drug allergy and drug sensitivity is important when you are "faced with limited therapeutic options."[16]

Unfortunately, excessive drug-to-allergy alerting is highly prevalent and causes a significant disruption to physician workflow.[16] A major reason for overriding this feature is related to the drug prescribing knowledge base; cross-sensitivity rules tend to be overly inclusive and generate many alerts with low clinical relevance. Consider inactivating some of the cross-sensitivities from the drug-to-allergy database based on what makes sense in your practice.

Critical Point

Stage 1 MU menu set measure #4 requires drug interaction checks.

- Drug-to-drug and drug-to-allergy interaction checks functionality needs to be turned on.

Depending on the EHR's capabilities regarding CPOE and CDS, you should consider exploring other types of CPOE-related alerts. For example, if your practice has developed an order set for patients with specific medical conditions (eg, patients with diabetes and hypertension), providing a suggested order set when entering the CPOE system may be appropriate. Not only can this approach improve CQMs and other outcome measures, it can improve efficiencies. Your practice will need to appropriately leverage CDS to its fullest capability and in a way that optimally supports its goals. Your practice's success in effectively doing this will directly affect clinical and business outcomes.

Communication and Data-Exchange Capabilities

Communication and data exchange with other health care providers and public-health entities are important to physicians in their goal to improve patient outcomes. This capability provides a source of data needed to deliver health care to patients and support public health. Data, as noted before, are critical to effectively improve outcomes. What follows is an overview of the data-exchange capabilities that will need to be implemented for MU. You should think about how these capabilities can be leveraged to support the priorities and needs of your practice. Chapter 6 discusses the topic of communication and clinical data exchange between the physician and the patients and their caregivers.

The capability to exchange clinical data becomes critical for the effective implementation of the Affordable Care Act and the operation of ACOs. For a physician's office, the following are important:

- Exchange of information regarding insurance coverage and payment, including drug formulary checks
- Exchange of clinical data from other providers and health care systems to enable continuity of care
    - Medication orders, updates, and reconciliation
    - Transition-of-care summaries (and consultations)
    - Test orders and results
    - CQMs and other measures
- Exchange of information to support public health and quality reporting

Many MU objectives (current and future) require data-exchange capabilities. These are:

- Medication-related
    - Drug-formulary checks
    - E-prescribing
    - Medication reconciliation
- Electronic exchange of clinical information
    - Clinical information
    - Transition of care
- Submitting data for public health and research
    - Immunization registries
    - Syndromic surveillance
    - Cancer registries
    - Specialized registries
- Patient-focused exchange of clinical information (covered in Chapter 6)

Medication-Focused Data Exchange

More than one-third of adults take five or more medicines, not including over-the-counter drugs, vitamins, herbs, and nutritional supplements. Medication errors are among the most common medical errors, harming at least 1.5 million people a year.[17] Given the magnitude of the problem, implementing interventions to minimize drug-related medical errors is an important goal for physician practices. Therefore, it is important for physicians to effectively leverage tools such as CPOE, e-prescribing, and clinical information exchange (medication lists) to support medication reconciliation.

What to Do: Assess and Optimize the EHR Capabilities Relating to Medication-Focused Data Exchange to Best Meet the Needs of the Practice

Formularies are intended to reduce the costs associated with medications. From the physician's perspective, the ability to check formulary coverage has direct implications for outcomes. If the medication is not on formulary and expensive, patients may choose not to fill the prescription, and no real improvements can be expected in the outcome. The benefits are also evident for supporting e-prescribing. Certified EHRs are required to enable a user to electronically generate and transmit prescriptions and prescription-related information and to electronically check if drugs are in a formulary or preferred drug list. You should ask EHR vendors how integrated this capability is. For example, does the EHR just provide a list that the physician can review or does the EHR incorporate this list into the CPOE system and flag whether a drug is covered during ordering? This difference can have a significant effect on your workflow and that of your practice.

The ability to electronically submit prescriptions to a pharmacy has many reported benefits. It can reduce the time you spend on pharmacy callbacks and faxing prescriptions to pharmacies, and it automates the prescription-renewal request and authorization process.[18] From the patients' perspective, making the process of filling prescriptions easier is likely to improve patients' compliance with their medications. E-prescribing can help decrease the number of unfilled prescriptions.

You can issue electronic controlled substance prescriptions only when the electronic prescription or EHR application you are using complies with the requirements in the interim final rule (see www.deadiversion.usdoj.gov/fed_regs/rules/2010/fr0331.htm). If the system does not comply, you can use an existing electronic prescription or EHR application to prepare and print a manual controlled substance prescription for signature. These prescriptions are subject to the existing requirements for paper prescriptions.[19]

To successfully implement e-prescribing, as with any of the other functionalities discussed in this chapter, you need to assess current state, articulate future state (including changes in workflow), obtain commitment, and monitor progress. There are many resources around e-prescribing, which can be useful for your practice, and examples of such resources include:

■ www.ama-assn.org/ama/pub/eprescribing/what-is-eprescribing.shtml

■ http://healthit.ahrq.gov/portal/server.pt/community/health_it_tools_and_resources/919/implementation_toolsets_for_e-prescribing/30593

Critical Point

Stage 1 MU core measure #4 requires e-prescribing.

■ The EHR must have the ability to generate and transmit permissible prescriptions electronically.

■ 40% of prescriptions must be electronically transmitted in Stage 1; 50% in Stage 2.

■ Exclusions exist for physicians who write fewer than 100 prescriptions and for those who do not have a pharmacy within 10 miles that accepts electronic prescriptions.

What to Do: Assess EHR Tools to Support Medication Reconciliation and Develop a Practice-Appropriate Plan to Optimize Them

Having an accurate medication list for a patient is important for managing the care of the patient. Studies have shown that more than half of patients admitted to the hospital have one or more unintended medication discrepancies at hospital admission, with more than one-third having a moderate to severe harm potential.[20] In one study, the major reason for an incorrect medication list was incorrect dose and frequency. Other challenges include medications listed that are no longer being taken by the patient and patients taking medications that are not listed in the EHR medication list.[21] Medication reconciliation remains a challenge, especially in the ambulatory setting.

To improve medication reconciliation overall in a physician practice, you must provide continuous education for clinicians and staff, increase patient participation in the process, and provide performance feedback. From an EHR perspective, it is critical that the medication list is populated from the CPOE application and edited as necessary. Resources providing approaches to medication reconciliation include:

- http://patientsafety.org/file_depot/0-10000000/20000-30000/24986/folder/65244/med toolkit.pdf
- www.macoalition.org/Initiatives/RMDiscussion.shtml

In the context of MU measures, medication reconciliation requires a physician to update a patient's medication list when receiving a patient from another setting or provider of care. This occurs not only at discharge from a setting (eg, hospital, nursing home, long-term care facility), but also when a patient receives clinical care outside of the clinical practice (eg, physician consult). The information included in the medication reconciliation is determined by the provider and patient.

Critical Point

Stage 1 MU menu set measure #7 requires medication reconciliation.

- The physician *receiving* the patient is responsible for performing the medication reconciliation.
- The medication reconciliation has to be done for 50% of patients having transition of care.
- Stage 3 and beyond may expand information to include medication allergies, problem list, and contraindications.

You will need to assess the capabilities of the EHR around the capture and maintenance of the active medication and allergy lists. Moreover, the ability to link medications to the patient's problem list is also a helpful capability. For medication reconciliation, you should understand how problem lists sent from other health care providers (eg, transition-of-care summaries) are treated within the EHR. Do you need to open up a transition-of-care document and flip back and forth to reconcile? Does the EHR have a tool that supports the reconciliation process? Refer back to Chapter 6 to assess how patients may provide input electronically (eg, via portal) to facilitate the process. You should also reflect on how to address information about orders that were not filled by the patient or his or her caregiver. Being able to differentiate between a medication being prescribed and a medication being prescribed but not taken by the patient because he or she did not fill the prescription is important to more accurately project and improve outcomes.

In the context of assessing your practice and the EHR capabilities, developing clear processes that are tailored for your practice should be developed and implemented. As noted earlier, medication errors account for a significant number of negative outcomes, and mitigating them, as appropriate and relevant to the practice, will improve outcomes.

ELECTRONIC EXCHANGE OF CLINICAL INFORMATION

As noted earlier, the electronic exchange of clinical information for transitions of care, public health, and other entities is important to health outcomes. For example, the process of transitioning patients with complex conditions from one setting of care to another (eg, hospital to home or nursing home to hospital) is shown to be prone to errors. For Medicare recipients, nearly one in five discharged from the hospital is readmitted within 30 days.[22]

What to Do: Assess EHR Data-Exchange Capabilities to Support Care Transitions in the Context of Your Practice

You should be familiar with elements for safe, effective, and efficient care transitions,[22] as they will have a direct effect on outcomes. Examples of these elements include:

- Training patients and/or caregivers for increased self-care/advocacy
- Working with patients and family, in the context of medical and social service resources, to develop patient-centered care plans
- Standardized information exchange, including data elements such as:
  - Primary diagnoses and major health problems
  - Care plan that includes patient goals and preferences, diagnosis and treatment plan, and community care and/or service plan (if applicable)
  - Patient's goals of care, advance directives, and power of attorney
  - Emergency plan and contact number and person
  - Reconciled medication list
  - Follow-up with the patient and/or caregiver within 48 hours after discharge from a setting
  - Identification of, and contact information for, transferring clinician and institution
  - Patient's cognitive and functional status
  - Test results and/or pending results and planned interventions
  - Follow-up appointment schedule with contact information
  - Formal and informal caregiver status and contact information
  - Designated community-based care provider, long-term services, and social supports as appropriate
- Medication reconciliation and safe medication practices
- Ensured transportation for health care–related travel
- Procurement of timely delivery of durable medical equipment
- Ensuring the sending provider maintains responsibility for care of the patient until the receiving clinician and/or location confirms the transfer and assumes responsibility

Your practice assessment should provide insight into the expected number of patients who may undergo care transitions based on historical trends (if available). You should assess the EHR's capability to produce transition-in-care summaries and how the summaries can be received and acted upon to improve outcomes. For example, if a patient of yours is seen in the emergency room and is then discharged home, how would you be notified? What are the policies and processes regarding follow-up that are appropriate for your practice? What EHR capabilities can be leveraged to support these workflows?

Additional resources supporting care transitions include:

■ Resources for transition care coordination: www.cfmc.org/integratingcare/provider
_resources.htm and www.healthcare.gov/news/factsheets/2011/04/partnership
04122011a.html

■ General tools and information for providers around transitions: www.ntocc.org/Portals
/0/PDF/Resources/TransitionsOfCare_Measures.pdf

■ For training caregivers: www.caretransitions.org/caregiver_resources.asp

---

Critical Point

Stage 1 MU menu set measure #8 requires the exchange of transition-of-care summaries.

■ The physician who transitions a patient to another setting or provider of care should provide
a summary-of-care record.

■ The summary-of-care record can be sent by paper or electronically for Stage 1; for Stage 2,
it has to be sent electronically.

■ 50% of patients transitioned should have a summary-of-care record sent with them to the
provider or setting receiving the patient.

The Health IT Policy Committee MU workgroup has made Stage 3 recommendations to
add the following MU measures to support transitions of care:

■ The addition of care-plan information for each transition-of-care site with the following
elements (as applicable):
  ■ Medical diagnoses and stages
  ■ Functional status, including advanced daily living skills
  ■ Relevant social and financial information (free text)
  ■ Relevant environmental factors affecting patient's health (free text)
  ■ Most likely course of illness or condition, in broad terms (free text)
  ■ Cross-setting care team member list, including the primary contact from each active
  provider setting, including primary care, relevant specialists, and caregiver
  ■ The patient's long-term goal(s) for care, including timeframe (not specific to setting)
  and initial steps toward meeting these goals
  ■ Specific advance-care plan, such as physician orders for life-sustaining treatment
  (POLST), and the care setting in which it was executed. The POLST is a standardized medical order form that indicates the specific types of life-sustaining treatment
  a seriously ill patient does or does not want. (To read more, go to: www.chcf.org
  /practical-progress/catalyst-culture-change-endoflife-care#ixzz28OCVLEH9.)

Under this proposed Stage 3 measure, the physician who transitions or refers a patient to
another site of care or provider of care must provide the electronic care-plan information
to the receiving site or provider and to the patient and/or caregiver. To ensure that the
transition is complete, another MU measure is being proposed for Stage 3 that would require a physician to whom a patient is referred to acknowledge receipt of external information and provide referral results to the requesting provider, thereby closing the loop on
information exchange.

Some of the Stage 3 recommendations are focused on coordination of care. One proposed objective would require any licensed health care professional who can enter orders
into the medical record per state, local, and professional guidelines to use CPOE to create
the first record of an order for referral and/or transition-of-care.

For physician practices whose patients move from one care setting to another and/or require collaboration of other physicians (eg, specialists) to support their care, leveraging EHR capabilities to more effectively share the data and implement care-plan recommendations will significantly improve outcomes. You should assess current workflows and EHR functionalities to better leverage capabilities in the context of your practice. The approach and priority will likely be different for a practice where 1 or 2 patients a month have some transition in care vs a practice that transitions 100 patients. You should assess how much of the data that are being proposed for future stages are currently being captured and how you might leverage those data to optimize outcomes. Data are key, but how the information is acted upon determines outcomes.

SUBMITTING DATA FOR THE PUBLIC GOOD (PUBLIC HEALTH AND RESEARCH)

There are state and local health-related reporting requirements that physician practices need to abide by. Many are necessary to support public-health monitoring activities, such as immunization registries and syndromic surveillance,[23] which will inform the public-health department's reaction to a disease outbreak. Other reporting requirements address disease registries, which are focused on chronic diseases and cancers.

As discussed earlier in the chapter, preventive services such as immunization are an important strategy for improving outcomes. In the early stages of MU, data relevant to immunizations will be directed to the immunization registries. Physicians should assess the ordering and documentation of immunizations within their practice and how those actions are supported within the EHR. The physician should determine whether the relevant immunization registry or system is able to receive electronic submissions and, if so, if other physicians have successfully submitted data using the same EHR system. Determine if there are additional costs incurred to develop the interface and who is responsible for supporting it if there are changes to either system.

As is clear from Table 7-7, one objective of Stage 3 is to provide bidirectional exchange of information to physicians, which could help prevent unnecessary immunizations and potentially provide information to providers on other recommendations (eg, availability of new vaccines).

TABLE 7-7

MU Menu Set Measure #9: Immunization Registries Data Submission

Clinical Decision Support Rule	Stage 1	Stage 2	Direction for Stage 3
Objective	Capability to submit electronic data to immunization registries or immunization information systems and actual submission according to applicable law and practice	Same as Stage 1	*Capability to receive a patient's immunization history supplied by an immunization registry or immunization information system and to enable health care professionals to use structured historical immunization events in the clinical workflow, except where prohibited and in accordance with applicable law and practice (Beyond Stage 3—addition of submission of vaccine contraindication(s) and reason(s) for refusal)*

The required data elements for syndromic surveillance are being developed through the International Society for Disease Surveillance, which will inform the requirements for Stage 3 MU.[24] The Centers for Disease Control and Prevention (CDC) Web site (www.cdc.gov /ehrmeaningfuluse) is a good place to track this topic. The current elements align with those already covered by other MU objectives, with the addition of an initial pulse oximetry reading.

There are two new MU measures that support population and public health. The two new measures require data submission to cancer registries and to disease registries (summarized in Tables 7-8 and 7-9). A potential third measure would automate the reporting of vaccine adverse events to the Food and Drug Administration (FDA) and/or CDC. Most of these measures are not focused on supporting the physician practice directly. However, the physician should assess the data elements and capabilities in context of the practice priorities for future business opportunities. For example, physician practices that treat patients with cancer may be able to leverage potentially more detailed cancer registries for clinical trials or as a benchmark around outcomes. Much of the public-health data, if reported, may

TABLE 7-8

Stage 2 MU Menu Set Measure #5: Cancer Registries Data Submission

Clinical Decision Support Rule	Stage 1	Stage 2	*Direction for Stage 3*
Objective	None	Capability to identify and report cancer cases to a state cancer registry, except where prohibited and in accordance with applicable law and practice	*Capability to electronically send standardized, commonly formatted reports to a mandated jurisdictional registry (eg, cancer, children with special needs, early hearing detection and intervention) from a certified EHR to either local or state health departments, except where prohibited and in accordance with applicable law and practice. This objective is in addition to prior requirements for submission to an immunization registry.*

TABLE 7-9

Stage 2 MU Menu Set Measure #6: Disease Registries Submission Data

Clinical Decision Support Rule	Stage 1	Stage 2	*Direction for Stage 3*
Objective	None	Capability to identify and report specific cases to a specialized registry (other than a cancer registry), except where prohibited and in accordance with applicable law and practice	*Capability to electronically submit standardized reports to an additional registry beyond any prior MU requirements (eg, immunizations, cancer, early hearing detection and intervention, children with special needs) from a certified EHR to a jurisdictional, professional, or other aggregating resources (eg, health information exchange, ACO), except where prohibited and in accordance with applicable law and practice. Registry examples include hypertension, diabetes, body mass index, devices, and/or other diagnoses/ conditions.*

Abbreviations: ACO indicates accountable care organization; and EHR, electronic health record.

be leveraged to assess business opportunities to provide clinical services meeting specific needs in the community. The ability to automate adverse-event reporting to the FDA (beyond vaccines) would allow potentially dangerous adverse effects of products to be identified earlier so those products could quickly be removed from the market. The patient-list capability mentioned earlier could facilitate rapid outreach to relevant patients to discontinue use of such products. Although these activities may not directly enhance the outcomes at the physician-practice level, they will improve outcomes at the local and national levels.

LEVERAGING CHANGE MANAGEMENT TO ENHANCE SUCCESS

Data and tools available through the EHR can aid physicians and their practices to identify clinical areas of focus that will most benefit their patients and their practice. However, data and tools are not sufficient to improve outcomes. Physician practices that are committed to improving patient outcomes will need to institute a change-management process within their practice (see Figure 7-1). This is because EHR capabilities only support the delivery of the services, they do not change them—the practice does. The approach shown in Figure 7-1 is just one way to support change management within a practice. The key components for success are a clear understanding and shared vision of the future state and the path forward from the current state, commitment from all involved, implementation, and continued assessment and improvement.

This last section of the chapter provides a high-level overview of a change-management process that will be critical to successfully improve outcomes. This approach can be applied to the specific priorities identified by your practice. The steps are discussed in more detail below, along with a case study.

F I G U R E 7-1

The Change-Management Process

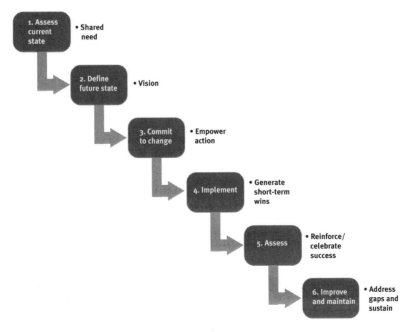

1. Assess Current State

The first step before moving forward with implementing a change is to understand the current state of the practice. This assessment can cover a broad range of practice information or can have a narrow focus around a specific goal (eg, improving a quality-performance measure related to the percentage of patients with hypertension with adequate blood pressure control). To manage a patient population, you would assess the patient demographics, chief complaints, diseases and medical problems, orders, treatments, and outcomes. If there's more than one physician in the practice, this information can be further parsed by physician. This is a critical activity for a practice; the actual data inform the prioritization of the practice around MU and help the practice target the most relevant CQMs. For example, the CQMs chosen for a practice serving primarily younger women would be different from those serving older adults with chronic diseases.

2. Define Future State

Defining the future state is a multistep process in that it charts the course from current state to one based on the vision and goals of the clinical practice. With that end in mind, you must be able to articulate how it will be met. One step would be defining the internal processes within the practice needed to meet the goal, such as defining roles and responsibilities and refining practice workflows for relevant staff. In the context of the EHR, another step would be the creation or customization of appropriate tools such as order sets, physical exam templates, education materials, and reports. In addition, an implementation plan needs to be created. Remember to include processes to celebrate achievements, such as giving awards, as they are important to staff engagement and commitment.

3. Commit to Change

After articulating the future state and how it will be achieved, it is critical to obtain a commitment to make these changes within the clinical practice. One approach to develop commitment, beyond just cursory approval, is to include the members of the practice in the development of the first two steps. This helps ensure buy-in throughout the process. Work with the members of the clinical practice to come up with the method to reinforce this commitment throughout the process.

4. Implement

Implementation of the plan moves the process from discussion to action. Throughout the implementation process, it is important to celebrate successes, address issues in a proactive way, provide open channels of communication, and allow for a process to integrate improvements as they present themselves.

5. Assess

Assessing the impact of the plan on the desired goal is important for a variety of reasons. It helps you identify areas that are working while flagging any gaps. It also provides each participant in the plan with a measure as to how well they're doing. In this stage, it is important to be open and nonjudgmental and to provide a mechanism to work together to address any gaps, apply lessons learned, and celebrate successes.

6. Improve and Maintain

You must ensure that the practice supports the improvement and maintenance of the processes put in place to facilitate continued performance and improvement. As additional goals are added to the practice, integrate activities to ensure optimal workflow and maximize outcomes and benefits to the practice.

Case Study

The following case study focuses on a practice with three physicians serving over 6000 patients.

Step 1: Assess Current State
- Overall assessment
  - 6150 patients seen during the last 18 months (patient panel)
  - Top five diagnosis codes:
    - 21% hypertension (*ICD-9-CM* [*Clinical Modification*] 401-05); 40% are documented to have well-controlled blood pressure
    - 20% nonspecific diagnosis (*ICD-9-CM* 780-89)
    - 20% overweight, obesity (*ICD-9-CM* 278)
    - 12% acute respiratory (*ICD-9-CM* 460-66)
    - 10% diabetes (*ICD-9-CM* 250); 65% are documented to have HbA_{1c} less than 7%
- The first step is to select the focus of the intervention. From the list, the three major diagnosis codes that align most readily to a population health/preventive services approach are hypertension, obesity, and diabetes. When targeting an intervention, consider the availability of effective interventions, patient benefit, availability of appropriate resources, business drivers (eg, incentives), and how quickly outcomes can be improved. Of the three, hypertension provides the biggest opportunity for the practice given the findings of poorly controlled blood pressure, relevance to a practice selected CQM (see Table 7-2: Controlling High Blood Pressure, 0018), and availability of national evidence-based treatment guides. With this focus, collecting more data is necessary so that a future stage can be appropriately developed for the practice.
- Evaluate the population of patients with hypertension who match the information relevant to best practices:
  - Blood pressure classes (normal, prehypertensive, stage 1, and stage 2)
  - Assess documentation relevant to the diagnostic workup (eg, urinalysis, blood glucose, hematocrit, risk factors, causes)
  - Assess treatments against best practices
  - Compare the data for patients who have well-managed blood pressure with those who do not (for diabetes/chronic kidney disease, blood pressure needs to be <130/80 mm Hg; otherwise, 140/90 mm Hg)
  - Run a report for each physician in the practice

Step 2: Define Future State
- Goal: Follow best-practice guidelines of the Seventh Report of the Joint National Committee on Prevention, Detection, Evaluation, and Treatment of High Blood Pressure (JNC 7) for managing patients with hypertension (Figure 7-2)

Here is a list of tools for managing the care of patients with hypertension that can be leveraged by the practice:

Treatment tools:

- Clinical practice guidelines and report (cardiovascular): www.nhlbi.nih.gov/guidelines /current.htm

- Reference card on JNC 7 guidelines: www.nhlbi.nih.gov/guidelines/hypertension /jnc7card.htm

- JNC home page: www.nhlbi.nih.gov/guidelines/hypertension

Documentation forms and tools (consider using these to guide your EHR templates):

- American Academy of Family Physicians hypertension encounter form: www.aafp.org/ fpm/2004/0300/p79.html[25]

  - Short-term goal: Improve percentage of patients with well-controlled blood pressure from 40% to 80% in 1 year

- Define future state and how to get there:

  - Define workflow for all relevant staff, and highlight changes to current workflow.

  - Cross-walk all activities to where the data will be captured within the EHR and how it will be leveraged (see Table 7-10).

  - Create appropriate tools:

    - Order sets for the appropriate hypertensive patient groups (eg, heart failure, post–myocardial infarction, high cardiovascular disease risk, diabetes, chronic kidney disease, recurrent stroke prevention)

    - Hypertensive patient examination template

    - Patient education materials and external resources available within the community

  - Internal processes within the practice to better manage hypertensive patients:

    - Monitoring (at home and drop-ins)

    - Obtaining patient input around treatment side effects and other factors that would affect treatment

  - Award structure for staff based on improvements in patient hypertension management

  - Implementation plan

Step 3: Commit to Change

- The physicians and staff need to agree to:

  - Follow the guidelines of the JNC 7. For more details, go to www.nhlbi.nih.gov /guidelines/hypertension/express.pdf.

  - Commit to the defined future state.

  - Commit to implementation plan.

Step 4: Implement

- Implement and assess continually; modify as necessary.

Step 5: Assess

- Assess progress through a monthly report, and meet to discuss strategies to address any gaps, apply lessons learned, and celebrate improvements.

Step 6: Improve and Maintain

- Evolve the processes, order sets, etc based on feedback and lessons learned from the practice.

- Sustain performance.

- Report measures as part of MU.

FIGURE 7-2

Reference Card from the JNC 7 Guidelines on Prevention, Detection, Evaluation, and Treatment of High Blood Pressure[26]

EVALUATION

CLASSIFICATION OF BLOOD PRESSURE (BP)*

CATEGORY	SBP mmHg		DBP mmHg
Normal	<120	and	<80
Prehypertension	120–139	or	80–89
Hypertension, Stage 1	140–159	or	90–99
Hypertension, Stage 2	≥160	or	≥100

* See *Blood Pressure Measurement Techniques* (reverse side)
Key: SBP = systolic blood pressure   DBP = diastolic blood pressure

DIAGNOSTIC WORKUP OF HYPERTENSION

- Assess risk factors and comorbidities.
- Reveal identifiable causes of hypertension.
- Assess presence of target organ damage.
- Conduct history and physical examination.
- Obtain laboratory tests: urinalysis, blood glucose, hematocrit and lipid panel, serum potassium, creatinine, and calcium. Optional: urinary albumin/creatinine ratio.
- Obtain electrocardiogram.

ASSESS FOR MAJOR CARDIOVASCULAR DISEASE (CVD) RISK FACTORS

- Hypertension
- Obesity (body mass index ≥30 kg/m²)
- Dyslipidemia
- Diabetes mellitus
- Cigarette smoking
- Physical inactivity
- Microalbuminuria, estimated glomerular filtration rate <60 mL/min
- Age (>55 for men, >65 for women)
- Family history of premature CVD (men age <55, women age <65)

ASSESS FOR IDENTIFIABLE CAUSES OF HYPERTENSION

- Sleep apnea
- Drug induced/related
- Chronic kidney disease
- Primary aldosteronism
- Renovascular disease
- Cushing's syndrome or steroid therapy
- Pheochromocytoma
- Coarctation of aorta
- Thyroid/parathyroid disease

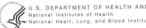 U.S. DEPARTMENT OF HEALTH AND HUMAN SERVICES
National Institutes of Health
National Heart, Lung, and Blood Institute

BLOOD PRESSURE MEASUREMENT TECHNIQUES

METHOD	NOTES
In-office	Two readings, 5 minutes apart, sitting in chair. Confirm elevated reading in contralateral arm.
Ambulatory BP monitoring	Indicated for evaluation of "white coat hypertension." Absence of 10–20 percent BP decrease during sleep may indicate increased CVD risk.
Patient self-check	Provides information on response to therapy. May help improve adherence to therapy and is useful for evaluating "white coat hypertension."

CAUSES OF RESISTANT HYPERTENSION

- Improper BP measurement
- Excess sodium intake
- Inadequate diuretic therapy
- Medication
  - Inadequate doses
  - Drug actions and interactions (e.g., nonsteroidal anti-inflammatory drugs (NSAIDs), illicit drugs, sympathomimetics, oral contraceptives)
  - Over-the-counter (OTC) drugs and herbal supplements
- Excess alcohol intake
- Identifiable causes of hypertension (see reverse side)

COMPELLING INDICATIONS FOR INDIVIDUAL DRUG CLASSES

COMPELLING INDICATION	INITIAL THERAPY OPTIONS
• Heart failure	THIAZ, BB, ACEI, ARB, ALDO ANT
• Post myocardial infarction	BB, ACEI, ALDO ANT
• High CVD risk	THIAZ, BB, ACEI, CCB
• Diabetes	THIAZ, BB, ACEI, ARB, CCB
• Chronic kidney disease	ACEI, ARB
• Recurrent stroke prevention	THIAZ, ACEI

Key: THIAZ = thiazide diuretic, ACEI= angiotensin converting enzyme inhibitor, ARB = angiotensin receptor blocker, BB = beta blocker, CCB = calcium channel blocker, ALDO ANT = aldosterone antagonist

STRATEGIES FOR IMPROVING ADHERENCE TO THERAPY

- Clinician empathy increases patient trust, motivation, and adherence to therapy.
- Physicians should consider their patients' cultural beliefs and individual attitudes in formulating therapy.

The National High Blood Pressure Education Program is coordinated by the National Heart, Lung, and Blood Institute (NHLBI) at the National Institutes of Health. Copies of the JNC 7 Report are available on the NHLBI Web site at http://www.nhlbi.nih.gov or from the NHLBI Health Information Center, P.O. Box 30105, Bethesda, MD 20824-0105; Phone: 301-592-8573 or 240-629-3255 (TTY); Fax: 301-592-8563.

TREATMENT

PRINCIPLES OF HYPERTENSION TREATMENT

- Treat to BP <140/90 mmHg or BP <130/80 mmHg in patients with diabetes or chronic kidney disease.
- Majority of patients will require two medications to reach goal.

ALGORITHM FOR TREATMENT OF HYPERTENSION

LIFESTYLE MODIFICATIONS

Not at Goal Blood Pressure (<140/90 mmHg)
(<130/80 mmHg for patients with diabetes or chronic kidney disease)
See Strategies for Improving Adherence to Therapy

INITIAL DRUG CHOICES

Without Compelling Indications | **With Compelling Indications**

Stage 1 Hypertension (SBP 140–159 or DBP 90–99 mmHg)	Stage 2 Hypertension (SBP ≥160 or DBP ≥100 mmHg)	Drug(s) for the compelling indications
Thiazide-type diuretics for most. May consider ACEI, ARB, BB, CCB, or combination.	2-drug combination for most (usually thiazide-type diuretic and ACEI, or ARB, or BB, or CCB).	See *Compelling Indications for Individual Drug Classes*. Other antihypertensive drugs (diuretics, ACEI, ARB, BB, CCB) as needed.

NOT AT GOAL BLOOD PRESSURE

Optimize dosages or add additional drugs until goal blood pressure is achieved. Consider consultation with hypertension specialist.
See Strategies for Improving Adherence to Therapy

PRINCIPLES OF LIFESTYLE MODIFICATION

- Encourage healthy lifestyles for all individuals.
- Prescribe lifestyle modifications for all patients with prehypertension and hypertension.
- Components of lifestyle modifications include weight reduction, DASH eating plan, dietary sodium reduction, aerobic physical activity, and moderation of alcohol consumption.

LIFESTYLE MODIFICATION RECOMMENDATIONS

MODIFICATION	RECOMMENDATION	AVG. SBP REDUCTION RANGE†
Weight reduction	Maintain normal body weight (body mass index 18.5–24.9 kg/m²).	5–20 mmHg/10 kg
DASH eating plan	Adopt a diet rich in fruits, vegetables, and lowfat dairy products with reduced content of saturated and total fat.	8–14 mmHg
Dietary sodium reduction	Reduce dietary sodium intake to ≤100 mmol per day (2.4 g sodium or 6 g sodium chloride).	2–8 mmHg
Aerobic physical activity	Regular aerobic physical activity (e.g., brisk walking) at least 30 minutes per day, most days of the week.	4–9 mmHg
Moderation of alcohol consumption	Men: limit to ≤2 drinks* per day. Women and lighter weight persons: limit to ≤1 drink* per day.	2–4 mmHg

* 1 drink = 1/2 oz or 15 mL ethanol (e.g., 12 oz beer, 5 oz wine, 1.5 oz 80-proof whiskey).
† Effects are dose and time dependent.

U.S. DEPARTMENT OF HEALTH AND HUMAN SERVICES
National Institutes of Health
National Heart, Lung, and Blood Institute
National High Blood Pressure Education Program

NIH Publication No. 03-5231
May 2003

FIGURE 7-3

JNC 7 Guidelines on Prevention, Detection, Evaluation, and Treatment of High Blood Pressure[27]

COMPELLING INDICATION*	RECOMMENDED DRUGS						CLINICAL TRIAL BASIS†
	DIURETIC	BB	ACEI	ARB	CCB	ALDO ANT	
Heart failure	●	●	●	●		●	ACC/AHA Heart Failure Guideline,[132] MERIT-HF,[133] COPERNICUS,[134] CIBIS,[135] SOLVD,[136] AIRE,[137] TRACE,[138] ValHEFT,[139] RALES,[140] CHARM[141]
Postmyocardial infarction		●	●			●	ACC/AHA Post-MI Guideline,[142] BHAT,[143] SAVE,[144] Capricorn,[145] EPHESUS[146]
High coronary disease risk	●	●	●		●		ALLHAT,[109] HOPE,[110] ANBP2,[112] LIFE,[102] CONVINCE,[101] EUROPA,[114] INVEST[147]
Diabetes	●	●	●	●	●		NKF-ADA Guideline,[88,89] UKPDS,[148] ALLHAT[109]
Chronic kidney disease			●	●			NKF Guideline,[89] Captopril Trial,[149] RENAAL,[150] IDNT,[151] REIN,[152] AASK[153]
Recurrent stroke prevention	●		●				PROGRESS[111]

Drug abbreviations: ACEI, angiotensin converting enzyme inhibitor; Aldo ANT, aldosterone antagonist; ARB, angiotensin receptor blocker; BB, beta blocker; CCB, calcium channel blocker.
*Compelling indications for antihypertensive drugs are based on benefits from outcome studies or existing clinical guidelines; the compelling indication is managed in parallel with the BP.
†Conditions for which clinical trials demonstrate the benefit of specific classes of antihypertensive drugs used as part of an antihypertensive regimen to achieve BP goal to test outcomes.
[For names of study groups and the cited references, see the full report.[27]]

TABLE 7-10

Data Needed for Implementing and Assessing Effectiveness of the Physician Practice Hypertension Intervention

Focus	Specifics	Where Captured	How Leveraged
Physician	Primary, consulting, or covering physician	Visit data	The ability to segregate at the physician level enables physicians to assess how well they are managing their hypertensive patients and learn from each other. Capability of separating CQMs by physician is required for reporting.
Patient	Age, ethnicity, gender, insurance, frequency of visits	Demographics Scheduling	Some aspects of patient information, such as gender, are important for clinical decision support, while others, such as frequency of visits, provide insight into practice patterns.

(continued)

TABLE   7-10 (continued)

Data Needed for Implementing and Assessing Effectiveness of the Physician Practice Hypertension Intervention

Focus	Specifics	Where Captured	How Leveraged
Diagnosis	Hypertension	Diagnosis	The diagnosis of hypertension is a critical data element, is the focus of the intervention, and is needed for clinical decision support, a core reporting requirement for CQMs.
Diagnosis-level risk factors	Diabetes mellitus, dyslipidemia, obesity	Diagnosis	The ability to easily flag comorbidities that will affect treatment approaches is important for effective treatment, clinical decision support, and CQM reporting.
Identifiable causes of hypertension	Sleep apnea, chronic kidney disease, primary aldosteronism, renovascular disease, long-term steroid therapy and Cushing syndrome, pheochromocytoma, coarctation of the aorta, thyroid or parathyroid disease	Diagnosis	Treatment and assessment value
Risk factors	Cigarette smoking, physical inactivity, age, gender, family history of premature cardiovascular disease (men <55 years or women <65 years)	Social history (mixed standards; for CQM CPT codes queried or reported) Demographic information Family history (flagging risks)	Treatment and assessment value. Important for clinical decision support and other intervention processes; data relevant for reporting CQMs
Target organ damage	Left ventricular hypertrophy, angina or prior myocardial infarction, prior coronary revascularization, heart failure, stroke or transient ischemic attack, peripheral arterial disease, retinopathy	Past medical history Past surgical history Diagnosis	Treatment and assessment value

(*continued*)

T A B L E　7-10 (continued)

Data Needed for Implementing and Assessing Effectiveness of the Physician Practice Hypertension Intervention

Focus	Specifics	Where Captured	How Leveraged
Physical exam	Blood pressure, verification in the contralateral arm; examination of the optic fundi; BMI, waist circumference; auscultation for carotid, abdominal, and femoral bruits; palpation of the thyroid gland; thorough examination of the heart and lungs; examination of the abdomen for enlarged kidneys, masses, and abnormal aortic pulsation; palpation of the lower extremities for edema and pulses; neurological assessment	Physical exam Vital signs	Blood pressure is the core measure for determining effective management of hypertensive patients; the other findings are important for their treatment and assessment value; some of the best values are relevant for CQM reporting.
Tests	Electrocardiogram; urinalysis; blood glucose, hematocrit; serum potassium, creatinine (GFR), and calcium, lipid profile; optional: urinary albumin/creatinine ratio	Laboratory results	Treatment and assessment value; some data relevant for reporting CQMs; may be leveraged for clinical decision support around treatment and medications.
Treatment	Lifestyle modifications: counseling patient on: weight reduction, adopting the DASH eating plan, dietary sodium reduction, increased physical activity, moderation of alcohol consumption; oral antihypertensive drugs dependent on presence of compelling indications (ie, heart failure, post–myocardial infarction, high coronary disease risk, diabetes, chronic kidney disease, recurring stroke prevention), pharmacologic treatment	Treatment plan, visit note, CPOE	The ability to understand treatment patterns by clinician or at the practice level will help identify business opportunities and areas for improvement.

Abbreviations: BMI indicates body mass index; CPOE, computerized provider order entry; CPT, *current procedural terminology*; CQM, clinical quality measure; DASH, Dietary Approaches to Stop Hypertension; and GFR, glomerular filtration rate.

Adapted from the *Seventh Report of the Joint National Committee on the Prevention, Detection, Evaluation, and Treatment of High Blood Pressure (JNC 7)*. NIHPublication. 04-5230, August 2004. www.nhlbi.nih.gov/guidelines/hypertension/jnc7full.pdf. Accessed January 10, 2013.

REALIZING UNEXPECTED BENEFITS

When developing your goals and the processes to achieve those goals, you may find your practice has also achieved unexpected and additional benefits. In the case study targeting hypertensive treatment at a physician practice, improving the care patients are receiving may also provide an opportunity to provide more covered services. For example, if the practice sees a large number of patients with hypertension and diabetes who can benefit from a nutritional consult, the office may consider hiring a nutritionist part time to provide those services. This will help improve outcomes at no additional cost to the practice—and perhaps increase revenues.

The challenge for a physician practice will be to cost-effectively leverage these tools to improve outcome measures and identify opportunities for business growth. It has been estimated that if all preventive services were implemented for each patient, for a practice size of 2500 patients, it could add 7.4 hours to a physician's work each day (assuming no automation and that the physician performs all preventive services, such as sigmoid-oscopy).[28] Although this number is likely inflated, it is not practical for a physician to implement everything at one time. It is critical that the practice make decisions about its priorities and how best to streamline the provision of some of these services. This priority-based approach, which considers different workflows to gain efficiencies, will help practices be successful, especially around quality measures. As discussed earlier, many of the preventive services are related to many of the CQMs.

Critical Point

Leverage the data to improve business efficiencies and improve care.

- Consider providing patients the capability to document their risk factors and social history through a patient portal. This allows for a more streamlined approach to getting information about topics such as alcohol use, cigarette smoking, and the like.

- For special services such as nutrition counseling, consider organizing a class and inviting the appropriate patients to attend as part of a "physician-prescribed" activity. This would allow a nutritionist to provide nutritional services to 10 to 20 patients at a time. Patients would receive an important service relevant to improving their health. Although these activities are generally not payable, there may be other financial incentives that would offset any costs accrued. Moreover, it might be possible to leverage external resources (eg, American Health Association).

- Identify patients who require immunizations. Organize immunization activities at certain points during the year. Provide educational materials to patients needing the service on the importance of these immunizations with their immunization appointment.

SUMMARY

In the fast-paced clinical environment that physicians often operate in, there are not many chances to assess what goes on within the practice. The implementation of an EHR allows for a reflection point to articulate practice goals and to select the EHR that most closely supports those goals. It is clear that, given the move to pay for performance and CQM reporting, demonstrating positive outcomes will become increasingly critical to the success of the physician practice. The first step to ensure success of the physician practice is to complete a comprehensive assessment of the practice. The results of this assessment will inform the direction taken by the practice (eg, EHR selection, how it's implemented, which CQMs). PBPH provide the needed approaches and tools to optimize outcomes. Leveraging

MU requirements to maximize the benefit to the practice is the goal. Physicians need to fully understand the capabilities and limitations of the relevant EHR capabilities (eg, CDS, measure reports) needed to support outcome improvement. Decisions should be made in the context of practice realities and implications to workflow, resource needs, and benefits. Physicians should look beyond the check-box of meeting the MU requirement and take advantage of the infrastructure developed for MU to position the practice for long-term success.

What's in It for Physicians?

■ The EHR will be a helpful tool in improving both the quality of the care delivered and the ability of a physician to be more effective in managing the care of patients at a population level. This latter capability will become increasingly important to physicians as they seek to integrate and expand their services to support their role as being the medical home for patients. It will also enable participation in clinical trials, support research, and provide disease management. However, this requires capture of structured data, such as demographics, family history, problem lists, test results, and medication lists.

■ It is clear that physicians are affected significantly by the addition of these MU objectives. How physicians in the practice implement the EHR and leverage it to align the MU measures to those that will most directly and positively affect their practice is a critical factor for success. If physicians and their practices are able to successfully focus their efforts, effectively implement change management, and leverage their EHRs, they will benefit greatly. Clinical practice efficiency will improve along with outcome measures, resulting in increased incentive payments, reduced liability, and opportunities for business expansion.

What's in It for Staff?

■ The physician office staff will participate in many of the changes that could result from a more outcomes-focused approach. This includes establishing workflows covering patient reminders, ensuring that transition-of-care information is routed appropriately, and documenting appropriate clinical data to support CDS. For the staff supporting the business side of the practice, having available data upon which to base resource decisions is always beneficial.

What's in It for Patients?

■ The MU measures that are relevant to outcomes have a direct, positive impact on patients and their health. As a result of numerous tools to support the physician, patients will experience fewer drug-to-drug and drug-to-allergy adverse events, benefit from improved care coordination, and be more likely to receive preventive and follow-up care.

ACTION ITEMS

1. Clearly articulate your practice goals, and understand individual goals of staff who works within the practice.
2. Assess the nature of your patient population in the context of your practice type (eg, specialty).

3. Align the CQMs with your practice goals, practice type, and population.
4. Understand the details of data that are needed for meeting CQMs, achieving practice priorities, and supporting CDS. Assess the EHR's abilities to support these needs.
5. Determine how robust your EHR reporting capabilities are or what you will want in a new EHR.
6. Determine which CQMs are most aligned with your practice.
7. Assess the EHR functionality needed to support the CQMs and what is needed by the practice.
8. Assess what data are needed to better evaluate your practice. Determine strategies to capture the needed information (consider embedding it in a targeted intervention). An example of this would be providing a documentation option next to a link to a stop-smoking resource. This would allow the physician to select "Doesn't smoke" or "Advised to stop smoking." The latter would provide a link to smoking-cessation resources for the patient (sending the link electronically to the patient or to print as "Information prescription" for the patient to pick up when checking out). This approach enables the collection of data while providing tools to improve the outcome.
9. Review data on your patient population monthly to assess care gaps.
10. Learn how to analyze your patient population and business processes from the data available.
11. Assess your EHR as to how it can best support your needs to ensure compliance with MU attestation requirements.
12. Assess how your EHR can help you improve your CQMs.
13. If your EHR does not support your ability to manage your practice from a population-health perspective, consider your options. This capability will become increasingly important to your business.

REFERENCES

1. Patient Protection and Affordable Care Act of 2010, Pub L 111-148, 124 Stat 119 (2010).
2. Gallegos A, Glendinning D. What's next for physicians after Affordable Care Act ruling. Amednews. Posted June 29, 2012. www.ama-assn.org/amednews/2012/06/25/gvsf0629.htm Accessed January 30, 2013.
3. Mangione-Smith R, DeCristofaro AH, Setodji CM, et al. The quality of ambulatory care delivered to children in the United States. *N Engl J Med*. 2007;357(15):1515-1523.
4. McGlynn EA, Asch SM, Adams J, et al. The quality of health care delivered to adults in the United States. *N Engl J Med*. 2003;348(26):2635-2645.
5. Schuster MA, McGlynn EA, Brook RH. How good is the quality of health care in the United States? *Milbank Q*. 1998;76(4):509, 517-563.
6. The Office of the National Coordinator for Health Information Technology (ONC). How to Attain Meaningful Use. www.healthit.gov/providers-professionals/how-attain-meaningful-use. Accessed January 4, 2013.
7. ———. Standards & Certification Criteria Final Rule. http://healthit.hhs.gov/portal/server.pt?open=512&objID=1195&parentname=CommunityPage&parentid=97&mode=2&in_hi_userid=11673&cached=true. Accessed August 12, 2012.
8. Cusack CM, Knudson AD, Kronstadt JL, Singer RD, Brown AL. *Practice-Based Population Health: Information Technology to Support Transformation to Proactive Primary Care*. Rockville, MD: Agency for Healthcare Quality and Research; 2010.
9. The Ottawa Hospital Research Institute (OHRI). Patient Decision Aids 2012: Implementation Toolkit. http://decisionaid.ohri.ca/implement.html. Accessed August 12, 2012.
10. Osheroff JA, Teich JM, Levick D, et al. *Improving Outcomes With Clinical Decision Support: An Implementer's Guide*. Chicago, IL: HIMSS Press; 2012.

11. Roshanov PS, Misra S, Gerstein HC, et al. Computerized clinical decision support systems for chronic disease management: a decision-maker-researcher partnership systematic review. *Implement Sci.* 2011;6:92. doi:10.1186/1748-5908-6-92.

12. Beaulieu ND, Horrigan DR. Putting smart money to work for quality improvement. *Health Serv Res.* 2005;40(5 pt 1):1318-1334.

13. Casalino LP. Disease management and the organization of physician practice. *JAMA.* 2005; 293(4):485-488.

14. Souza NM, Sebaldt RJ, Mackay JA, et al. Computerized clinical decision support systems for primary preventive care: a decision-maker-researcher partnership systematic review of effects on process of care and patient outcomes. *Implement Sci.* 2011;6:87. doi:10.1186/1748-5908-6-87.

15. Centers for Medicare & Medicaid Services (CMS). Eligible Hospital and Critical Access Hospital Meaningful Use Core Measures. Measure 10 of 14. Stage 1. November 7, 2010. www.cms.gov /Regulations-and-Guidance/Legislation/EHRIncentivePrograms/downloads/10_Clinical_Decision _Support_Rule.pdf. Accessed February 5, 2013.

16. Kuperman GJ, Bobb A, Payne TH, et al. Medication-related clinical decision support in computerized provider order entry systems: a review. *J Am Med Inform Assoc.* 2007;14(1):29-40.

17. Committee on Identifying and Preventing Medication Errors, Board on Health Care Services; Aspden P, Wolcott J, Bootman JL, Cronenwett LR, Eds. *Preventing Medication Errors: Quality Chasm Series.* Washington, DC; The National Academies Press; 2007.

18. Health Resources and Services Administration (HRSA). What are some of the benefits of e-prescribing? www.hrsa.gov/healthit/toolbox/HealthITAdoptiontoolbox/ElectronicPrescribing /benefitsepres.html. Accessed August 28, 2012.

19. Department of Justice. Electronic Prescriptions for Controlled Substances. www.deadiversion .usdoj.gov/ecomm/e_rx/faq/faq.htm. Accessed September 1, 2010.

20. Cornish PL, Knowles SR, Marchesano R, et al. Unintended medication discrepancies at the time of hospital admission. *Arch Intern Med.* 2005;165(4):424-429.

21. Nassaralla CL, Naessens JM, Hunt VL, et al. Medication reconciliation in ambulatory care: attempts at improvement. *Qual Saf Health Care.* 2009;18(5):402-407.

22. HealthCare.gov. Partnership for Patients: Better Care, Lower Costs. www.healthcare.gov/news /factsheets/2011/04/partnership04122011a.html. Accessed February 11, 2013.

23. Centers for Disease Control and Prevention (CDC). Meaningful Use Fact Sheet. Syndromic Surveillance: Submission of Electronic Syndromic Surveillance Data to Public Health Agencies. www.cdc.gov/phin/library/PHIN_Fact_Sheets/FS_MU_SS.pdf. Accessed February 2, 2013.

24. International Society for Disease Surveillance (ISDS). Revised Guidelines for Syndromic Surveillance Using Inpatient and Ambulatory Clinical Care EHR Data. www.syndromic.org/uploads /files/GuidelinesFAQ.pdf. Accessed June 15, 2012.

25. Ebell MH. Improving Patient Care: a tool for evaluating hypertension. *Fam Pract Manag.* 2004;11(3):79.

26. US Department of Health and Human Services. Reference Card from the Seventh Report of the Joint National Committee on Prevention, Detection, Evaluation, and Treatment of High Blood Pressure (JNC7). www.nhlbi.nih.gov/guidelines/hypertension/phycard.pdf. Accessed February 30, 2013.

27. ———. *The Seventh Report of the Joint National Committee on Prevention, Detection, Evaluation, and Treatment of High Blood Pressure (JNC7).* Bethesda, MD: NIH Publication No. 04-5230, August 2004. www.nhlbi.nih.gov/guidelines/hypertension/jnc7full.pdf. Accessed January 30, 2013.

28. Yarnall KS, Pllak KI, Ostbye T, Krause KM, Michener JL. Primary care: is there enough time for prevention? *Am J Public Health.* 2003;93(4):635-641.

active medication list. A list of medications that a given patient is currently taking.

active medication allergy list. A list of medications to which a given patient has known allergies.

accountable care organization. A group of health care providers who provide coordinated care and chronic disease management, and thereby, improve the quality of care patients receive. The organization's payment is tied to achieving health care quality goals and outcomes that result in cost savings. (For more information, go to www.healthit.gov/policy-researchers-implementers/technology-standards-certification-glossary.)

Agency for Healthcare Research and Quality (AHRQ). The Agency for Healthcare Research and Quality's (AHRQ) mission is to improve the quality, safety, efficiency, and effectiveness of health care for all Americans. As 1 of 12 agencies within the Department of Health and Human Services, AHRQ supports research that helps people make more informed decisions and improves the quality of health care services. (For more information, go to www.ahrq.gov/about/mission/glance/index.html.)

allergy. An exaggerated immune response or reaction to substances that are generally not harmful.

allowed amount. Maximum amount on which payment is based for covered health care services. This may be called "eligible expense," "payment allowance," or "negotiated rate." If the physician charges more than the allowed amount, the patient may have to pay the difference. (For more information, go to www.healthit.gov/policy-researchers-implementers/technology-standards-certification-glossary.)

analytic application. A type of business intelligence tool used to measure and improve business operations. For Meaningful Use, an analytic application could help physicians determine if they are accurately entering data for quality reporting purposes. For example, the application may serve as a dashboard or scorecard, or offer a report.

attestation. The process by which eligible professionals or eligible hospitals legally states through Medicare or Medicaid that they have demonstrated Meaningful Use with certified electronic health record technology. (For more information, go to www.healthit.gov/policy-researchers-implementers/technology-standards-certification-glossary.)

attestation calculator. An online tool that lets physicians determine whether they will meet Meaningful Use before submitting live data to complete their attestation.

base electronic health record (EHR). EHR technology that includes fundamental capabilities that all physicians would need to have. (For more information, go to www.healthit.gov/policy-researchers-implementers/technology-standards-certification-glossary.)

BATHE technique. A psychotherapeutic procedure and serves as a rough screening test for anxiety, depression, and situational stress disorders. The BATHE technique consists of four specific questions about the patient's background, affect, troubles, and handling of the current situation, followed by an empathic response; the procedure takes approximately 1 minute and must be practiced. Physicians may use the BATHE technique to connect meaningfully with patients, screen for mental health problems, and empower patients to handle many aspects of their life in a more constructive way. (For more information, go to www.psychiatrist.com/pcc/pccpdf/v01n02/v01n0202.pdf.)

business days. Business days are defined as Monday through Friday, excluding federal and state holidays in which the eligible professionals or their respective administrative staff is unavailable.

certified electronic health record (EHR) technology (CEHRT) for FY/CY 2013. A complete EHR that meets the requirements included in the definition of a qualified EHR and has been tested and certified in accordance with the certification program established by the Office of the National Coordinator for Health Information Technology (ONC) or a combination of EHR modules in which each module has been tested and certified in accordance with the certification program established by the ONC. (For more information, go to www.healthit.gov/policy-researchers-implementers/technology-standards-certification -glossary.)

certified electronic health record (EHR) technology (CEHRT) for FY/CY 2014. EHR technology certified under the Office of the National Coordinator for Health Information Technology CEHRT program to the 2014 Edition EHR certification criteria, which has the capabilities required to meet the definition of a base EHR and all other capabilities that are necessary to meet the objectives and associated measures under 42 CFR 495.6 and successfully report the clinical quality measures selected by the Centers for Medicare & Medicaid Services. (For more information, go to www.healthit.gov/policy-researchers-implementers /technology-standards-certification-glossary for more information.)

Centers for Disease Control and Prevention. An agency in the Department of Health and Human Services that collaborates to create the expertise, information, and tools that people and communities need to protect their health through health promotion, prevention of disease, injury and disability, and preparedness for new health threats. (For more information, go to www.cdc.gov.)

clinical decision support (CDS). Information and tools to support professionals and others in making clinical decisions. CDS encompasses a variety of tools to enhance decision making in clinical workflow. These tools include computerized alerts and reminders to care providers and patients, clinical guidelines, condition-specific order sets, focused patient data reports and summaries, documentation templates, diagnostic support, and contextually relevant reference information, among other tools. (For more information, go to www.healthit.gov/policy-researchers-implementers/clinical-decision-support-cds.)

certified electronic health record (EHR) technology. A complete EHR that meets the requirements included in the definition of a qualified EHR and has been tested and certified in accordance with the certification program, such as the standards, implementation specifications, and certification criteria, established by the Office of the National Coordinator for Health Information Technology (ONC) as having met all applicable certification criteria adopted by the Department of Health and Human Services. EHR technology must be tested and certified by an ONC-authorized testing and certification body in order for a physician to qualify for EHR incentive payments. (For more information, go to http:// journal.ahima.org/2010/09/02/meaningful-use-and-ehr-certification/ and www.cms.gov /ehrincentiveprograms/25_Certification.asp.)

clinical quality measure (CQM). A tool that helps measure and track the quality of health care services provided by eligible professionals (EPs), eligible hospitals (EHs), and critical access hospitals (CAHs) within the health care system. The CQMs are based on specific evidence-based practices that have been shown to give the best results to the most people. To demonstrate Meaningful Use successfully, EPs, EHs, and CAHs are also required to report CQMs specific to EPs or EHs and CAHs. (For more information, go to www.cms .gov/Regulations-and-Guidance/Legislation/EHRIncentivePrograms/ClinicalQualityMeasures .html and www.cms.gov/EHRIncentivePrograms for more information.)

Clinical Laboratory Improvement Amendments (CLIA). Ensures quality laboratory testing. Established in 1988 by Congress, CLIA sets quality standards for all nonresearch laboratory testing performed on specimens derived from humans for the purpose of providing information for the diagnosis, prevention and treatment of disease, or impairment of, or assessment of health. CLIA requires that laboratories performing these types of tests to be certified by the secretary of the Department of Health and Human Services. (For more information, go to www.cms.gov/Regulations-and-Guidance/Legislation/CLIA/index .html?redirect=/clia/.)

clinical summary. An after-visit summary that provides a patient with relevant and actionable information and instructions containing the patient name; provider's office contact information; date and location of visit; an updated medication list; updated vitals; reason(s) for visit; procedures and other instructions based on clinical discussions that took place during the office visit; any updates to a problem list; immunizations or medications administered during visit; summary of topics covered and/or considered during visit; time and location of next appointment and/or testing, if scheduled, or a recommended appointment time if not scheduled; and a list of other appointments and tests that the patient needs to schedule with contact information, recommended patient decision aids, laboratory and other diagnostic test orders, test or laboratory results (if received sooner than 24 hours after visit), and symptoms. (For more information, go to www.cms.gov/Regulations-and-Guid ance/Legislation/EHRIncentivePrograms/downloads/13ClinicalSummaries.pdf.)

complete electronic health record (EHR). An EHR system that meets, at a minimum, all mandatory certification criteria (CC) of an edition of CC adopted by the secretary of Department of Health and Human Services (for an ambulatory setting or inpatient setting) that has been tested and certified for a qualified EHR, as opposed to a modular EHR system (see modular EHR system). (For more information, go to www.medhealthworld.com /?p =1072 and www.healthit.gov/policy-researchers-implementers/technology-standards -certification-glossary.)

computerized provider order entry (CPOE). Computer system that allows direct entry of medication and other orders by qualified providers, which is documented or captured in a digital, structured, and computable format for use in improving safety and organization. (For more information, go to www.connectopensource.org/about/faq and www.cpoe.org.)

CONNECT. An open source software gateway that organizations can use to securely link their existing health information technology systems into the health information exchanges (HIEs). The CONNECT solution enables secure and interoperable electronic HIEs with other Nationwide Health Information Network (NwHIN)–compliant organizations, including federal agencies; state, tribal, and local-level health organizations, and health care participants in the private sector. (For more information, go to www.connectopen source.org/about/faq.)

current state. When describing or managing workflows, this represents the way tasks are completed or information flows currently. Studying the current state allows a practice to measure what it is currently doing and compare it with how work would flow in an electronic or future state.

core measures (CMs). Mandatory objectives that eligible professionals (EPs) or eligible hospitals must meet in order to achieve quality incentive payments. EPs must meet 15 CMs in Stage 1 and 17 CMs in Stage 2.

covered entity. Individuals, organizations, and agencies that meet the definition of a covered entity under the Health Information Portability and Accountability Act (HIPAA) 1996 must comply with HIPAA requirements to protect the privacy and security of health information and must provide individuals with certain rights with respect to their health information. If a covered entity engages a business associate to help it carry out its health care activities and functions, the covered entity must have a written business associate contract or other arrangement with the business associate that establishes specifically what the business associate has been engaged to do and requires the business associate to comply with HIPAA requirements to protect the privacy and security of protected health information. In addition to these contractual obligations, business associates are directly liable for compliance with certain provisions of HIPAA. (For more information, go to www.hhs.gov/ocr/privacy/hipaa/understanding/coveredentities/.)

critical access hospitals (CAHs). Rural community hospitals that receive cost-based reimbursement. To be designated a CAH, a rural hospital must meet defined criteria that were outlined in the Conditions of Participation 42CFR485 and subsequent legislative refinements to the program. (For more information, go to www.aha.org/advocacy-issues/cah/index.shtml.)

data. In an electronic health record (EHR), data are pieces of information created, stored, used, disclosed, analyzed, and transmitted in a secure environment. Most EHRs require data to be entered into specific fields, so that when the same or different users choose to analyze data, the data are accessible from within the database to produce accurate reports. The types of data in an EHR include free-text fields, discrete or structured data, and image or scanned data. (For more information, go to www.merriam-webster.com/dictionary/data.)

data management. Development and execution of architectures, policies, practices, and procedures in order to manage the information life-cycle needs of an enterprise in an effective manner. (For more information, go to http://searchdatamanagement.techtarget.com/definition/data-management.)

denominator. A collection of data that is used to calculate a percentage to determine if Meaningful Use (MU) objectives are met according to a minimum threshold for the objectives. In the context of MU objectives, the denominator is based on:
- All patients seen or admitted during the electronic health record (EHR) reporting period. The denominator is all patients, regardless of whether their records are kept using certified EHR technology (CEHRT).
- Actions or subsets of patients seen or admitted during the EHR reporting period. The denominator includes only patients or actions taken on behalf of the patients whose records are kept using CEHRT. (For more information, go to https://questions.cms.gov/faq.php?id=5005&faqId=2813.)

Direct Project. The Direct Project focuses on the technical standards and services necessary to securely "push" content from a sender to a receiver. When these services are used by providers and organizations to transport and share qualifying clinical content, the combination of content and Direct Project–specified transport standards may satisfy some Stage 1 Meaningful Use requirements. For example, a primary care physician who is referring a patient to a specialist can use the Direct Project to provide a clinical summary of the patient's condition to the specialist, and, in turn, to receive a summary of the consultation from the specialist. (For more information, go to www.cms.gov/Regulations-and-Guidance /Legislation/EHRIncentivePrograms/index.html?redirect=/EHRIncentivePrograms.)

discrete or structured data. Individual pieces of information that are entered into a specific field in the electronic health record (EHR). Each piece of information has a unique place in the database. Example: If the patient's weight is entered into the individual field for patient weight in the EHR, each weight at each visit can be compared with the last and displayed as a graph, list, table, and so forth.

diagnostic test results. All data derived from tests used to diagnose and treat disease. Examples include, but are not limited to, blood tests, microbiology, urinalysis, pathology tests, radiology, cardiac imaging, nuclear medicine tests, and pulmonary function tests. (For more information, go to www.texmed.org/Template.aspx?id=21590.)

distinct certified electronic health record technology (CEHRT). CEHRTs can achieve certification and operate independently of other CEHRTs. Each instance of CEHRT must be certified and operate independently from all others in order to be considered as distinct. Therefore, separate instances of CEHRT that must link to a common database in order to gain certification would not be considered distinct. (For an example, go to www.emr approved.com/hitanswers/tag/cehrt/.)

electronic health record (EHR). An electronic version of a patient's medical history that is maintained by the provider over time and may include all of the key administrative clinical data relevant to that person's care under a particular provider, including demographics, progress notes, problems, medications, vital signs, past medical history, immunizations, laboratory data, and radiology reports. (EHR is sometimes referred to as an electronic medical record [EMR]). (For more information, go to www.cms.gov/Medicare/E-Health/EHealth Records/index.html?redirect=/ehealthrecords/.)

EHR certification standards. The standards, implementation specifications, and certification criteria adopted by the secretary of Department of Health and Human Services for EHRs in order to support the achievement of Meaningful Use (MU) Stage 1 or Stage 2 by eligible professionals and eligible hospitals under the Centers for Medicare & Medicaid Services EHR Incentive Programs. For all MU stages, the EHR certification standards are performance measures that a vendor must meet in order to achieve the Office of the National Coordinator for Health Information Technology (ONC) recognition. Standards are established by the ONC health information technology certification program. (For more information, go to www.healthit.gov/policy-researchers-implementers/onc-hit-certification -program.)

EHR incentive program. Program that provides incentive payments for eligible professionals, eligible hospitals, and critical access hospitals as they adopt, implement, upgrade, or demonstrate meaningful use of certified EHR technology in ways that can positively impact patient care. (For more information, go to www.cms.gov/Regulations-and-Guidance /Legislation/EHRIncentivePrograms/Downloads/beginners_guide.pdf and www.cms.gov /Regulations-and-Guidance/Legislation/EHRIncentivePrograms/Basics.html.)

electronic prescribing (e-Rx). Computer-based electronic generation, transmission, and filling of a medical prescription in which physicians may use handheld or personal computer devices, such as tablets and mobile phones, to electronically send accurate, error-free and understandable prescription directly to a pharmacy from the point of care. (For more information, go to www.cms.gov/Medicare/E-Health/Eprescribing/index.html ?redirect =/eprescribing/.)

eligible hospital. A hospital that is eligible to participate in the Centers for Medicare & Medicaid Services EHR [electronic health record] Incentive Program include the following: "Subsection (d) hospitals" in the 50 states and the District of Columbia that are paid under the inpatient prospective payment system, critical access hospitals, Medicare Advantage (MA-Affiliated) Hospitals.

eligible professional (EP). A qualified health care professional who is eligible to participate in the Centers for Medicare & Medicaid Services EHR [electronic health record] Incentive Programs. Medicare EPs include doctors of medicine or osteopathy; doctors of dental surgery or dental medicine; doctors of podiatry; doctors of optometry; and chiropractors; Medicaid EPs include physicians (primarily doctors of medicine and doctors of osteopathy); nurse practitioners, certified nurse-midwives, dentists, and physician assistants who furnish services in a federally qualified health center or rural health clinic that is led by a physician assistant. (For more information, go to www.hitechanswers.net/ehr-incentive-program /eligible-professionals/.)

exchange [of clinical information]. Exchange of key clinical information (for example, problem list, medication list, medication allergies, and diagnostic test results) among providers of care and patient authorized entities electronically. The exchange of information requires eligible professionals to use the Office of the National Coordinator for Health Information Technology standards for certified electronic health record technology (CEHRT), which enables clinical information to be sent between different legal entities with distinct CEHRT instead of between organizations that share a CEHRT. (For more information and an example, go to www.healthit.gov/providers-professionals/achieve-meaningful-use/core -measures/electronic-exchange-of-clinical-information, https://questions.cms.gov/faq.php ?faqId=7697, and www.emrapproved.com/hitanswers/tag/cehrt/.)

free-text fields. Used to add notes or comments about the patient visit, but free text is typically not searchable. Instead, free text or narrative is meant for the provider's use in order to document the patient's words or explanation, the provider's impression, and for reminders and notes. (For more information, go to www.merriam-webster.com/dictionary /data for more information.)

future state. A vision for how work would be completed or how information would move from one point to another. Future state may be based on what the electronic health record vendor recommends, how the practice believes it can offer services more efficiently, or a vision of how other practices have successfully managed a workflow that a practice wants to adopt.

health information technology (health IT or HIT). Comprehensive management of health information across computerized systems and its secure exchange among consumers, providers, government and quality entities, and insurers. The application of information processing involves both computer hardware and software that deals with the storage, retrieval, sharing, and use of health care information, data, and knowledge for communication and decision making. (For more information, go to www.healthit.gov/policy -researchers-implementers/technology-standards-certification-glossary.)

Health Information Technology for Economic and Clinical Health (HITECH) Act. Reinvestment Act of 2009, signed into law on February 17, 2009, to promote the adoption and meaningful use of health information technology. Subtitle D of the HITECH Act addresses the privacy and security concerns associated with the electronic transmission of health information, in part, through several provisions that strengthen the civil and criminal enforcement of the Health Information Portability and Accountability Act rules. (For more information, go to www.healthit.gov/policy-researchers-implementers/hitech-act-0 and www.hhs.gov/ocr/privacy/hipaa/understanding/coveredentities/hitechact.pdf.)

health information exchange (HIE). Electronic movement of health care information across organizations within a region, community, or hospital system according to nationally recognized standards. The goal of HIE is to facilitate access to and retrieval of clinical data to provide safer, timelier, efficient, effective, equitable, patient-centered care. Health information exchange organizations provide the capability to electronically move clinical information between disparate health care information systems while maintaining the meaning of the information being exchanged. (For more information, go to www.hrsa.gov/healthit /toolbox/RuralHealthITtoolbox/Collaboration/whatishie.html.)

Health Level Seven (HL7). A nonprofit, American National Standards Institute accredited standards–developing organization dedicated to providing a comprehensive framework and related standards for the exchange, integration, sharing, and retrieval of electronic health information that supports clinical practice and the management, delivery, and evaluation of health services. HL7's 2300 or more members include approximately 500 corporate members, which represent more than 90% of the information systems vendors serving the health care industry. (For more information, go to www.hl7.org/about/index.cfm?ref=nav.)

hybrid chart. Documentation of a person's health record that is stored in multiple formats or multiple locations, such as in a paper chart and an electronic health record (EHR), or in multiple EHRs, eg, when a practice is transitioning from one EHR to another. Also included in a hybrid chart are electronic documents, images, and audio and video files, all part of the legal EHR.

image or scanned data. Information that is entered into the electronic health record EHR) as a block of text or an image (picture), and it is filed in the EHR as a scanned document. Information entered into the computer by this method can be viewed and appear as it did when it was scanned. The information cannot be compared or graphed by the EHR, as it is only a picture of the information. Example: The patient's last physical exam report is scanned into the EHR. (For more information, go to www.merriam-webster.com/dictionary /data.)

interoperability standards. Integrated and technical standards that support the secure exchange of health information. The ONC's Office of Interoperability and Standards oversees US Health IT Initiatives, including the Standards & Interoperability (S&I) Framework, the Nationwide Health Information Network, the EHR Certification Program, the Direct Project, and Managing the Federal Health Architecture and CONNECT Program. (For more information, go to www.healthit.gov/sites/default/files/pdf/fact-sheets/onc-office-of-inter operability-and-standards.pdf.)

International Society for Disease Surveillance (ISDS). A 501(c)3 nonprofit organization founded in 2005, dedicated to the improvement of population health by advancing the science and practice of disease surveillance. The ISDS membership of 400 or more represents professional and academic subject-matter experts in the fields of public health surveillance, clinical practice, health informatics, health policy, and other areas related to national and global health surveillance. (For more information, go to www.syndromic.org/about-isds.)

measure [of objective]. A task to complete in order to demonstrate that the eligible professional or eligible hospital can successfully meet a Meaningful Use (MU) objective. For example, one of the MU *Objectives* is to "Report ambulatory clinical quality measure to CMS," and the corresponding *Measure* for this *Objective* is to "Successfully report to CMS ambulatory clinical quality measures selected by CMS in the manner specified by CMS. (For more information, go to www.healthit.gov/policy-researchers-implementers/technology -standards-certification-glossary for more information.)

Meaningful Use (MU). Sets specific objectives that eligible professionals and eligible hospitals must achieve to qualify for the Centers for Medicare & Medicaid Services EHR [electronic health record] Incentive Programs. Simply put, MU means providers need to show they are using certified EHR technology in ways that can be measured significantly in quality and in quantity. (For more information, go to www.cdc.gov/ehrmeaningfuluse /introduction.html and www.cms.gov/EHRIncentivePrograms/.)

meaningful users. Providers who demonstrate meaningful use of their electronic health records (EHRs) in ways that can positively affect the care of their patients and meet all of the Meaningful Use objectives, which are measured significantly in quality and quantity, as established by the Centers for Medicare & Medicaid Services EHR Incentive Program. (For more information, go to www.healthit.gov/policy-researchers-implementers /technology-standards-certification-glossary.)

medication reconciliation. The process of comparing a patient's medication orders (including the name, dosage, frequency, and route) with all of the medications that the patient has been taking. The process of comparison is performed by comparing a patient's medical record with an external list of medications obtained from a patient, hospital, or other provider. Medical reconciliation is done to avoid medication errors such as omissions, duplications, dosing errors, or drug interactions.

menu set measure. Meaningful Use (MU) includes a core set and a menu set of objectives that are specific to eligible professionals (EPs) or eligible hospitals (EHs) and critical access hospitals (CAHs). In order to embrace a flexible approach to meeting MU measures, EPs and EHs are required to meet core measures, but have the flexibility to select the menu set measures. Menu measures are required, but their selection is broader and features something of an "a la carte" approach. For example, in Stage 1, EPs must select 5 of the menu set measures, one of which must be a population and public-health objective.

modular electronic health record (EHR). An EHR system that can be assembled by combining several certified EHR modules so that together they meet all of the requirements for a qualified EHR. (For more information, go to www.medhealthworld.com/?p=1072.)

National Plan and Provider Enumeration Series (NPPES). The Administrative Simplification provisions of the Health Insurance Portability and Accountability Act of 1996 mandated the adoption of standard unique identifiers for health care providers and health plans. The purpose of these provisions is to improve the efficiency and effectiveness of the electronic transmission of health information. The Centers for Medicare & Medicaid Services has developed the NPPES to assign this unique identifiers. (For more information, go to https://nppes.cms.hhs.gov/NPPES/Welcome.do.)

National Quality Forum (NQF). The NQF reviews, endorses, and recommends the use of standardized health care performance measures. Performance measures, also known as quality measures, are essential tools that are used to evaluate how well health care services are being delivered. The NQF's endorsed measures are often "invisible" at the clinical bedside, but they quietly influence the care delivered to millions of patients every day. (For more information, go to www.qualityforum.org.)

numerator. A collection of data that is used to calculate a percentage to determine if Meaningful Use (MU) objectives are met according to a minimum threshold for the objectives. In the context of MU objectives, the numerator is defined as the number of activities, events, or patient records in the denominator recorded in the electronic health record (EHR). For example, when assessing the numerator and denominator for Stage 2 Core Measure 1, CPOE for Medication, Laboratory, and Radiology, the denominator would be the number of medication, orders created by the EP during the EHR reporting period. The numerator is the number of orders in the denominator recorded using CPOE. (For more information, go to www.cms.gov/ehrincentiveprograms, https://questions.cms.gov /faq.php?id=5005&faqId=2813, http://mycourses.med.harvard.edu/ec_res/nt/36980CA6 -E154-4820-A0ED-8B235138B79F/measures.pdf, and www.dpw.state.pa.us/ucmprd/groups /webcontent/documents/document/p_012312.pdf.)

Office of the National Coordinator for Health Information Technology (ONC). The ONC is the principal federal entity charged with the coordination of nationwide efforts to implement and use the most advanced health information technology and the electronic exchange of health information. The position of the National Coordinator was created in 2004, through an Executive Order, and legislatively mandated in the HITECH Act of 2009.

office visit. Office visits include separate, billable encounters that result from the evaluation and management services provided to the patient, which include the following: (1) concurrent care or transfer of care visits, (2) consultant visits, or (3) prolonged physician service without direct (face-to-face) patient contact (tele-health). A consultant visit occurs when a provider is asked to render an expert opinion and/or service for a specific condition or problem by a referring provider.

patient authorized entities. Any individual or organization to which a patient has granted access to his or her clinical information. Examples would include an insurance company that covers the patient, an entity facilitating health information exchange among providers, or a personal health record vendor identified by the patient. A patient would have to affirmatively grant access to these entities.

patient decision aids. Tools that help people become involved in decision making by providing information about the options and outcomes and by clarifying personal values. They are designed to complement, rather than replace, counseling from a health practitioner. (For more information, go to decisionaid.ohri.ca.)

Patient Protection and Affordable Care Act (Affordable Care Act or ACA). Landmark health reform legislation passed by the 111th Congress and signed into law by President Barack Obama in March 2010. In 2010, Congress enacted the Patient Protection and Affordable Care Act in order to increase the number of Americans covered by health insurance and decrease the cost of health care. One key provision is the individual mandate, which requires most Americans to maintain "minimum essential" health insurance coverage. Another key provision of the Act is the Medicaid expansion. The current Medicaid program offers federal funding to states to assist pregnant women, children, needy families, blind people, elderly people, and people with disabilities in obtaining medical care. (For more information, go to www.supremecourt.gov/opinions/11pdf/11-393c3a2.pdf.)

patient-specific education resources. Resources identified through logic built into certified electronic health record technology that evaluate information about the patient and to suggest education resources that would be of value to the patient.

permissible prescriptions. Permissible prescriptions refers to the current restrictions established by the Department of Justice on electronic prescribing for controlled substances in Schedules II through V. (For more information, go to https://questions.cms.gov/faq .php?id=5005&faqId=2763.)

personal health record (PHR). A record with information about a patient's health in which a patient maintains and manage his or her health information (or someone who is helping the patient and is authorized to have access) in a private, secure, confidential, and computerized environment, which is available for easy reference using a computer. The patient controls the health information in the PHR and can get to it anywhere at any time with Internet access.

permanent certification program (PCP). Certification program to authorize organizations to certify electronic health record (EHR) technology, such as complete EHRs and/or EHR modules issued under the final rule. The PCP could also be expanded to include the certification of other types of health information technology (HIT). The secretary of the Department of Health and Human Services issued the PCP Final Rule to establish a successor to the Temporary Certification Program. The Office of the National Coordinator (ONC) for the HIT Certification Program (formerly known as the PCP) was launched on October 4, 2012. The PCP Final Rule contains the policies and procedures that will regulate ONC HIT Certification Program operations. (For more information, go to www.gpo.gov/fdsys /pkg/FR-2011-01-07/pdf/2010-33174.pdf and www.healthit.gov/policy-researchers-imple menters/permanent-certification-program-faqs#a1.)

practice-based population health (PBPH). An approach to care that uses information on a group ("population") of patients within a clinical practice ("practice-based") to improve the care and clinical outcomes of patients within that practice. (For more information, see Cusack CM, Knudson AD, Kronstadt JL, Singer RF, Brown AL. *Practice-Based Population Health: Information Technology to Support Transformation to Proactive Primary Care.* AHRQ publication 10-0092-EF. Rockville, MD: AHRQ; July 2010.)

Physician Quality Reporting System (PQRS). A reporting program that uses a combination of incentive payments and payment adjustments to promote reporting of quality information by eligible professionals (EPs). The program provides an incentive payment to practices with EPs (identified on claims by their individual National Provider Identifier and Tax Identification Number) who satisfactorily report data on quality measures for covered Physician Fee Schedule services furnished to Medicare Part B Fee-for-Service beneficiaries (including Railroad Retirement Board and Medicare Secondary Payer). Beginning in 2015, the program also applies a payment adjustment to EPs who do not satisfactorily report data on quality measures for covered professional services. (For more information, go to www.cms.gov/Medicare/Quality-Initiatives-Patient-Assessment-Instruments/PQRS/index .html?redirect=/PQRI.)

prescription. The authorization by an eligible professional (EP) to a pharmacist to dispense a drug that the pharmacist would not dispense to the patient without such authorization.

problem list. A list of current and active diagnoses, as well as past diagnoses relevant to the current care of the patient.

public-health agency. An entity under the jurisdiction of the Department of Health and Human Services, tribal organization, state, and/or city or county administration that serves a public-health function.

regional extension center (REC). An organization that has received funding under the HITECH Act to assist health care providers with community-based education and technical support as they select and implement electronic health records technology. (For more information, go to www.ajmc.com/publications/issue/2013/2013-1-vol19-n3/Engaging

-Providers-in-Underserved-Areas-to-Adopt-Electronic-Health-Records and www.ajmc.com /publications/issue/2013/2013-1-vol19-n3/Engaging-Providers-in-Underserved-Areas-to -Adopt-Electronic-Health-Records.)

relevant encounter. An encounter during which an eligible professional (EP) performs a medication reconciliation because of new medication or long gaps in time between patient encounters or for other reasons determined appropriate by the EP. Essentially, an encounter is relevant if the EP judges it to be so. (For more information, go to www.cms.gov /Regulations-and-Guidance/Legislation/EHRIncentivePrograms/downloads/6_Medication _Reconciliation.pdf.)

separate legal entities. A separate or different legal entity is an entity that has its own separate legal existence. Indications that two entities are legally separate would include the following: (1) They are each separately incorporated. (2) They have separate boards of directors. and (3) Neither entity is owned or controlled by the other.

syndromic surveillance data. The ongoing, systematic collection, analysis, and interpretation of health-related data essential to the planning, implementation, and evaluation of public-health practice, closely integrated with the timely dissemination of these data to those responsible for the prevention and control of diseases, injuries, or other health problems. The term "surveillance system" describes the networks of people and procedures involved in conducting surveillance among populations within specific places or jurisdictions. Individual surveillance systems generally focus on particular health threats or problems as part of a prevention and control program. For example, as part of an HIV/AIDS prevention program, a public-health agency may conduct surveillance for HIV risk behaviors, asymptomatic HIV infection, or illnesses associated with HIV-related immune dysfunction. (For more information, go to www.cdc.gov/MMWR/preview/mmwrhtml /su5301a3.htm.)

temporary certification program (TCP). TCP was the first part of the Office of the National Coordinator for Health Information Technology two-part approach to establish a transparent and objective certification process. The TCP was established to ensure that certified EHR technology was available for adoption by health care providers seeking to qualify for the Medicare and Medicaid EHR incentive payments beginning in 2011. (For more information, go to www.healthit.gov/policy-researchers-implementers/temporary-certifica tion-program-faqs#a1.)

transition of care. The movement or referral of a patient from one setting of care (hospital, ambulatory primary care practice, ambulatory specialty care practice, long-term care, home health, rehabilitation facility) to another provider of care.

unique patient. If a patient is seen by an eligible professional more than once during the electronic health record (EHR) reporting period, then for purposes of measurement, the patient is counted only once in the denominator for the measure. All the measures relying on the term "unique patient" relate to what is contained in the patient's medical record. Not all of this information will need to be updated or even be needed by the provider at every patient encounter. This is especially true for patients whose encounter frequency is such that they would see the same provider multiple times in the same EHR reporting period.

up-to-date [problem list]. Problem list in the patient's electronic health record is maintained and populated with the most recent diagnosis known by the EP. This knowledge could be ascertained from previous records, transfer of information from other providers, diagnosis by the EP, or querying the patient. (For more information, go to www.cms.gov /Regulations-and-Guidance/Legislation/EHRIncentivePrograms/downloads/3_Maintain _Problem_ListEP.pdf.)

workflow. The process or steps to move people and information through an office to accomplish a task. Examples of workflows would be the check-in of patients or "rooming" the patient. Other workflows might be ordering medications or the order and results of laboratory tests. In one office, how the staff completes tasks when using paper medical records might be very efficient, but the process may change when a new paper form, test, or procedure is added to the current practice.

STAGE 1 VS STAGE 2 COMPARISON TABLE FOR ELIGIBLE PROFESSIONALS

Last updated: August 2012

CORE OBJECTIVES (17 total)

Stage 1 Objective	Stage 1 Measure	Stage 2 Objective	Stage 2 Measure
Use CPOE for medication orders directly entered by any licensed healthcare professional who can enter orders into the medical record per state, local and professional guidelines	More than 30% of unique patients with at least one medication in their medication list seen by the EP have at least one medication order entered using CPOE	Use computerized provider order entry (CPOE) for medication, laboratory and radiology orders directly entered by any licensed healthcare professional who can enter orders into the medical record per state, local and professional guidelines	More than 60% of medication, 30% of laboratory, and 30% of radiology orders created by the EP during the EHR reporting period are recorded using CPOE
Implement drug-drug and drug-allergy interaction checks	The EP has enabled this functionality for the entire EHR reporting period	*No longer a separate objective for Stage 2*	*This measure is incorporated into the Stage 2 Clinical Decision Support measure*
Generate and transmit permissible prescriptions electronically (eRx)	More than 40% of all permissible prescriptions written by the EP are transmitted electronically using certified EHR technology	Generate and transmit permissible prescriptions electronically (eRx)	More than 50% of all permissible prescriptions written by the EP are compared to at least one drug formulary and transmitted electronically using certified EHR technology
Record demographics: ■ Preferred language ■ Gender ■ Race ■ Ethnicity ■ Date of birth	More than 50% of all unique patients seen by the EP have demographics recorded as structured data	Record the following demographics ■ Preferred language ■ Gender ■ Race ■ Ethnicity ■ Date of birth	More than 80% of all unique patients seen by the EP have demographics recorded as structured data

Stage 1 Objective	Stage 1 Measure	Stage 2 Objective	Stage 2 Measure
Maintain an up-to-date problem list of current and active diagnoses	More than 80% of all unique patients seen by the EP have at least one entry or an indication that no problems are known for the patient recorded as structured data	*No longer a separate objective for Stage 2*	*This measure is incorporated into the Stage 2 measure of Summary of Care Document at Transitions of Care and Referrals*
Maintain active medication list	More than 80% of all unique patients seen by the EP have at least one entry (or an indication that the patient is not currently prescribed any medication) recorded as structured data	*No longer a separate objective for Stage 2*	*This measure is incorporated into the Stage 2 measure of Summary of Care Document at Transitions of Care and Referrals*
Maintain active medication allergy list	More than 80% of all unique patients seen by the EP have at least one entry (or an indication that the patient has no known medication allergies) recorded as structured data	*No longer a separate objective for Stage 2*	*This measure is incorporated into the Stage 2 measure of Summary of Care Document at Transitions of Care and Referrals*
Record and chart changes in vital signs: ■ Height ■ Weight ■ Blood pressure ■ Calculate and display BMI ■ Plot and display growth charts for children 2-20 years, including BMI	For more than 50% of all unique patients age 2 and over seen by the EP, blood pressure, height and weight are recorded as structured data	Record and chart changes in vital signs: ■ Height ■ Weight ■ Blood pressure (age 3 and over) ■ Calculate and display BMI ■ Plot and display growth charts for patients 0-20 years, including BMI	More than 80% of all unique patients seen by the EP have blood pressure (for patients age 3 and over only) and height and weight (for all ages) recorded as structured data
Record smoking status for patients 13 years old or older	More than 50% of all unique patients 13 years old or older seen by the EP have smoking status recorded as structured data	Record smoking status for patients 13 years old or older	More than 80% of all unique patients 13 years old or older seen by the EP have smoking status recorded as structured data

Stage 1 Objective	Stage 1 Measure	Stage 2 Objective	Stage 2 Measure
Implement one clinical decision support rule relevant to specialty or high clinical priority along with the ability to track compliance [with] that rule	Implement one clinical decision support rule	Use clinical decision support to improve performance on high-priority health conditions	1. Implement 5 clinical decision support interventions related to 4 or more clinical quality measures, if applicable, at a relevant point in patient care for the entire EHR reporting period. 2. The EP, eligible hospital, or CAH has enabled the functionality for drug-drug and drug-allergy interaction checks for the entire EHR reporting period
Report clinical quality measures (CQMs) to CMS or the states	Provide aggregate numerator, denominator, and exclusions through attestation or through the PQRS Electronic Reporting Pilot	*No longer a separate objective for Stage 2, but providers must still submit CQMs to CMS or the States in order to achieve meaningful use*	*Starting in 2014, all CQMs will be submitted electronically to the CMS*
Provide patients with an electronic copy of their health information (including diagnostic test results, problem list, medication lists, medication allergies), upon request	More than 50% of all patients of the EP who request an electronic copy of their health information are provided it within 3 business days	Provide patients the ability to view online, download and transmit their health information within four business days of the information being available to the EP	i. More than 50% of all unique patients seen by the EP during the EHR reporting period are provided timely (available to the patient within 4 business days after the information is available to the EP) online access to their health information ii. More than 5% of all unique patients seen by the EP during the EHR reporting period (or their authorized representatives) view, download, or transmit to a third party their health information
Provide clinical summaries for patients for each office visit	Clinical summaries provided to patients for more than 50% of all office visits within 3 business days	Provide clinical summaries for patients for each office visit	Clinical summaries provided to patients within one business day for more than 50% of office visits

Stage 1 Objective	Stage 1 Measure	Stage 2 Objective	Stage 2 Measure
Capability to exchange key clinical information (for example, problem list, medication list, medication allergies, diagnostic test results), among providers of care and patient authorized entities electronically	Performed at least one test of certified EHR technology's capacity to electronically exchange key clinical information	*This objective is eliminated from Stage 1 in 2013 and is no longer an objective for Stage 2*	*This measure is eliminated from Stage 1 in 2013 and is no longer a measure for Stage 2*
Protect electronic health information created or maintained by the certified EHR technology through the implementation of appropriate technical capabilities	Conduct or review a security risk analysis per 45 CFR 164.308 (a)(1) and implement security updates as necessary and correct identified security deficiencies as part of its risk management process	Protect electronic health information created or maintained by the certified EHR technology through the implementation of appropriate technical capabilities	Conduct or review a security risk analysis in accordance with the requirements under 45 CFR 164.308 (a)(1), including addressing the encryption/security of data at rest and implement security updates as necessary and correct identified security deficiencies as part of its risk management process
Implement drug-formulary checks	The EP has enabled this functionality and has access to at least one internal or external drug formulary for the entire EHR reporting period	*No longer a separate objective for Stage 2*	*This measure is incorporated into the e-Prescribing measure for Stage 2*
Incorporate clinical labtest results into certified EHR technology as structured data	More than 40% of all clinical lab tests results ordered by the EP during the EHR reporting period whose results are either in a positive/negative or numerical format are incorporated in certified EHR technology as structured data	Incorporate clinical lab-test results into certified EHR technology as structured data	More than 55% of all clinical lab-test results ordered by the EP during the EHR reporting period whose results are either in a positive/negative or numerical format are incorporated in certified EHR technology as structured data
Generate lists of patients by specific conditions to use for quality improvement, reduction of disparities, research, or outreach	Generate at least one report listing patients of the EP with a specific condition	Generate lists of patients by specific conditions to use for quality improvement, reduction of disparities, research, or outreach	Generate at least one report listing patients of the EP with a specific condition

Stage 1 Objective	Stage 1 Measure	Stage 2 Objective	Stage 2 Measure
Send reminders to patients per patient preference for preventive/follow up care	More than 20% of all unique patients 65 years or older or 5 years old or younger were sent an appropriate reminder during the EHR reporting period	Use clinically relevant information to identify patients who should receive reminders for preventive/follow-up care	Use EHR to identify and provide reminders for preventive/follow-up care for more than 10% of patients with two or more office visits in the last 2 years
Provide patients with timely electronic access to their health information (including lab results, problem list, medication lists, medication allergies) within 4 business days of the information being available to the EP	More than 10% of all unique patients seen by the EP are provided timely (available to the patient within four business days of being updated in the certified EHR technology) electronic access to their health information subject to the EP's discretion to withhold certain information	*This objective is eliminated from Stage 1 in 2014 and is no longer an objective for Stage 2*	*This measure is eliminated from Stage 1 in 2014 and is no longer a measure for Stage 2*
Use certified EHR technology to identify patient-specific education resources and provide those resources to the patient if appropriate	More than 10% of all unique patients seen by the EP are provided patient-specific education resources	Use certified EHR technology to identify patient-specific education resources and provide those resources to the patient if appropriate	Patient-specific education resources identified by CEHRT are provided to patients for more than 10% of all unique patients with office visits seen by the EP during the EHR reporting period
The EP who receives a patient from another setting of care or provider of care or believes an encounter is relevant should perform medication reconciliation	The EP performs medication reconciliation for more than 50% of transitions of care in which the patient is transitioned into the care of the EP	The EP who receives a patient from another setting of care or provider of care or believes an encounter is relevant should perform medication reconciliation	The EP performs medication reconciliation for more than 50% of transitions of care in which the patient is transitioned into the care of the EP

Stage 1 Objective	Stage 1 Measure	Stage 2 Objective	Stage 2 Measure
The EP who transitions their patient to another setting of care or provider of care or refers their patient to another provider of care should provide summary of care record for each transition of care or referral	The EP who transitions or refers their patient to another setting of care or provider of care provides a summary of care record for more than 50% of transitions of care and referrals	The EP who transitions their patient to another setting of care or provider of care or refers their patient to another provider of care should provide summary of care record for each transition of care or referral	1. The EP who transitions or refers their patient to another setting of care or provider of care provides a summary of care record for more than 50% of transitions of care and referrals 2. The EP who transitions or refers their patient to another setting of care or provider of care provides a summary of care record either a) electronically transmitted to a recipient using CEHRT or b) where the recipient receives the summary of care record via exchange facilitated by an organization that is a NwHIN Exchange participant or is validated through an ONC-established governance mechanism to facilitate exchange for 10% of transitions and referrals 3. The EP who transitions or refers their patient to another setting of care or provider of care must either a) conduct one or more successful electronic exchanges of a summary of care record with a recipient using technology that was designed by a different EHR developer than the sender's, or b) conduct one or more successful tests with the CMS-designated test EHR during the EHR reporting period

Stage 1 Objective	Stage 1 Measure	Stage 2 Objective	Stage 2 Measure
Capability to submit electronic data to immunization registries or immunization information systems and actual submission except where prohibited and in accordance with applicable law and practice	Performed at least one test of certified EHR technology's capacity to submit electronic data to immunization registries and follow up submission if the test is successful (unless none of the immunization registries to which the EP submits such information have the capacity to receive the information electronically)	Capability to submit electronic data to immunization registries or immunization information systems and actual submission except where prohibited and in accordance with applicable law and practice	Successful ongoing submission of electronic immunization data from certified EHR technology to an immunization registry or immunization information system for the entire EHR reporting period
New	New	Use secure electronic messaging to communicate with patients on relevant health information	A secure message was sent using the electronic messaging function of certified EHR technology by more than 5% of unique patients seen during the EHR reporting period

MENU OBJECTIVES (EPs must select 3 of 6 menu objectives)

Stage 1 Objective	Stage 1 Measure	Stage 2 Objective	Stage 2 Measure
Capability to submit electronic syndromic surveillance data to public health agencies and actual submission except where prohibited and in accordance with applicable law and practice	Performed at least one test of certified EHR technology's capacity to provide electronic syndromic surveillance data to public health agencies and follow-up submission if the test is successful (unless none of the public health agencies to which an EP, eligible hospital or CAH submits such information have the capacity to receive the information electronically)	Capability to submit electronic syndromic surveillance data to public health agencies and actual submission except where prohibited and in accordance with applicable law and practice	Successful ongoing submission of electronic syndromic surveillance data from certified EHR technology to a public health agency for the entire EHR reporting period
New	New	Record electronic notes in patient records	Enter at least one electronic progress note created, edited and signed by an EP for more than 30% of unique patients

Stage 1 Objective	Stage 1 Measure	Stage 2 Objective	Stage 2 Measure
New	New	Imaging results consisting of the image itself and any explanation or other accompanying information are accessible through CEHRT	More than 10% of all scans and tests whose result is an image ordered by the EP for patients seen during the EHR reporting period are incorporated into or accessible through certified EHR technology
New	New	Record patient family health history as structured data	More than 20% of all unique patients seen by the EP during the EHR reporting period have a structured data entry for one or more first-degree relatives or an indication that family health history has been reviewed
New	New	Capability to identify and report cancer cases to a state cancer registry, except where prohibited, and in accordance with applicable law and practice	Successful ongoing submission of cancer case information from certified EHR technology to a cancer registry for the entire EHR reporting period
New	New	Capability to identify and report specific cases to a specialized registry (other than a cancer registry), except where prohibited, and in accordance with applicable law and practice	Successful ongoing submission of specific case information from certified EHR technology to a specialized registry for the entire EHR reporting period

Abbreviations: BMI indicates body mass index; CAH, critical access hospital; CEHRT, certified electronic health record technology; CMS, Centers for Medicare & Medicaid Services; CQM, clinical quality measure; EHR, electronic health record; EP, eligible professional; NwHIN, Nationwide Health Information Network; ONC, Office of the National Coordinator for Health Information Technology; and PQRS, Physician Quality Reporting System.
From: www.cms.gov/Regulations-and-Guidance/Legislation/EHRIncentivePrograms/Downloads/Stage1vs2Comp TablesforEP.pdf.

STAGE 2 OVERVIEW TIPSHEET

Last updated: August 2012

Overview

CMS recently published a final rule that specifies the Stage 2 criteria that eligible professionals (EPs), eligible hospitals, and critical access hospitals (CAHs) must meet in order to continue to participate in the Medicare and Medicaid Electronic Health Record (EHR) Incentive Programs.

If you have not participated in the Medicare or Medicaid EHR Incentive Programs previously, or if you have never achieved meaningful use under the Stage 1 criteria, please visit the CMS EHR Incentive Programs website (www.cms.gov/EHRIncentivePrograms) for more information about how to take part in the program.

Stage 2 Timeline

In the Stage 1 meaningful use regulations, CMS had established a timeline that required providers to progress to Stage 2 criteria after two program years under the Stage 1 criteria. This original timeline would have required Medicare providers who first demonstrated meaningful use in 2011 to meet the Stage 2 criteria in 2013.

However, we have delayed the onset of Stage 2 criteria. The earliest that the Stage 2 criteria will be effective is in fiscal year 2014 for eligible hospitals and CAHs or calendar year 2014 for EPs. The table below illustrates the progression of meaningful use stages from when a Medicare provider begins participation in the program.

1st Year	Stage of Meaningful Use										
	2011	2012	2013	2014	2015	2016	2017	2018	2019	2020	2021
2011	1	1	1	2	2	3	3	TBD	TBD	TBD	TBD
2012		1	1	2	2	3	3	TBD	TBD	TBD	TBD
2013			1	1	2	2	3	3	TBD	TBD	TBD
2014				1	1	2	2	3	3	TBD	TBD
2015					1	1	2	2	3	3	TBD
2016						1	1	2	2	3	3
2017							1	1	2	2	3

Note that providers who were early demonstrators of meaningful use in 2011 will meet three consecutive years of meaningful use under the Stage 1 criteria before advancing to the Stage 2 criteria in 2014. All other providers would meet two years of meaningful use under the Stage 1 criteria before advancing to the Stage 2 criteria in their third year.

In the first year of participation, providers must demonstrate meaningful use for a 90-day EHR reporting period; in subsequent years, providers will demonstrate meaningful use for a full year EHR reporting period (an entire fiscal year for hospitals or an entire calendar year for EPs) except in 2014, which is described below. Providers who participate in the Medicaid EHR Incentive Programs are not required to demonstrate meaningful use in consecutive years as described by the table above, but their progression through the stages of meaningful use would follow the same overall structure of two years meeting the criteria of each stage, with the first year of meaningful use participation consisting of a 90-day EHR reporting period.

For 2014 only

All providers regardless of their stage of meaningful use are only required to demonstrate meaningful use for a three-month EHR reporting period.

- For Medicare providers, this 3-month reporting period is fixed to the quarter of either the fiscal (for eligible hospitals and CAHs) or calendar (for EPs) year in order to align with existing CMS quality measurement programs, such as the Physician Quality Reporting System (PQRS) and Hospital Inpatient Quality Reporting (IQR).
- For Medicaid providers only eligible to receive Medicaid EHR incentives, the 3-month reporting period is not fixed, where providers do not have the same alignment needs.

CMS is permitting this one-time three-month reporting period in 2014 only so that all providers who must upgrade to 2014 certified EHR technology will have adequate time to implement their new certified EHR systems.

Core and Menu Objectives

Stage 1 established a core and menu structure for objectives that providers had to achieve in order to demonstrate meaningful use. Core objectives are objectives that all providers must meet. There are also a predetermined number of menu objectives that providers must select from a list and meet in order to demonstrate meaningful use.

For many of the core and menu objectives, exclusions were provided that would allow providers to achieve meaningful use without having to meet those objectives that were outside of their normal scope of clinical practice. Under the Stage 1 criteria, EPs had to meet 15 core objectives and 5 menu objectives that they selected from a total list of 10. Eligible hospitals and CAHs had to meet 14 core objectives and 5 menu objectives that they selected from a total list of 10.

Stage 2 retains this core and menu structure for meaningful use objectives. Although some Stage 1 objectives were either combined or eliminated, most of the Stage 1 objectives are now core objectives under the Stage 2 criteria. For many of these Stage 2 objectives, the threshold that providers must meet for the objective has been raised. We expect that providers who reach Stage 2 in the EHR Incentive Programs will be able to demonstrate meaningful use of their certified EHR technology for an even larger portion of their patient populations.

Some new objectives were also introduced for Stage 2, and most of these were introduced as menu objectives for Stage 2. As with the previous stage, many of the Stage 2 objectives have exclusions that allow providers to achieve meaningful use without having to meet objectives outside their normal scope of clinical practice.

To demonstrate meaningful use under Stage 2 criteria—

- EPs must meet 17 core objectives and 3 menu objectives that they select from a total list of 6, or a total of 20 core objectives.
- Eligible hospitals and CAHs must meet 16 core objectives and 3 menu objectives that they select from a total list of 6, or a total of 19 core objectives.

The end of this tipsheet contains a complete list of the Stage 2 core and menu objectives for both EPs and eligible hospitals and CAHs. Providers can also download a table of the Stage 2 core and menu objectives and measures by clicking on the links below:

- Stage 1 vs Stage 2 Comparison Table for Eligible Professionals
- Stage 1 vs Stage 2 Comparison Table for Eligible Hospitals and CAHs

New Objectives & New Measures

Though most of the new objectives introduced for Stage 2 are menu objectives, EPs and eligible hospitals each have a new core objective that they must achieve. CMS believes that both of these objectives will have a positive impact on patient care and safety and are therefore requiring all providers to meet the objectives in Stage 2.

New Stage 2 Core Objectives:

Use secure electronic messaging to communicate with patients on relevant health information (for EPs only)
Automatically track medications from order to administration using assistive technologies in conjunction with an electronic medication administration record (eMAR) (for eligible hospitals/CAHs only)

Stage 2 also replaces the previous Stage 1 objectives to provide electronic copies of health information or discharge instructions and provide timely access to health information with objectives that allow patients to access their health information online.

Stage 2 Patient Access Objectives:

Provide patients the ability to view online, download and transmit their health information within four business days of the information being available to the EP (for EPs only)
Provide patients the ability to view online, download and transmit their health information within 36 hours after discharge from the hospital (for eligible hospitals/CAHs only)

In addition, the Stage 2 criteria place an emphasis on health information exchange between providers to improve care coordination for patients. One of the core objectives for both EPs and eligible hospitals and CAHs requires providers who transition or refer a patient to another setting of care or provider of care to provide a summary of care record for more than 50% of those transitions of care and referrals. Additionally, there are new requirements for the electronic exchange of summary of care documents:

- For more than 10% of transitions and referrals, EPs, eligible hospitals, and CAHs that transition or refer their patient to another setting of care or provider of care must provide a summary of care record electronically.
- The EP, eligible hospital, or CAH that transitions or refers their patient to another setting of care or provider of care must either a) conduct one or more successful electronic exchanges of a summary of care record with a recipient using technology that was designed by a different EHR developer than the sender's, or b) conduct one or more successful tests with the CMS-designated test EHR during the EHR reporting period.

There are also new Stage 2 menu objectives for EPs, eligible hospitals, and CAHs:

Record electronic notes in patient records
Imaging results accessible through CEHRT
Record patient family health history
Identify and report cancer cases to a state cancer registry (for EPs only)
Identify and report specific cases to a specialized registry (other than a cancer registry) (for EPs only)
Generate and transmit permissible discharge prescriptions electronically (eRx) (new for eligible hospitals and CAHs only)
Provide structured electronic lab results to ambulatory providers (for eligible hospitals and CAHs only)

Finally, there are new Stage 2 measures for several objectives that require patients to use health information technology [IT] in order for providers to achieve meaningful use. CMS believes that EPs, eligible hospitals, and CAHs are in the best position to encourage the use of health IT by patients to further their own health care.

Under the Stage 2 core objectives to provide patients the ability to view online, download and transmit their health information, more than 5 percent of patients seen by the EP or admitted to an inpatient (Place of Service 21) or emergency department (Place of Service 23) of an eligible hospital or CAH view, download, or transmit to a third party their health information.

Under the Stage 2 core objective to use secure electronic messaging to communicate with patients on relevant health information, a secure message must be sent using the electronic messaging function of certified EHR technology by more than 5 percent of unique patients seen by an EP during the EHR reporting period.

Clinical Quality Measures for 2014 and Beyond

Although clinical quality measure (CQM) reporting has been removed as a core objective for both EPs and eligible hospitals and CAHs, all providers are required to report on CQMs in order to demonstrate meaningful use. Beginning in 2014, all providers regardless of their stage of meaningful use will report on CQMs in the same way.

■ EPs must report on 9 out of 64 total CQMs.

■ Eligible hospitals and CAHs must report on 16 out of 29 total CQMs.

In addition, all providers must select CQMs from at least 3 of the 6 key health care policy domains recommended by the Department of Health and Human Services' National Quality Strategy:

1. Patient and Family Engagement
2. Patient Safety
3. Care Coordination
4. Population and Public Health
5. Efficient Use of Healthcare Resources
6. Clinical Processes/Effectiveness

A complete list of 2014 CQMs and their associated National Quality Strategy domains will be posted on the CMS EHR Incentive Programs website (www.cms.gov/EHRIncentive Programs) in the future. CMS will also post a recommended core set of CQMs for EPs.

Beginning in 2014, all Medicare-eligible providers beyond their first year of demonstrating meaningful use must electronically report their CQM data to CMS. (Medicaid EPs and hospitals that are eligible only for the Medicaid EHR Incentive Program will electronically report their CQM data to their state.) There will be a variety of options for providers to electronically report their CQMs.

EPs can electronically report CQMs either individually or as a group using the following methods:

■ Physician Quality Reporting System (PQRS)—Electronic submission of samples of patient-level data in the Quality Reporting Data Architecture (QRDA) Category I format. EPs can also report as group using the PQRS GPRO tool. EPs who electronically report using this PQRS option will meet both their EHR Incentive Program and PQRS reporting requirements.

■ CMS-designated transmission method—Electronic submission of aggregate-level data in QRDA Category III format.

Eligible hospitals and CAHs will electronically report their CQMs in the QRDA Category I format through the infrastructure similar to the EHR Reporting Pilot for hospitals, which will be the basis for an EHR-based reporting option in the Hospital Inpatient Quality Reporting program. They may also submit aggregate-level data in QRDA III format.

For more detailed information on 2014 CQMs and electronic reporting options, click to download our 2014 Clinical Quality Measures Tip sheet.

More Information

If you are interested in learning more about the Medicare payment adjustments and hardship exceptions for EPs, eligible hospitals, and CAHs, take a look at our Payment Adjustments & Hardship Exceptions Fact Sheet.

If you are interested in learning more about changes to the Medicaid patient volume calculations, review the FAQs here https://questions.cms.gov/.

Stage 2 Core and Menu Objectives

Eligible Professionals

Report on all 17 Core Objectives:

1. Use computerized provider order entry (CPOE) for medication, laboratory and radiology orders
2. Generate and transmit permissible prescriptions electronically (eRx)
3. Record demographic information
4. Record and chart changes in vital signs
5. Record smoking status for patients 13 years old or older
6. Use clinical decision support to improve performance on high-priority health conditions
7. Provide patients the ability to view online, download and transmit their health information
8. Provide clinical summaries for patients for each office visit
9. Protect electronic health information created or maintained by the certified EHR technology
10. Incorporate clinical lab-test results into certified EHR technology
11. Generate lists of patients by specific conditions to use for quality improvement, reduction of disparities, research, or outreach
12. Use clinically relevant information to identify patients who should receive reminders for preventive/follow-up care
13. Use certified EHR technology to identify patient-specific education resources
14. Perform medication reconciliation
15. Provide summary of care record for each transition of care or referral
16. Submit electronic data to immunization registries
17. Use secure electronic messaging to communicate with patients on relevant health information

Report on 3 of 6 Menu Objectives:

1. Submit electronic syndromic surveillance data to public health agencies
2. Record electronic notes in patient records
3. Imaging results accessible through CEHRT
4. Record patient family health history
5. Identify and report cancer cases to a state cancer registry
6. Identify and report specific cases to a specialized registry (other than a cancer registry)

Eligible Hospitals and CAHs

Report on all 16 Core Objectives:

1. Use computerized provider order entry (CPOE) for medication, laboratory and radiology orders
2. Record demographic information
3. Record and chart changes in vital signs
4. Record smoking status for patients 13 years old or older
5. Use clinical decision support to improve performance on high-priority health conditions
6. Provide patients the ability to view online, download and transmit their health information within 36 hours after discharge.
7. Protect electronic health information created or maintained by the certified EHR technology
8. Incorporate clinical lab-test results into certified EHR technology
9. Generate lists of patients by specific conditions to use for quality improvement, reduction of disparities, research, or outreach
10. Use certified EHR technology to identify patient-specific education resources and provide those resources to the patient if appropriate
11. Perform medication reconciliation
12. Provide summary of care record for each transition of care or referral
13. Submit electronic data to immunization registries
14. Submit electronic data on reportable lab results to public health agencies
15. Submit electronic syndromic surveillance data to public health agencies
16. Automatically track medications with an electronic medication administration record (eMAR)

Report on 3 of 6 Menu Objectives:

1. Record whether a patient 65 years old or older has an advance directive
2. Record electronic notes in patient records
3. Imaging results accessible through CEHRT
4. Record patient family health history
5. Generate and transmit permissible discharge prescriptions electronically (eRx)
6. Provide structured electronic lab results to ambulatory providers

Abbreviations: CEHRT indicates certified electronic health record technology; CMS, Centers for Medicare & Medicaid Services; GPRO, group practice reporting option; and TBD, to be determined.
From: www.cms.gov/Regulations-and-Guidance/Legislation/EHRIncentivePrograms/Downloads/Stage2Overview_Tip sheet.pdf.

ELIGIBLE PROFESSIONAL (EP) ATTESTATION WORKSHEET FOR STAGE 1 OF THE MEDICARE ELECTRONIC HEALTH RECORD (EHR) INCENTIVE PROGRAM

The EP Attestation Worksheet is for EPs in Stage 1 of meaningful use and allows them to log their meaningful use measures on this page to use as a reference when attesting for the Medicare EHR Incentive Program in the CMS system.

Numerator, denominator, and exclusion information for clinical quality measures (CQMs) must be reported directly from information generated by certified EHR technology and are not included in this worksheet. However, information for the remaining meaningful use core and menu set measures does not necessarily have to be entered directly from information generated by certified EHR technology. For each objective with a percentage-based measure, certified EHR technology must include the capability to electronically record the numerator and denominator and generate a report including the numerator, denominator, and resulting percentage for these measures. However, EPs may use additional data to calculate numerators and denominators and to generate reports on all measures of the core and menu set meaningful use objectives except CQMs. In order to provide complete and accurate information for certain of these measures, EPs may also have to include information from paper-based patient records or from records maintained in uncertified EHR technology.

EPs can enter their meaningful use criteria in the blue boxes [of the CMS system]. Each measure's objective is included to help EPs enter the correct criteria. Certain measures do not require a numerator and denominator, but rather a yes/no answer, and are marked as such. Measures with exclusions have the exclusion description listed in the measure information section.

Note: Claiming an exclusion for a specific measure qualifies as submission of that measure. If an EP claims an exclusion for which they qualify, indicate this in the Attestation System by clicking "yes" under the exclusion part of the measure question.

EPs must meet report on the following:

1. All 15 of the core measures
   Note: One of the required core measures is that EPs report clinical quality measures (CQMs)
2. 5 out of 10 of the menu measures; at least 1 public health measure must be selected
3. A sum total of up to 9 CQMs; 3 core, up to 3 alternate core, and 3 additional CQMs. If an EP reports a denominator of 0 for any of the 3 core measures, the EP must record for an alternate core CQM to supplement the core measure. Therefore, an EP may report a minimum of 6 and a maximum of 9 CQMs depending on the resulting values in the denominators for the core measures as reported from their certified EHR.

Reporting Period: For an EP the reporting period must be at least 90 consecutive days within calendar year 2011 (January 1, 2011, through December 31, 2011).

Meaningful Use Core Measures—EPs must fill out all 15 core measures

#	Measure Information	Measure Values
1	Objective: Use computerized provider order entry (CPOE) for medication orders directly entered by a licensed healthcare professional who can enter orders into the medical record per state, local and professional guidelines Measure: More than 30 percent of all unique patients with at least one medication in their medication list seen by the EP have at least one medication order entered using CPOE Exclusion: Any EP who writes fewer than 100 prescriptions during the EHR reporting period would be excluded from this requirement	
	Does this exclusion apply to you?	Yes No
	Numerator: The number of patients in the denominator that have at least one medication order entered using CPOE	
	Denominator: Number of unique patients with at least one medication in their medication list seen by the EP during the EHR reporting period	
2	Objective: Implement drug-drug and drug-allergy interaction checks Measure: The EP has enabled this functionality for the entire EHR reporting period Note: This measure only requires a yes/no answer	
	Numerator: N/A	YES NO
	Denominator: N/A	
3	Objective: Maintain an up-to-date problem list of current and active diagnoses Measure: More than 80 percent of all unique patients seen by the EP have at least one entry or an indication that no problems are known for the patient recorded as structured data	
	Numerator: Number of patients in the denominator who have at least one entry or an indication that no problems are known for the patient recorded as structured data in their problem list	
	Denominator: Number of unique patients seen by the EP during the EHR reporting period	
4	Objective: Generate and transmit permissible prescriptions electronically (eRx) Measure: More than 40 percent of all permissible prescriptions written by the EP are transmitted electronically using certified EHR technology Exclusion: Any EP who writes fewer than 100 prescriptions during the EHR reporting period would be excluded from this requirement	
	Does this exclusion apply to you?	Yes No
	Numerator: Number of prescriptions in the denominator generated and transmitted electronically	
	Denominator: Number of prescriptions written for drugs requiring a prescription in order to be dispensed other than controlled substances during the EHR reporting period	

#	Measure Information	Measure Values
5	Objective: Maintain active medication list	
	Measure: More than 80 percent of all unique patients seen by the EP have at least one entry (or an indication that the patient is not currently prescribed any medication) recorded as structured data	
	Numerator: Number of patients in the denominator who have a medication (or an indication that the patient is not currently prescribed any medication) recorded as structured data	
	Denominator: Number of unique patients seen by the EP during the EHR reporting period	
6	Objective: Maintain active medication allergy list	
	Measure: More than 80 percent of all unique patients seen by the EP have at least one entry (or an indication that the patient has no known medication allergies) recorded as structured data	
	Numerator: Number of unique patients in the denominator who have at least one entry (or an indication that the patient has no known medication allergies) recorded as structured data in their medication allergy list	
	Denominator: Number of unique patients seen by the EP during the EHR report period	
7	Objective: Record all of the following demographics: preferred language, gender, race, ethnicity, and date of birth	
	Measure: More than 50 percent of all unique patients seen by the EP have demographics recorded as structured data	
	Numerator: Number of patients in the denominator who have all the elements of demographics (or a specific exclusion if the patient declined to provide one or more elements or if recording an element is contrary to state law) recorded as structured data	
	Denominator: Number of unique patients seen by the EP during the EHR reporting period	
8	Objective: Record and chart changes in vital signs: height, weight, blood pressure, calculate and display body mass index (BMI), plot and display growth charts for children 2-20, including BMI	
	Measure: More than 50 percent of all unique patients age 2 and over seen by the EP, height, weight, and blood pressure are recorded as structured data	
	Exclusion 1: Any EP who does not see patients 2 years or older would be excluded from this requirement	
	Exclusion 2: An EP who believes that all three vital signs of height, weight, and blood pressure have no relevance to scope of practice would be excluded from this requirement	
	Does exclusion 1 apply to you?	Yes No
	Does exclusion 2 apply to you?	Yes No
	Numerator: Number of patients in the denominator who have at least one entry of their height, weight and blood pressure are recorded as structured data. [BMI and growth charts will be automatically calculated by certified EHR and do not need to be included in the numerator calculation.]	
	Denominator: Number of unique patients age 2 or over seen by the EP during the EHR reporting period	

#	Measure Information	Measure Values
9	Objective: Record smoking status for patients 13 years old or older Measure: More than 50 percent of all unique patients 13 years old or older seen by the EP have smoking status recorded as structured data Exclusion: An EP who did not see patients 13 years or older would be excluded from this requirement	
	Does this exclusion apply to you?	Yes No
	Numerator: Number of patients in the denominator with smoking status recorded as structured data	
	Denominator: Number of unique patients age 13 or older seen by the EP during the EHR reporting period	
10	Objective: Report ambulatory clinical quality measures to CMS Measure: Successfully report to CMS ambulatory clinical quality measures selected by CMS in the manner specified by CMS Note: This measure only requires a yes/no answer	
	Numerator: N/A	
	Denominator: N/A	YES NO
11	Objective: Implement one clinical decision support rule relevant to specialty or high clinical priority along with the ability to track compliance with that rule Measure: Implement one clinical decision support rule relevant to specialty or high clinical priority along with the ability to track compliance to that rule Note: This measure only requires a yes/no answer	
	Numerator: N/A	YES NO
	Denominator: N/A	
12	Objective: Provide patients with an electronic copy of their health information (including diagnostics test results, problem list, medication lists, medication allergies) upon request Measure: More than 50 percent of all patients who request an electronic copy of their health information are provided it within three business days Exclusion: An EP who has no requests from patients or their agents for an electronic copy of patient health information during the EHR reporting period would be excluded from this requirement	
	Does this exclusion apply to you?	Yes No
	Numerator: Number of patients in the denominator who receive an electronic copy of their electronic health information within three business days	
	Denominator: Number of patients of the EP who request an electronic copy of their electronic health information four business days prior to the end of the EHR reporting period	
13	Objective: Provide clinical summaries for patients for each office visit Measure: Clinical summaries provided to patients for more than 50 percent of all office visits within three business days Exclusion: Any EP who has no office visits during the EHR reporting period would be excluded from this requirement	
	Does this exclusion apply to you?	Yes No

#	Measure Information	Measure Values
	Numerator: Number of office visits in the denominator for which the patient is provided a clinical summary within three business days	
	Denominator: Number of office visits by the EP during the EHR reporting period	
14	Objective: Capability to exchange key clinical information (for example, problem list, medication list, medication allergies, and diagnostic test results), among providers of care and patient authorized entities electronically Measure: Performed at least one test of certified EHR technology's capacity to electronically exchange key clinical information Note: This measure only requires a yes/no answer	
	Numerator: N/A	YES NO
	Denominator: N/A	
15	Objective: Protect electronic health information created or maintained by the certified EHR technology through the implementation of appropriate technical capabilities Measure: Conduct or review a security risk analysis in accordance with the requirements under 45 CFR 164.308(a)(1) and implement security updates as necessary and correct identified security deficiencies as part of its risk management process Note: This measure only requires a yes/no answer	
	Numerator: N/A	YES NO
	Denominator: N/A	

Meaningful Use Menu Measures—EPs must fill out 5 out of 10 measures (at least 1 of these must be a public health measure, which are noted with an asterisk)

#	Measure Information	Measure Values
1*	Objective: Capability to submit electronic data to immunization registries or immunization information systems and actual submission in accordance with applicable law and practice Measure: Performed at least one test of certified EHR technology's capacity to submit electronic data to immunization registries and follow up submission if the test is successful (unless none of the immunization registries to which the EP submits such information has the capacity to receive the information electronically) Exclusion 1: An EP who does not perform immunizations during the EHR reporting period would be excluded from this requirement Exclusion 2: If there is no immunization registry that has the capacity to receive the information electronically, an EP would be excluded from this requirement Note: This measure only requires a yes/no answer	
	Does this exclusion 1 apply to you?	Yes No
	Does this exclusion 2 apply to you?	Yes No
	Numerator: N/A	YES NO
	Denominator: N/A	

#	Measure Information	Measure Values
2*	Objective: Capability to submit electronic syndromic surveillance data to public health agencies and actual submission in accordance with applicable law and practice Measure: Performed at least one test of certified EHR technology's capacity to provide electronic syndromic surveillance data to public health agencies and follow-up submission if the test is successful (unless none of the public health agencies to which an EP submits such information have the capacity receive the information electronically) Exclusion 1: If an EP does not collect any reportable syndromic information on their patients during the EHR reporting period, then the EP is excluded from this requirement Exclusion 2: If there is no public health agency that has the capability to receive the information electronically, then the EP is excluded from this requirement Note: This measure only requires a yes/no answer	
	Does exclusion 1 apply to you?	Yes No
	Does exclusion 2 apply to you?	Yes No
	Numerator: N/A	YES NO
	Denominator: N/A	
3	Objective: Implement drug formulary checks Measure: The EP has enabled this functionality and has access to at least one internal or external formulary for the entire EHR reporting period Exclusion: Any EP who writes fewer than 100 prescriptions during the EHR reporting period would be excluded from this requirement Note: This measure only requires a yes/no answer	
	Does this exclusion apply to you?	Yes No
	Numerator: N/A	YES NO
	Denominator: N/A	
4	Objective: Incorporate clinical lab test results into EHR as structured data Measure: More than 40 percent of all clinical lab test results ordered by the EP during the EHR reporting period whose results are either in a positive/negative or numerical format are incorporated in certified EHR technology as structured data Exclusion: Any EP who orders no lab tests whose results are either in a positive/negative or numeric format during the EHR reporting period would be excluded from this requirement	
	Does this exclusion apply to you?	Yes No
	Numerator: Number of lab test results whose results are expressed in a positive or negative affirmation or as a number which are incorporated as structured data	
	Denominator: Number of lab tests ordered during the EHR reporting period by the EP whose results are expressed in a positive or negative affirmation or as a number	
5	Objective: Generate lists of patients by specific conditions to use for quality improvement, reduction of disparities, research, or outreach Measure: Generate at least one report listing patients of the EP with a specific condition Note: This measure only requires a yes/no answer	
	Numerator: N/A	YES NO
	Denominator: N/A	

#	Measure Information	Measure Values
6	Objective: Send reminders to patients per patient preference for preventive/follow-up care Measure: More than 20 percent of all patients 65 years or older or 5 years old or younger were sent appropriate reminders during the EHR reporting period Exclusion: Any EP who has no patients 65 years or older or 5 years old or younger with records maintained using certified EHR technology is excluded from this requirement	
	Does this exclusion apply to you?	Yes No
	Numerator: Number of patients in the denominator who were sent the appropriate reminder	
	Denominator: Number of unique patients 65 years old or older or 5 years old or younger	
7	Objective: Provide patients with timely electronic access to their health information (including lab results, problem list, medication lists, and allergies) within four business days of the information being available to the EP Measure: At least 10 percent of all unique patients seen by the EP are provided timely (available to the patient within four business days of being updated in the certified EHR technology) electronic access to their health information subject to the EP's discretion to withhold certain information Exclusion: Any EP that neither orders nor creates lab tests or information that would be contained in the problem list, medication list, medication allergy list (or other information as listed at 45 CFR 170.304(g)) during the EHR reporting period would be excluded from this requirement	
	Does this exclusion apply to you?	Yes No
	Numerator: Number of patients in the denominator who have timely (available to the patient within four business days of being updated in the certified EHR technology) electronic access to their health information online	
	Denominator: Number of unique patients seen by the EP during the EHR reporting period	
8	Objective: Use certified EHR technology to identify patient-specific education resources and provide those resources to the patient if appropriate Measure: More than 10 percent of all unique patients seen by the EP are provided patient-specific education resources	
	Numerator: Number of patients in the denominator who are provided patient-specific education resources	
	Denominator: Number of unique patients seen by the EP during the EHR reporting period	
9	Objective: The EP who receives a patient from another setting of care or provider of care or believes an encounter is relevant should perform medication reconciliation Measure: The EP performs medication reconciliation for more than 50 percent of transitions of care in which the patient is transitioned into the care of the EP Exclusion: An EP who was not the recipient of any transitions of care during the EHR reporting period would be excluded from this requirement	
	Does this exclusion apply to you?	Yes No
	Numerator: Number of transitions of care in the denominator where medication reconciliation was performed	
	Denominator: Number of transitions of care during the EHR reporting period for which the EP was the receiving party of the transition	

#	Measure Information	Measure Values
10	Objective: The EP who transitions their patient to another setting of care or provider of care or refers their patient to another provider of care should provide summary care record for each transition of care or referral Measure: The EP who transitions or refers their patient to another setting of care or provider of care provides a summary of care record for more than 50 percent of transitions of care and referrals Exclusion: An EP who does not transfer a patient to another setting or refer a patient to another provider during the EHR reporting period would be excluded from this requirement	
	Does this exclusion apply to you?	Yes No
	Numerator: Number of transitions of care and referrals in the denominator where a summary of care record was provided	
	Denominator: Number of transitions of care and referrals during the EHR reporting period for which the EP was the transferring or referring provider	

PAYMENT ADJUSTMENTS AND HARDSHIP EXCEPTIONS TIPSHEET FOR ELIGIBLE PROFESSIONALS

Last updated: August 2012

Overview

As part of the American Recovery and Reinvestment Act of 2009 (ARRA), Congress mandated payment adjustments to be applied to Medicare eligible professionals (EPs) who are not meaningful users of certified electronic health record (EHR) technology under the Medicare EHR Incentive Programs. These payment adjustments will be applied beginning on January 1, 2015, for Medicare EPs. Medicaid EPs who can only participate in the Medicaid EHR Incentive Program and do not bill Medicare are not subject to these payment adjustments.

EPs who can participate in either the Medicare or Medicaid EHR Incentive Programs will be subject to the payment adjustments unless they are meaningful users under one of the EHR Incentive Programs in the time periods specified below.

Payment Adjustments for Medicare EPs

Medicare EPs who are not meaningful users will be subject to a payment adjustment beginning on January 1, 2015.

This payment adjustment will be applied to the Medicare physician fee schedule (PFS) amount for covered professional services furnished by the EP during the year (including the fee schedule amount for purposes of determining a payment based on the fee schedule amount). The payment adjustment is 1% per year and is cumulative for every year that an EP is not a meaningful user. Depending on the total number of Medicare EPs who are meaningful users under the EHR Incentive Programs after 2018, the maximum cumulative payment adjustment can reach as high as 5%. The table below illustrates the potential application of payment adjustments to covered professional services for a Medicare EP who is not a meaningful user beginning in 2014.

% ADJUSTMENT ASSUMING LESS THAN 75 PERCENT OF EPs ARE MEANINGFUL USERS						
	2015	2016	2017	2018	2019	2020+
EP is not subject to the payment adjustment for the e-Rx in 2014	99%	98%	97%	96%	95%	95%
EP is subject to the payment adjustment for the e-Rx in 2014	98%	98%	97%	96%	95%	95%

% ADJUSTMENT ASSUMING MORE THAN 75 PERCENT OF EPs ARE MEANINGFUL USERS						
	2015	2016	2017	2018	2019	2020+
EP is not subject to the payment adjustment for the e-Rx in 2014	99%	98%	97%	97%	97%	97%
EP is subject to the payment adjustment for the e-Rx in 2014	98%	98%	97%	97%	97%	97%

Because payment adjustments are mandated to begin on the first day of the 2015 calendar year, CMS will apply a prospective determination for payment adjustments. Therefore Medicare EPs must demonstrate meaningful use prior to the 2015 calendar year in order to avoid the adjustments.

EPs who first demonstrated meaningful use in 2011 or 2012 must demonstrate meaningful use for a full year in 2013 to avoid payment adjustments in 2015. They must continue to demonstrate meaningful use every year to avoid payment adjustments in subsequent years. The table below illustrates the timeline to avoid payment adjustments for EPs who must demonstrate meaningful use for a full year in 2013.

Payment Adjustment Year	2015	2016	2017	2018	2019	2020
Full Year EHR Reporting Period	2013	2014	2015	2016	2017	2019

EPs who first demonstrate meaningful use in 2013 must demonstrate meaningful use for a 90-day reporting period in 2013 to avoid payment adjustments in 2015. They must continue to demonstrate meaningful use every year to avoid payment adjustments in subsequent years. The table below illustrates the timeline to avoid payment adjustments for EPs who demonstrate meaningful use for a 90-day reporting period in 2013.

Payment Adjustment Year	2015	2016	2017	2018	2019	2020
90 day EHR Reporting Period	2013					
Full Year EHR Reporting Period		2014	2015	2016	2017	2019

EPs who first demonstrate meaningful use in 2014 must demonstrate meaningful use for a 90-day reporting period in 2014 to avoid payment adjustments in 2015. This reporting period must occur in the first 9 months of calendar year 2014, and EPs must attest to meaningful use no later than October 1, 2014, in order to avoid the payment adjustments. EPs must continue to demonstrate meaningful use every year to avoid payment adjustments in subsequent years. The table below illustrates the timeline to avoid payment adjustments for EPs who first demonstrate meaningful use in 2014.

Payment Adjustment Year	2015	2016	2017	2018	2019	2020
90 day EHR Reporting Period	2013					
Full Year EHR Reporting Period		2014	2015	2016	2017	2019

EPs who first demonstrate meaningful use in 2014 must demonstrate meaningful use for a 90-day reporting period in 2014 to avoid payment adjustments in 2015. This reporting period must occur in the first 9 months of calendar year 2014, and EPs must attest to meaningful use no later than October 1, 2014, in order to avoid the payment adjustments. EPs must continue to demonstrate meaningful use every year to avoid payment adjustments in subsequent years. The table below illustrates the timeline to avoid payment adjustments for EPs who first demonstrate meaningful use in 2014.

Payment Adjustment Year	2015	2016	2017	2018	2019	2020
90 day EHR Reporting Period	2014*	2014				
Full Year EHR Reporting Period			2015	2016	2017	2019

*EPs must attest to meaningful use no later than October 1, 2014.

Hardship Exceptions for Medicare EPs

EPs may apply for hardship exceptions to avoid the payment adjustments described above. Hardship exceptions will be granted only under specific circumstances and only if CMS determines that providers have demonstrated that those circumstances pose a significant barrier to their achieving meaningful use. Information on how to apply for a hardship exception will be posted on the CMS EHR Incentive Programs website (www.cms.gov /EHRIncentiveProgram) in the future.

EPs can apply for hardship exceptions in the following categories:

- Infrastructure — EPs must demonstrate that they are in an area without sufficient Internet access or face insurmountable barriers to obtaining infrastructure (eg, lack of broadband).
- New EPs — Newly practicing EPs who would not have had time to become meaningful users can apply for a 2-year limited exception to payment adjustments. Thus EPs who begin practice in calendar year 2015 would receive an exception to the penalties in 2015 and 2016, but would have to begin demonstrating meaningful use in calendar year 2016 to avoid payment adjustments in 2017.
- Unforeseen Circumstances — Examples may include a natural disaster or other unforeseeable barrier.
- Patient Interaction:
  1. Lack of face-to-face or telemedicine interaction with patients
  2. Lack of follow-up need with patients
- Practice at Multiple Locations: Lack of control over availability of CEHRT for more than 50% of patient encounters

Frequently Asked Questions

Do I have to be a meaningful user each year to avoid the payment adjustments or can I avoid the payment adjustments by achieving meaningful use only once?

You must demonstrate meaningful use every year according to the timelines detailed above in order to avoid Medicare payment adjustments. For example, an EP who demonstrates meaningful use for the first time in 2013 will avoid the payment adjustment in 2015, but will need to demonstrate meaningful use again in 2014 in order to avoid the payment adjustment in 2016.

If I am an EP who is eligible for both the Medicare and Medicaid EHR Incentive Programs, but I register to participate in the Medicaid EHR Incentive Program, do I still have to be a meaningful user to avoid the payment adjustments?

Yes. If you are eligible to participate in both the Medicare and Medicaid EHR Incentive Programs, you must demonstrate meaningful use according to the timelines detailed above to avoid the payment adjustments. You may demonstrate meaningful use under either Medicare or Medicaid.

If I am an EP who is eligible for both the Medicare and Medicaid EHR Incentive Programs, will I avoid the payment adjustments during a calendar year when I receive an incentive payment for adopting, implementing, or upgrading my certified EHR technology?

No. Congress mandated that an EP must be a meaningful user in order to avoid the payment adjustment; therefore receiving a Medicaid EHR incentive payment for adopting, implementing, or upgrading your certified EHR technology would not exempt you from the payment adjustments. You must demonstrate meaningful use according to the timelines detailed above to avoid the payment adjustments. You may demonstrate meaningful use under either Medicare or Medicaid.

How do I demonstrate meaningful use in order to avoid a payment adjustment?

You demonstrate meaningful use by successfully attesting through either the CMS Medicare EHR Incentive Programs Attestation System (https://ehrincentives.cms.gov/) or through your state's attestation system.

If I am a hospital-based Medicare EP, am I subject to the payment adjustments?

No. If you perform 90% or more of your covered professional services in either the inpatient (Place of Service 21) or emergency department (Place of Service 23) of a hospital, then you will be determined to be hospital-based and are not eligible to receive an EHR incentive and will not be subject to the payment adjustments.

However, your hospital-based status can change from year to year. For example, an EP who is determined to be hospital-based for the 2015 program year would not be subject to the payment adjustments in 2017. But if that EP is determined not to be hospital-based for the 2016 and the 2017 program year, then he or she could be subject to the payment adjustments in 2018 if the EP does not demonstrate meaningful use. Therefore it is important to check your hospital-based status at the beginning of each year. You can check your hospital-based status by visiting the Medicare EHR Incentive Programs Registration System (https://ehrincentives.cms.gov/).

Abbreviations: CEHRT indicates certified electronic health record technology; CMS, Centers for Medicare & Medicaid Services; and e-Rx, electronic prescribing.
From: www.cms.gov/Regulations-and-Guidance/Legislation/EHRIncentivePrograms/Downloads/Payment_Hardship ExcepTipsheetforEP.pdf.

INDEX